Arnold P. Gol[illegible]
Leonard Krasner, *SUNY at S[illegible]*

Achieving Patient Compliance

The Psychology of the Medical Practitioner's Role

M. Robin DiMatteo
University of California, Riverside

D. Dante DiNicola
University of California, Los Angeles, School of Medicine

New York [illegible] [illegible]kfurt

Pergamon Press Offices:

U.S.A.	Pergamon Press Inc., Maxwell House, Fairview Park, Elmsford, New York 10523, U.S.A.
U.K.	Pergamon Press Ltd., Headington Hill Hall, Oxford OX3 0BW, England
CANADA	Pergamon Press Canada Ltd., Suite 104, 150 Consumers Road, Willowdale, Ontario M2J 1P9, Canada
AUSTRALIA	Pergamon Press (Aust.) Pty. Ltd., P.O. Box 544, Potts Point, NSW 2011, Australia
FRANCE	Pergamon Press SARL, 24 rue des Ecoles, 75240 Paris, Cedex 05, France
FEDERAL REPUBLIC OF GERMANY	Pergamon Press GmbH, Hammerweg 6 6242 Kronberg/Taunus, Federal Republic of Germany

Library of Congress Cataloging in Publication Data

DiMatteo, M. Robin.
Achieving patient compliance.

(Pergamon general psychology series ; no. 110)
Bibliography: p.
Includes index.
Patient compliance. 2. Physician and patient.
I. DiNicola, D. Dante (David Dante), 1957-
II. Title. III. Series.
R726.5.D55 1982 615.5 82-3644
ISBN 0-08-027552-4 AACR2
ISBN 0-08-027551-6 (pbk.)

Printed in the United States of America

For
Devonne Dominique,
Deanna Donna,
Denise Diana,
Deborah Dawn,
and
Mom and Dad D.,
and
Mom and Dad D.

"Because suffering has more than academic interest, social theory should be more than a matter of academic curiosity."

H. Waitzkin and B. Waterman, *The Exploitation of Illness in Capitalist Society*, Indianapolis: Bobbs Merrill, 1974, p. 34.

Contents

Foreword

As a physician, I become daily more convinced of the psychophysiological nature of illness. I recognize in the behavior of patients what is so often borne out by empirical research—that illness is a function of both psychological and physiological processes. When our bodies are taxed (for example, by the environment or by poor nutrition) they respond (usually maladaptively) with disease. Likewise, when emotional stresses are high, the maladaptive response of psychosis may ensue. Physical and psychological aspects of health overlap in many cases, such that disease itself can become a mode of coping with psychological conflict and stress. Headaches, ulcers, back pains, ulcerative colitis, hypertension, as well as a host of other diseases may become channels for the expression of more basic problems such as depression, anxiety, and unresolved conflicts from the past or present. Physical illness can serve as a "socially acceptable" outlet for psychological distress.

In the light of the complexity of this phenomenon known as illness, we are sometimes hard-pressed to define precisely what a patient is looking for when he or she seeks the help of a physician or other medical practitioner. Certainly at the surface the patient is looking for medical advice and treatment. A "medico-logical" problem is presented, although it often masks a more complex form of distress involving the whole person. The practitioner, who is expertly trained to deal with physical findings proceeds to formulate a diagnosis and devise an effective treatment regimen.

Practitioner and patient are, however, quite often engaged in a *folie a deux*. The patient presents only the physical manifestations of the many stresses and conflicts he or she is experiencing, unaware of or hiding the emotional manifestations. The practitioner responds in kind to the medical issue from the framework he or she knows best. Yet the very crux of the matter may be overlooked, for in fact between 50 and 75% of patients who seek medical care have no positive physical findings—their problems are primarily psychosocial. Although these psychosocial issues are seldom addressed, patients are provided prescriptions for treatment. A large proportion of these recommendations (an average of 40%) are not followed.

I first began to do research on patient compliance in 1960, writing my dissertation on the subject under Robert Eichhorn at Purdue University. At that time, I was hard-pressed to find a sociological theory to help me understand the problem of noncompliance. During a year at the Harvard School of Public Health, I focused on the epidemiological aspects of noncompliance but found that a public health approach also could not explain this phenomenon adequately. Working at Cornell University with George Reader and Mary Goss and later at the University of Southern California with Barbara Korsch I came to view the problem of patient noncompliance as a function of the practitioner-patient relationship. Our systematic observations of physician-patient interactions revealed to me the enormous complexity of the phenomenon of noncompliance, for it involved maladaptive behavior not only on the part of the patient but on the part of the practitioner as well. I still believe that *the practitioner-patient relationship is the most important variable in the study of noncompliance.*

After shifting gears from social scientist to physician, I found myself in the new position of attempting to elicit compliance from my own patients. It has become clear to me over these years of caring for patients that the compliance issue is primarily psychological in nature. As a practicing psychiatrist, I also recognize the illogical or unconscious motivations which prevail among patients who respond in maladaptive ways to illness and to the practitioners to whom they turn for help. Practitioners may respond in maladaptive ways as well. Hence, patient noncompliance is but one of many maladaptive responses in a much larger picture of health-seeking behavior.

The study of compliance is desperately in need of an approach which is broad in base and takes into account both the medical and psychological aspects of disease and medical care. This book by DiMatteo and DiNicola represents an approach to patient compliance based on the merging of psychology and medicine—the disciplines in which they were respectively trained. I would venture to suggest from my own experience that one problem in unraveling the puzzle of patient noncompliance is the conflict often apparent between social scientists and medical professionals who feel, perhaps not unfoundedly, that they do not understand one another. The marriage of these two approaches in this book is an important step toward solving the noncompliance problem.

A note of optimism pervades this book. The medical practitioner and the patient are given the opportunity for self-directed change. There is a great deal of emphasis (and appropriately so) on the role of negotiation in the practitioner-patient relationship and on helping the patient to internalize a more adaptive response to illness. Intrapsychic factors such as beliefs and attitudes as well as behavioral factors are taken into account. The intrapsychic factors posit that people are essentially rational in their choice of behaviors. The authors review some compelling research support for their approach to achieving patient compliance. Their organizing scheme can be applied in clinical and research settings alike.

One important issue that receives minimal recognition in this book is a factor that I believe will prove important to the future of this field. It involves the basic question of motivation for human behavior in general and patient compliance in particular. Do people decide how they will act (or adapt) or do they operate under the influence of unconscious processes? Does their behavior reflect their attempts to work through conflicts, present since early childhood, by acting out and exhibiting transferences and resistances of which they are vaguely or not at all aware? The noncompliance literature provides support for the approach emphasizing "rational man" (and the authors have done an excellent job of reviewing this literature). The empirical research which would bring to light the relevance of more irrational intrapsychic influences has yet to be undertaken. Perhaps because I am a psychiatrist, I trust that these factors will emerge with the power to fill in the "unexplainable gaps" in the very comprehensive model presented in this book. A logical and scientific examination of seemingly illogical issues (without dismissing them as merely illogical, as medical professionals are wont to do) is, in my opinion, an important next step to understanding even more about compliance behavior. In the meantime, this book by DiMatteo and DiNicola, which I am happy to introduce, is a new and exciting approach to understanding the practitioner-patient relationship. I am sure that it will help practitioners, patients, and scientists to understand and overcome this serious maladaptive response to illness.

Milton S. Davis, Ph.D., M.D.
Director of Adult Outpatient Psychiatry
Thalians, Cedars-Sinai Medical Center
Los Angeles

and

Adjunct Associate Professor
Department of Psychiatry, U.C.L.A.

Preface

In part because of the human actions that they might motivate, scientific theories are often judged on the basis of their pragmatic potential. Lately, this has become particularly true of the contributions of the social and behavioral sciences—sociology, psychology, and anthropology. Important questions regarding their applicability have been raised as the theories and empirical research findings from these fields have begun to play an increasingly important role in the everyday practice of medicine.

Our goal in this book is to examine in some depth, from the viewpoint of these sciences, a problem that has plagued medicine in modern times. This problem—patient noncompliance—involves patients' failure (because of resistance and/or unwillingness) to fulfill the requirements of a prescribed medical regimen or to engage in preventive health care. Patient noncompliance involves a number of social and behavioral science issues from thoughts and feelings to interpersonal relationships to the influence of social class and culture.

Many factors have been shown to influence patient compliance with preventive and curative regimens, not the least of which is the health professional himself or herself. In fact, as we will consider in this book, the practitioner (physician, nurse, nurse practitioner, physician's assistant) is probably the most important link between patient compliance and the other factors that can affect it. Thus, in a careful examination of the many factors that have been found to affect patients' cooperation, we have remained constantly aware of the practitioner's role in communicating with the patient, in establishing trust and rapport, in assessing cooperation and the attitudes and beliefs that support or inhibit it, in changing these beliefs and attitudes, and in altering the behaviors that result from them. While examining issues of interpersonal influence, we have encouraged the practitioner's emphasis on the patient's capacity to be personally responsible, to exercise self-control, and to be self-determining. We have taken the view that while the patient is guided, motivated, and cared for by the health professional, he or she remains in ultimate control of his or her own health actions. Acceptance of this fact is critical to the patient's success at internalizing health recommendations.

We have attempted to appeal to a broad readership. This book presupposes no background in the problem of medical noncompliance or in social psychology, although some basic familiarity with social science terms (such as "relationship," "personality," "social class," and "correlation") will be helpful. This book will most likely be used by advanced undergraduate students and beginning graduate students in the social sciences who are interested in health care applications of their fields. It is also broadly applicable to health science students and medical practitioners (especially those with primary patient care responsibilities) because it presents a comprehensive overview of the vast literature on patient cooperation within a heuristic framework which is at once intuitively appealing and clinically applicable. Finally, we have reviewed a great deal of empirical research and theory on the topic of patient compliance with medical recommendations, and have been careful to state which findings are strong and thus might be trusted to generate clinical applications, and which are more sparse in their empirical support. We also note important areas for future social science research.

This book has evolved slowly over the last four years. When one of us (DiMatteo) first began doing research on the practitioner-patient relationship, she was primarily interested in the factors that comprise the art of medicine. The expansion of this interest to include a focus on the interpersonal effects of the art of medicine was natural for someone who was trained as a social psychologist. On the other hand, DiNicola was initially enchanted with the classic sociological formulations of the practitioner-patient relationship. His early research on the effects of ambient temperature on the osmolality and pH of jackrabbit urine did not easily give way to this somewhat drier topic, but in time evolved to an interest in the health practitioner as influencer and agent of social control. Our collaboration on the material presented here began rather soon after our serendipitous meeting in early 1978 at the University of California at Riverside. At that time, the cages housing DiNicola's experimental pigs were leaking into DiMatteo's office, precariously close to the empirical data on practitioner-patient relationships presented in Chapter 3. Our joint efforts to retrieve and restore these data led to a research collaboration which has produced a number of papers as well as this book. Interestingly, it led to another collaboration—our marriage, which took place about half-way through Chapter 4.

Therefore, while it would certainly be in keeping with tradition for us to dedicate this book to our spouses who suffered long absences from us as we completed the manuscript, this was in fact not the case. We spent virtually all of our writing time together and found it extremely enjoyable. We dedicate this book instead to our family, who saw us very little during the last year, and who graciously and lovingly settled for abbreviated phone calls.

We would also like to acknowledge colleagues who encouraged us in this endeavor: Cathie Atkins and Bob Kaplan, Bert Raven, Michele Lunieski, and Karen Hartman. Special thanks go to Professor Mary Ann Baker of the Department of Biomedical Sciences at U.C. Riverside for standing as an enduring example of energy, intelligence, and dedication, and for the opportunity she provided DiNicola to work with experimental pigs.

We are also very grateful to UCR psychology department chairman, Professor Marvin Nachman, for his continuing support, and to UCR students, Ron Hays, Alan Stacy, Rob McArthur, Karen Hartman, Steve Ecoff, Brad Chew, Kent Swanson, Lee Stone, Jeremy Kaslow, and Inez Urie, who were helpful in reviewing research materials for the book. We also thank the reference librarians at the UCR Bioagricultural and General Libraries, UCLA, Biomedical Library, and Harvard Medical School Countway Library.

Finally, we would like to thank Malinda Fulmer of UCR who typed the entire manuscript, and Deanna DiNicola, who prepared the references.

M.R.D.
D.D.D.

Sunnymead, California
December, 1981

1

The Compliance Problem: An Introduction

Every day in their role as healers, medical practitioners provide their patients with specific treatment recommendations. They advise some patients to stop smoking in order to reduce the risks of heart attack or lung disease. They suggest that others adhere to a strict diet and course of insulin therapy in order to delay the vascular ravages of diabetes as long as possible. For still others they prescribe a simple ten-day course of penicillin to eradicate bacterial infections. In practice, nearly all medical encounters culminate in advice to the patient. What's more, it is widely held that these recommendations are made in the interest of the patient's own good.

In giving medical advice, clinicians call upon the many advances in patient care that have brought medicine to the scientific forefront in recent years. Patients with heart disease, once sure to die in early middle age, are now offered treatments that prolong their lives and restore in some measure their health and vigor. Diabetic patients can now enjoy essentially normal and productive lives by faithfully taking insulin and regulating their diet and exercise. Patients with acute infections are quickly and easily cured by merely adhering to a ten-day course of medication. Typically, patients who receive these sound medical recommendations have come in search of them and have invested considerable time, money, energy, and emotion. They have withstood detailed questioning and sometimes obnoxious physical examination in the process of seeking help. Their practitioners have in turn puzzled through elaborate and sometimes complicated differential diagnosis. At the end of the medical visit a specific treatment recommendation is usually formulated, but despite the considerable investment of both parties and the serious health consequences that might result, the chances are really quite good that the patient will fail to follow the hard-earned medical advice.

Attempts by medical practitioners to gain compliance, concession, obedience, allegiance, acquiescence, adherence, or self-control from their patients very often meet with failure. Deliberately or not, many patients ignore, totally forget, or erroneously implement their treatment recommendations. These recommendations can involve such diverse actions as following a restricted diet, taking a pill daily, or returning for follow-up appointments. Occasionally, patients creatively substitute their own particular treatment regimen in place of the one that was medically prescribed. In essence, noncompliance is the patient's failure to fulfill the clinical prescription (Haynes, 1979). It stands to reason, then, that in order for a patient to be noncompliant, a specific treatment recommendation must have been offered and received at some point. That this is not always the case is a problem which is investigated further in Chapter 2.

Empirical studies of patient compliance have shown that it occurs among patients of all ages, social classes, and ethnic groups, and amidst patients participating in various forms of health care delivery (for example, health maintenance organizations, private visits, specialty referral visits). Noncompliance is a common response of patients who are without symptoms, only slightly ill, or already seriously ill (Haynes, 1979; Sackett & Snow, 1979). In sum, it can be said that patient noncompliance thrives wherever and whenever medical recommendations are generated.

While certain complex recommendations, such as those involving major life-style changes, are somewhat less likely to be followed than are simpler assignments (like taking medication twice a day), adherence to either type of regimen is surprisingly poor. Regardless of its curative or preventive potential, the regular taking of *prescribed* medications is avoided to an alarming degree. Patients fail to follow short-term medication regimens at rates of 20–30 percent when the regimen is curative (resulting in the relief of symptoms) and 30–40 percent when the regimen is preventive (Sackett & Snow, 1979). With lifetime medication regimens and with long-term behavioral scheduling, such as eating a restricted diet to prevent or control symptoms in diabetes or hypertension, noncompliance is usually about 50 percent initially and increases as the therapy continues (Sackett & Snow, 1979; Haynes, 1979; Luntz & Austin, 1960).

Compliance is also very important in preventive health measures—those that seek to forestall or completely prevent the occurrence of disease. Despite knowledge of health risks for cancer, heart disease, stroke, and other serious illnesses, and despite direct medical advice against risky behaviors, people continue to smoke, overeat, drink too much, and avoid exercise (Knowles, 1977; Henderson, Hall & Lipton, 1979). Moreover, people often engage in combinations of these unhealthy behaviors (Langlie, 1977). This latter "preventive" category of noncompliance is the most problematic in terms of adherence because the required regimens extend into virtually every aspect of the patient's life (Surgeon General, 1979).

Noncompliance is increasingly regarded as an important issue, both because it jeopardizes patients' health and well-being, and because of the concomitant cost to the health care system. Patients' failure to keep medical appointments is expensive because clinician and clerical staff time is wasted. Research on appointment keeping in medical settings (reviewed by Sackett & Snow, 1979) has shown that only 40–50 percent of patients comply with appointments for preventive regimens and only 60–70 percent comply with appointments for curative regimens. If patients drop out of treatment, their histories, physical exams, and tests must be repeated when they seek care in other medical settings (Kasteler, Kane, Olsen, & Thetford, 1976; DiMatteo, Prince, & Taranta, 1979).

Noncompliance interferes with the practitioner's theraupeutic efforts, and in addition to exacerbating the already poor health of the patient, prompts the practitioner to order a renewed round of diagnostic evaluations and/or to prescribe another (second-choice) treatment regimen. These maneuvers are likely to bring discomfort to the patient and confusion to the practitioner. They enhance the cost, risk, and uncertainty of the patient's care. If the patient remains ill and the practitioner continually frustrated, the therapeutic relationship is likely to be jeopardized. Noncompliance also poses a threat to the accuracy of clinical research efforts, for the measurement of the effectiveness of a new drug or treatment is based upon the assumption that patients have followed the conditions of administration.

A HISTORICAL PERSPECTIVE ON THE MEDICAL RECOMMENDATIONS OF TODAY

Prior to the twentieth century, patients and practitioners had considerably less control over matters of medical concern than is currently the case. Whether or not patients adhered to their physicians' recommendations probably mattered little in days of old. In fact, because of the widespread use of such dangerous treatments as cupping, purging, trephining, and the ingestion of arsenic and strychnine tonics, it is quite likely that before this century patients who ignored their physicians' recommendations were much the better for it (Shapiro, 1960). Throughout the 1800s, the primary causes of morbidity were such diseases as tuberculosis, typhoid, pneumonia, and influenza (Torrens, 1978). In those days, scientifically efficacious cures, such as antibiotics, were unavailable and unsophisticated public health standards made widespread infection of the population a not uncommon reality (Torrens, 1978). While many hardy and fortunate individuals were able to avoid or fully recover from these infectious diseases, many others died in young adulthood or early middle age. Few lived long enough to experience today's

Table 1.1. Leading Causes of Death in the United States in 1900 and 1972.

1900 — Death Rate: 1.7% of U.S. population died in 1900

Rank	Cause of Death	Percentage of Total Deaths
1	Pneumonia and Influenza	11.8
2	Tuberculosis	11.3
3	Dysentery, enteritis, intestinal ulcer	8.3
4	Heart disease	8.0
5	Senility (ill defined)	6.8
6	Intracranial lesions (vascular)	6.2
7	Nephritis	5.2
8	All accidents	4.2
9	Cancer; malignant tumors	3.7
10	Diphtheria	2.3

1972 — Death Rate: 0.9% of U.S. population died in 1972

Rank	Cause of Death	Percentage of Total Deaths
1	Heart disease	38.4
2	Cancer; malignancies	17.7
3	Cerebrovascular disease (stroke)	10.7
4	Accidents	5.8
5	Influenza and pneumonia	3.1
6	Suicide and homicide	2.2
7	Diabetes mellitus	2.0
8	Diseases of early infancy	1.7
9	Arteriosclerosis	1.7
10	Cirrhosis of the liver	1.7
11	Bronchitis, emphysema, and asthma	1.5

Source: U.S. National Center for Health Statistics, *Vital Statistics of the United States*, Washington, D.C., August 1973.

more insidious killers—heart disease, stroke, and cancer—or to reproduce and pass on such genetically linked chronic diseases as diabetes.

Since 1900, patterns of morbidity and mortality have changed significantly in the industrialized countries of Western Europe and in the United States (see Table 1.1). Our primary health concerns have shifted from the acute infectious epidemics of the nineteenth century to the chronic, degenerative conditions treated by present-day medical practitioners (Dubos, 1959; McKeown, 1976; Torrens, 1978). The prevalence of today's chronic conditions may easily be taken to demonstrate the overwhelming success of early sociopolitical and public health endeavors (Dubos, 1959), as well as later medical developments of antibiotics and vaccines (Ingelfinger, 1978). Overcoming those early health problems required primarily responsible social and political action on the part of society's leaders and public health experts.

PREVENTION AND CONTROL OF TODAY'S DISEASES

Unlike the diseases of the 1800s, today's most prevalent health problems are not preventable through such mass measures as sanitation and vaccination, or curable with powerful "magic bullets," such as antibiotics. While the magic bullets for the cure of today's major afflictions—cardiovascular disease, cancer, diabetes, stroke, cirrhosis of the liver, to name but a few—may merely be as yet undiscovered (Thomas, 1979), our present state of knowledge points only to prevention and control as current viable solutions. (Of course there may never be magic bullets developed to treat most of today's chronic conditions. Many believe, in fact, that these conditions are multifactorial in nature and hence are not amenable to cure by magic bullets [Dubos, 1959]. Thomas [1979] reminds us, however, that at one time before their causes were known, syphilis and Vitamin B_{12} deficiency were also thought to be multifactorial diseases.)

Yet, constrained as we are by our present level of medical knowledge, the chronic health problems of today needn't wreak havoc on our population. The tremendous physical, emotional, and financial cost (including the high death rate) brought about by these diseases is, in part, avoidable. A significant percentage of the instances of heart disease, cancer (primarily certain forms such as lung, bladder, and throat), and cerebrovascular stroke, are believed to occur prematurely or to have significantly more damaging effects than are necessary (Pelletier, 1979). Let us consider this issue in more detail.

Heart disease is the most common cause of death of Americans over the age of 40. It is also the primary cause of permanent disability in this older population. For example, of the two million deaths that occurred in America in 1969, 40 percent were the direct result of heart disease. It has been estimated that 80 percent of all deaths owing to cardiovascular disease occur prematurely and are facilitated by adherence to unhealthy habits—primarily cigarette smoking, overweight, and a sedentary lifestyle (Knowles, 1977). The Surgeon General's report of 1964 officially implicated cigarette smoking as a direct cause of lung cancer (Surgeon General, 1964). Yet, today lung cancer remains our most common lethal malignancy, accounting for at least one-quarter of all cancer deaths. It has been estimated that 80 percent of all lung cancer deaths are directly caused by cigarette smoking. In 1964, 52 percent of the American male population smoked. In 1974, after ten years of an intense antismoking campaign in the United States, 42 percent of males smoked. Accompanying this small but favorable 10-percent decline in smoking among men was an unfortunate and signficant rise in teenage smoking and in smoking among women. Public health statistics estimate that by 1983, lung cancer will surpass breast cancer as the most common malignancy among women (Surgeon General, 1979). Other dangers are very real as well, for smoking not only leads directly to premature deaths from lung cancer, but is directly associated with mortality and morbidity from emphysema, chronic bronchitis, cardiovascular disease (stroke and heart attack), bladder cancer, and oropharyngeal cancer.

The recurring theme in this list of gruesome statistics is that a significant proportion of the morbidity and mortality in our society occurs prematurely. Much of it may even be completely preventable. The diseases enumerated above represent avoidable sources of suffering. Considerable evidence suggests that these conditions might be forestalled or prevented completely by people's control of their personal habits and behaviors (Belloc, 1973; Fuchs, 1975; Knowles, 1977, Carlson & Bollinger, 1972). Thus, today more than ever before, the maintenance of healthy habits and compliance with medical recommendations can contribute significantly to prevention and/or cure of disease.

Medical recommendations themselves can take a number of forms. Practitioners may *prescribe* certain behaviors such as exercise to their patients (and hope that their patients will carry out the behaviors), or they may *proscribe* behaviors such as smoking (and hope that their patients will refrain from engaging in them). Medical prescriptions and proscriptions may be made for the short-term (for a few days to a few weeks) or for the long-term (many months to a lifetime). The practitioner's intervention may also occur at any point in the disease process and so prevention can take one of three basic forms—primary, secondary, or tertiary. Primary prevention involves the prevention of disease *before* any symptoms are present. It may include widespread programs to promote healthy behaviors for everyone. Primary prevention involves taking such action as maintaining normal weight, exercising, not smoking, and participating in screening (to detect abnormalities such as early stages of cancer or essential hypertension) and immunization (such as for poliomyelitis). Secondary prevention involves the enactment of some preventive regimen by a person who has been defined as "at risk." An example of this is the maintenance by the hypertensive patient (at risk for a stroke or heart attack) of a lifetime regimen of medication and low-sodium diet in order to control his blood pressure. Another example is the yearly electrocardiogram taken by a man who has a family history of heart disease. Tertiary prevention involves strategies designed specifically to control the progress of disease (such as the self-injection of insulin by the diabetic, the cooperation with treatment by the cancer patient, and the faithful taking of medication by the patient with an acute infection). This category includes curative regimens.

Throughout this book we shall see that despite variance in the precise character of the required regimen and the disease which is to be prevented or controlled, the phenomenon of noncompliance can be understood in terms of a limited number of factors. We shall also see that medical care takes place within a complex interpersonal relationship between practitioner and patient. If medical care involved merely making decisions and giving advice in the format of a purely technical enterprise, diagnoses would be made by weighing the appropriate evidence, and treatment regimens would be planned solely in terms of optimal biomedical considerations. Advice would be put into practice by patients and illness would be cured or preventive care consistently managed. Purely technical medicine rarely exists, however. The patient is a person who, for many and varied reasons, may resist efforts to care for him/herself (DiMatteo & Friedman, 1982). Because of the complexity inherent in medical care, compliance requires attention to many psychological and social issues.

SEMANTICS AND THE CONCEPT OF COMPLIANCE

Any detailed analysis of compliance should at least consider the meaning of the word "compliance." The dictionary definition of compliance suggests yielding to the wish, request, or command of another. Researchers who have studied health behavior have employed a number of other words in lieu of compliance—terms such as adherence, obedience, cooperation, concordance, collaboration, and therapeutic alliance. Sackett and Haynes (1976) have argued that these terms are best used interchangeably, whereas other writers (one of us included; see DiMatteo & Friedman, 1982) have suggested that compliance reflects an overly authoritative approach to patient care which implies an obligation on the part of the patient to follow the practitioner's orders blindly. Some researchers have taken this a step further and have used various of these terms to refer to differing degrees or stages of power sharing in the practitioner-patient relationship (Barofsky, 1978). Others have justified the use of one term (adherence) over the other (compliance) by reference to the Whorf-Sapir hypothesis that "the nature of the words used to describe events has a powerful influence upon how those events are understood" (Dunbar & Stunkard, 1979, p. 392). Still others have justified the use of exactly the opposite term (compliance over adherence) since the "unhealthy connotations [of compliance] . . . keep ethical and social issues in compliance research and management up front where they belong" (Haynes, 1979, p. 2). The issue of when each term is best may be difficult to resolve since it reflects, at bottom, the user's philosophic orientation. We feel that it is rather unlikely that empirical demonstration that the term for a patient's following of medical advice either influences or reflects the power relationship between practitioner and patient will be obtained.

In order to remain consistent with the most accepted term in the literature, we have chosen to refer here primarily to patient compliance. We do, however, occasionally employ the terms adherence and cooperation as well. We use these terms interchangeably, and in so doing we do not wish to imply varying power relationships between the practitioner and patient. When we are dealing with issues of power and control, we shall identify them explicitly. In Chapter 6, we consider this semantic issue further, and suggest that the most appropriate goal for the pursuit of medical recommendations may in fact involve a different term altogether—that of internalization. (We are certainly not suggesting that compliance be forthwith called internalization. We believe that there already exists an abundance of words that refer to compliance. We offer the term internalization for heuristic purposes only.) This term has rarely if ever been used in the literature to describe the goal of the practitioner-patient influence process, yet internalization is precisely the most appropriate end point of such an attempt. Understandably difficult to achieve, internalization requires the patient's continued self-control and internally motivated commitment to adhere to the treatment regimen. During the process of internalization, the patient's positive beliefs about the regimen become a part of his entire system of beliefs; his behavior becomes self-reinforcing. He relates to the medical practitioner maturely, as a partner, and not as a cooperative subordinate or controlling superordinate. The goal of this book is to analyze the factors within the therapeutic relationship that promote initial cooperation and then give rise to and maintain patients' self-motivation and internalization.

ON ASSESSING PATIENT COMPLIANCE

The issue of assessment brings to the forefront some methodological and conceptual issues in compliance. As we shall see in this section, compliance is a very difficult parameter to measure accurately. This suggests some important questions about the practitioner-patient relationship and about patients' monitoring or awareness of their own behavior with respect to what has been prescribed. Specifically, do patients know what they are supposed to do? Are they aware enough of their own behavior to determine whether or not it measures up to criterion? If it does not, do patients feel free to admit their compliance difficulties to their practitioners? Answers to these and other questions are critically important for a complete understanding of the compliance phenomenon.

The Importance of Assessment

> Keep a watch also on the faults of the patients, which often make them lie about the taking of things prescribed. For through not taking disagreeable drinks, purgative or other, they sometimes die. What they have done never results in a confession, but the blame is thrown upon the physician.
>
> —Hippocrates, *On Decorum*

As far back as Hippocrates, the difficulty inherent in relying on patients' personal reports of their medical compliance has been understood. Patients, it seems, do not always tell the truth. They typically report that they have followed their health practitioner's advice when, in fact, sometimes they have not.

Monitoring patients' follow-through with prescribed regimens is important for several obvious—and some not so obvious—reasons. The patient may be dangerously following an incorrect schedule of administration, having misunderstood or forgotten the specific directions. Checking, in this case, can save a patient's life. Also monitoring by the practitioner allows him or her to modify the treatment regimen in the light of the patient's difficulty in following it or as a result of the effect of the regimen on the patient's medical condition. In the face of obvious compliance difficulties, the practitioner may need to provide more convincing evidence to the patient regarding the value of following a particular regimen, or provide suggestions to aid the patient in carrying the regimen through. Monitoring of the patient's level of compliance also provides an opportunity for the practitioner and patient to resolve conflicts that arise between them—conflicts stemming from the regimen itself or from aspects of the practitioner-patient interaction. One researcher found that if practitioners neglected to question their patients about compliance, the patients tended to conclude that the practitioners did not attach much importance to the regimen or did not believe in its efficacy (Svarstad, 1976). As we shall see later, practitioners are very often unaware of their patients' compliance and often fail to assess it. It is hardly surprising to note, then, that the accurate assessment of patients' cooperation is an important, though often neglected, task.

Some studies have addressed the issue of practitioners' monitoring and its effect on enhancing patients' commitment to the therapeutic regimen. Svarstad (1976) categorized the behavior of physicians according to the degree to which they engaged in monitoring patients and later assessed the patients' conformance to physicians' advice. She found that when physicians verbally checked with their patients regarding compliance, patients were more likely to comply. In addition, Svarstad found that physicians who engaged in more extensive follow-up monitoring of their patients received more *accurate* feedback from them. When physicians were concerned over a long period of time about their patients' compliance, patients were more honest. When physicians monitored patients' compliance, patients were more likely to express complaints and to admit to having had problems conforming to the regimen. On the other hand, when physicians did not explicitly question them, patients were much less likely to express dissatisfaction with the regimen, and were much more apt to conceal their noncompliance. Svarstad also found that when patients admitted to having had difficulty following their regimens, physicians were very likely to respond appropriately and to follow through with efforts to enhance their patients' motivation (for example, by expressing friendly concern).

Practitioners' Lack of Awareness

Despite the compelling beneficial effects of being aware of their patients' compliance, practitioners are somewhat unlikely to engage in patient monitoring. Physicians in general tend to believe that compliance is high enough to render monitoring unnecessary. Davis (1966) surveyed 131 junior and senior physicians (medical students and attending faculty physicians) from an academic medical center who were seeing patients in a general medical clinic. These physicians were asked to estimate the percentage of their patients who were compliant. Forty-two percent of the physicians claimed that almost all of their patients adhered to the medical advice prescribed. Another 47 percent claimed that three-fourths of their patients were cooperative. Only 11 percent felt that about half their patients were compliant (which was closest to the correct figure). Davis concluded that, in contrast to the findings in the literature on patient compliance, physicians' estimates were generally grossly exaggerated. Practitioners in this study were, for the most part, unable to recognize noncompliance among their patients.

Caron and Roth (1968, 1971) also studied physicians' awareness of patient compliance. After working on a gastrointestinal subspecialty ward for three months, 27 medical residents rated their patients' compliance. Each resident was given a list of patients (19 patients, on the average) who had been prescribed a liquid antacid. The patients had been in the hospital an average of three to four weeks at some time during the physician's rotation on the ward. Each physician was interviewed about his or her patients' compliance, and asked to estimate the amount of antacid each patient actually took. Physicians were also asked to rate their degree of confidence in their ratings. (Only the ratings made with a high degree of confidence were used in the analyses.) The physicians did not know that the actual dosage of antacid taken by the patient had been measured by nurses and other workers on the project. Twenty-two of the 27 resident physicians significantly overestimated their patients' compliance. Similar research with the senior faculty physicians indicated that they too overestimated their patients' compliance. A further finding concerned the resident physicians' knowledge of which of their patients were compliant and which were not. Residents were asked to rank their patients by level of adherence to the antacid regimen, and ranks were correlated with the patients' actual adherence. The median rank order correlation was .01, indicating that physicians were not able to discriminate at greater than chance level between patients who were good or bad compliers. To determine whether physicians had formed definite impressions of their patients, nine of them were asked to form new impressions two weeks after the original ratings. The high coefficients of correlation between the original and follow-up ratings showed that most physicians did hold definite ideas about their patients' actual rate of adherence to the medical regimen.

Other research (Moulding, Onstad & Sbarbaro, 1970; Mushlin & Appel, 1977; McClellan & Cowan, 1970; Norell, 1981) has also suggested that physicians typically overestimate rates of compliance among their patients, and that they are inaccurate in identifying noncompliant individuals. In their review of the compliance literature, Sackett and Snow (1979) noted that the gap between the regimen prescribed by the clinician and that adhered to by the patient is often distressingly wide, and that, tragically, the clinician is often the last to know about noncompliance.

The Causes of Practitioner Unawareness. Why are practitioners so unaware of their patients' compliance? Davis (1966) has suggested a psychological explanation—that the primary cause is the practitioner's ego involvement. The physician is particularly invested in the success of his treatment, and in his authority, status, and sense of importance. This investment prevents the physician from recognizing that patients are not following the prescribed treatment. This explanation seems to emphasize an adversarial position between practitioner and patient.

An equally plausible reason for the discrepancy is a lack of knowledge of the problem of compliance in general, and a low index of suspicion among physicians because of their own future orientation and belief in the importance of rational action (Gillum & Barsky, 1974). This explanation emphasizes the need for physicians' awareness of the general problem of compliance, and of the compliance of their own patients in particular. That the physician's lack of knowledge is an important factor related to the compliance issue is supported by a study by Inui, Yourtee, and Williamson (1976), who showed that compliance could be enhanced by simply increasing physicians' awareness of the problem. Despite the disadvantages of the physicians' unawareness, there exists no single simple explanation for it nor is there a simple rationale underlying difficulties in assessing patient compliance. Assessment is always complicated by the diverse determinants of compliance, the many issues related to patient motivation, and the multifarious nature of the practitioner-patient relationship. Because of this, assessment accuracy will depend heavily upon the extent to which the factors examined throughout this book are meticulously taken into account.

Patients' Withholding of the Truth

Practitioners often remain unaware of their patients' noncompliance because patients rarely spontaneously reveal their difficulties with the regimen to their physicians. Patients' withholding of information is understandable when physicians do not question patients specifically about the difficulties they may be having following their regimen. Patients, however, have been found to withhold information—to lie, as Hippocrates noted—even when directly asked whether or not they have complied. One of the earliest studies of compliance (Feinstein et al., 1959) noted discrepancies between compliance reported in interviews and that determined by the method of "pill count" among over 100 mothers of children on penicillin prophylaxis. To form a pill count, the practitioner must count the number of pills remaining in the pill bottle at some point in the regimen and compare it with the number that should be there if the patient has followed the regimen correctly. There was good agreement between the two measurement methods among those patients classified as poor compliers but there was a considerable discrepancy between interviews and pill counts among those classified as good compliers. While pill counts classified only 55 percent as good compliers and 35 percent as questionable, interviews presented 73 percent of patients as good compliers and only 19 percent as questionable. Thus, patients whose compliance was questionable (as measured by the more objective means of pill count) tended, in their self-reports, to "err" in the direction of presenting themselves as fully compliant. Other studies (such as Park & Lipman, 1964; and Rickels & Briscoe, 1970) have noted discrepancies between pill counts and self-reports in interviews, and found that the greatest discrepancy between the two methods occurred when the actual deviation from the prescribed dosage was small. Interview responses tended to be more in line with the objective measure when the deviation from prescribed dosage was large, perhaps owing to patients' inability to hide a truly serious deviation from the prescribed regimen, or to their lack of awareness of a small deviation.

In a study of mothers' compliance with medication regimens prescribed by pediatricians, Francis, Korsch, and Morris (1969) found a surprisingly close agreement between pill counts and interview self-reports of compliance. Out of 129 patients, only 11 (8.5 percent) exhibited a discrepancy between pill count and interview. In all 11 cases the patient implied compliance, while the pill count suggested noncompliance. Using urine tests of penicillin excretion as the objective criterion measure, Gordis et al. (1969) found mothers' responses to interview questions regarding their childrens' taking of penicillin to be considerably less accurate. They tended to exaggerate (or overstate) compliance. This was also found in studies of long-term compliance by adult patients on digitalis (Sheiner et al., 1974) and by ambulatory tuberculosis patients (Preston & Miller, 1964).

Researchers who study patient compliance often conclude that because of the discrepancies that exist between interview responses from patients and more "objective" measures (such as pill counts and direct assay of medication in the body), interview data from patients cannot be trusted (Gordis et al., 1969). Patients' reports are likely to be influenced by so many factors that they will not present a true picture of their compliance. We feel that such a conclusion is misleading for the very factors that bring about the discrepancies in measures of compliance are of interest in themselves. The reasons for patients' inaccuracy in interview reporting should be explored since they are likely to suggest methods for enhancing patients' interview accuracy. It is important to keep in mind that the simple conclusion that patients' reports "cannot be trusted" is imprecise and incorrect, and may present a serious barrier to the measurement and understanding of patient compliance. Instead, we should seek to understand patients' reporting of their compliance fully just as we must seek to understand compliance behavior itself. The factors that influence both are actually parallel in many ways.

Barriers to Patient Reporting of Noncompliance

Exaggerated statements by patients concerning the degree of their compliance conceivably involve two phenomena: (1) purposeful omission of the truth, and (2) failure of memory or understanding. Some might argue that these are one and the same phenomenon, but we do not take this view here. In the first case, the patient knows that he has not taken the medication as prescribed by the practitioner, but states that he has done so. He may do this in order to avoid recrimination, punishment, or rejection by the practitioner. He may attempt to fulfill the practitioner's expectations and desires, and seek to please the practitioner (who perhaps appears to need the cooperation of patients). The patient himself may be in need of emotional support and approval, and is aware that reporting compliance (instead of noncompliance) is an excellent way to receive it. In the second case, the patient intends to tell the truth, but just as he often cannot remember to take his medication, so too he cannot remember how much of it he has actually taken. His report of compliance is in error. Or, the patient may have misunderstood the regimen in the first place and thought he fulfilled its requirements completely.

There are no foolproof methods for determining which factor—deliberate misrepresentation of compliance or simple forgetting—motivates a given patient's responses regarding compliance. A failure of memory becomes that much easier to maintain if it is socially desirable to do so—that is, if it presents the patient as appropriately compliant even though he is not. Since accurate measurement of patients' compliance to their treatment is necessary for the delivery of effective medical care, the development of methods to enhance the accuracy of compliance reporting is of major importance. There are methods to enhance the patients' motivations to be truthful as well as to increase their ability to report on their behavior accurately. In the following paragraphs, we briefly examine theory and research which pertains directly to increasing patient honesty and improving patient memory. These methods derive from many of the issues we consider in this book, particularly the art of medicine (in Chapter 3) and communication (in Chapter 2).

Solutions for the Accurate Measurement of Patient Compliance

The need for secretive or probing strategies (such as pill counts, direct urine or blood assay, questioning a family member, and others) to gauge patient compliance has been seriously criticized by some compliance researchers (Sackett, 1979; Stone, 1979). They have noted that factors in the practitioner-patient relationship may interfere with the accurate interview reporting of patients' compliance with their medical regimens. If barriers to patient truthfulness are removed, a patient's report of his own difficulties and successes with the treatment regimen may become quite accurate and trustworthy and may be the most valuable source of information available regarding the patient's compliance. The important reason is that open and successful disclosure about compliance is both a product of and a catalyst for a practitioner-patient relationship of high quality. Open disclosure stems from and motivates a therapeutic partnership.

A Practitioner-Patient Partnership

In his presentation of the Health Transactions Model, psychologist George Stone (1979) has emphasized the importance of viewing compliance not as something a patient has or does not have, but rather as a property that arises in the transaction between two people. In the former, conventional view, compliance is considered the total responsibility of the patient:

> Acknowledgment of noncompliance constitutes an admission of failure, even moral culpability, on the part of the client. Such acknowledgment is, therefore, relatively unlikely to occur, even in response to a direct question. On the other hand, if the entire transaction between expert and client were construed in terms of shared responsibility, with difficulties in following recommendations accepted as normal, evaluation of the success of the treatment could deal objectively with all aspects of the compliance process. [Stone, 1979, pp. 48–49]

Open communication between practitioner and patient regarding the latter's compliance demands a relationship based on mutual understanding, rapport, and trust—factors considered in detail in Chapter 3. Other aspects of practitioner-patient communication are also important, such as the clarity of their verbal interchange (Chapter 2). How the practitioner responds to the patient can certainly influence the patient's willingness and ability to communicate information, particularly about compliance problems. Apparent criticism (for example, "You did *what*? You should have known better!") can turn an accurate, trusting patient-historian into a defensive, monosyllabic respondent who is afraid to voice concerns lest he be criticized. Further, the practitioner must maintain an air of objectivity and open-mindedness regarding the patient's beliefs and cultural norms related to health issues (see Chapters 4 and 5, respectively). The practitioner should accept, in a nonjudgmental way, the patient's frame of reference (for example, reluctance to take any kind of medication) without imposing his own particular value system on the patient. The practitioner should explore and attempt to fulfill (or to explain why he or she is not fulfilling) the patient's expectations for treatment (Korsch et al., 1968). The accurate gauging of patient compliance requires attempts at the reduction in social distance between practitioner and patient (Plaja, Cohen, & Samora, 1968), and a bridging of barriers that are due to differences in education, social class, occupational status, and ethnic identification. The basic concerns that plague all patients ("Will I be alright?" "What caused my illness?" "Am I responsible for my illness?") must be appropriately recognized and considered by the practitioner. In all cases, the patient should feel that he or she is being treated with dignity and respect.

Aiding the Patient's Memory

Crucial to the accurate assessment of patient compliance is the process of obtaining accurate answers. Interviews in health settings, as we discuss further in Chapter 2, are seldom conducive to patients' accurate recall of information. The setting itself typically provokes anxiety, and the material is usually difficult to recall or to express. Survey researchers (Marquis, 1970; Cannell, Oksenberg, & Converse, 1977) have studied health interviews extensively—particularly the accuracy of patients' reporting of their health behaviors. Two aspects of this research are important to enhancing the accurate reporting of compliance in the context of the practitioner-patient relationship: (1) the effects of social reinforcement on reporting of health events and health behaviors, and (2) specific techniques to enhance respondents' recall of health issues.

Social Reinforcement. The personal interview is used in nearly every health professional-patient interaction. It is not, however, a straightforward, simple method of collecting information about individuals. Interviewing people about facts and about opinions relies heavily upon both verbal transactions and human memory, motivation, and understanding. Because the interaction between health professional and patient is a *social* exchange, social variables affect the course of the interview.

Research on health reporting has shown that people tend to underreport health incidents in their lives. Between 12 and 17 percent of documented hospital episodes are not reported by patients when they are specifically questioned about their past hospital visits. Between 23 and 36 percent of medical visits with a physician are not mentioned, even in interviews that take place soon (one to two weeks) after the medical visit. Interestingly, at least 50 percent of chronic and acute conditions that are documented in medical records are not reported by patients in health interviews (Marquis, 1970). Yet this underreporting (probably owing primarily to forgetting) does not occur to the same degree under all conditions. Forgetting is greatest when the content issues have personal significance for the individual. Memory and recall also depend upon the behavior of the interviewer. In regard to this latter factor, research has shown that "response bias" in interviews is common. That is, interviewers tend to reinforce specific classes of behavior among respondents by using subtle signs of approval (such as nodding or saying "Mm-hmm" or "good" or "fine"). Studies of health interviews have shown that patients are consistently reinforced for the worst possible response—evasion of the question or direct refusal to answer it.

Medical interviewers can significantly influence the accuracy of the answers that they receive from their patients. Social reinforcement can be used to increase the accuracy of patients' reporting of difficulties encountered in following treatment regimens. For example, reinforcing statements can be used to enhance the reporting of problems by stating "Yes, that's the kind of information I need to know about," or "Tell me all the other things like that so we can figure out some solutions." The interactive character of patient interviewing points to the importance of health professionals' behavior in the interview process. Because of their tendency unknowingly to reinforce poor patient responding (perhaps, as they believe, to avoid confronting or distressing the patient), health professionals should be acutely aware of their own behavior in interviews with patients, and seek to reinforce only the types of responses that they wish to increase (and perhaps remain totally neutral regarding the rest).

Specific Techniques Enhancing Recall. Research by Cannell and colleagues has suggested that the practitioner can do a number of things to improve the accuracy of patients' reporting in the health care interview. Most patients can accurately report information if it is available in their memory and if it is not too threatening. The health professional's task is to enhance the retrievability of the information by supporting patients' attempts to recall the information, and by assuring patients by words and behaviors that they will not experience even "a minimal risk of embarrassment" (Cannell et al., 1977, p. 309). According to these researchers, practitioners should clarify what is expected of each patient in order that the task of gathering information may be properly performed. This means that patients should be given clear instructions regarding the kind of information needed from them (for example, the exact dosage of medication taken, precisely when it was taken, how the patient felt about the regimen, what specific side effects resulted). Instructions are needed to clarify the goals of the interview, to point out that the patient's best interest is foremost to the practitioner, and to spell out precisely what the patient's contribution to the provision of information should be. Instructions should tell the patient how he or she can most effectively perform the task of informing the practitioner about compliance. The health practitioner should provide clues through feedback to the patient regarding the quality of his or her responses. Feedback also provides attention and social reinforcement to the patient. In addition, the elicitation of commitment from the patient to provide as much accurate information as possible to the practitioner might also motivate the patient to work diligently to recall information that may be difficult to bring to memory. Commitment, formally stated, helps to enhance patients' efforts and hence the quality of the health reporting.

As we shall discuss later, the factors reviewed here that enhance patients' accurate reporting of compliance (factors such as social reinforcement, trust in the practitioner-patient relationship, and commitment) are the very same factors that serve to enhance patient compliance itself.

Assessment: A Conclusion

The assessment of patient compliance is multifaceted and complex. It requires accuracy and care in the formulation and delivery of questions. It also requires a degree of sensitivity in response to patients' disclosures. The assessment of compliance requires interpersonal rapport in the practitioner-patient relationship. Thus, medical practitioners must be constantly aware of the social and psychological factors that affect patients' willingness and ability to report on their own compliance. As we have considered, many common factors in the health care situation are likely to attenuate the reliability of patients' responses. With careful attention to the therapeutic relationship and to methods for enhancing patients' recall of their health behaviors, the interview can become very effective in gauging patient compliance. Alternative approaches such as pill counts and biochemical assay may not then be needed. In many places throughout this book, we consider in more detail the accomplishment of the goal of accurate assessment during the therapeutic encounter.

NONCOMPLIANCE: A PLETHORA OF EXPLANATORY FACTORS

Researchers and practitioners who have examined the issue of noncompliance have provided a number of competing theories to explain the phenomenon. Their explanations tends to fall into three broad categories.

Intrapsychic Factors

Many theories of compliance posit that thoughts, feelings, or attitudes may favorably or unfavorably dispose patients toward specific treatments or specific practitioners. Motivational theories tend toward psychodynamic explanations and suggest that patient resistance can be understood in terms of rejection of authority (Appelbaum, 1977; Stimson, 1974; see Chapter 8). Other approaches explain noncompliance in terms of disease denial or rationalization of unhealthy behavior (Podell, 1975). Beliefs and attitudes about one's susceptibility to disease and the severity of potential disease influence compliance, as do patients' beliefs about the costs versus the benefits of treatment (Becker, 1974; see Chapter 4). Misinformation and inaccurate beliefs (such as those derived from culturally accepted, nonmedical sources) are also implicated in the search for causes of noncompliance (Stone, 1979; see Chapter 5). It is further hypothesized that patients resist medical advice in an attempt to achieve control in a situation in which they have lost control. They may engage in an active search to restore lost freedom (called psychological reactance; Brehm, 1966) or they may try to avoid developing a dependency to which past experience has shown them they are prone (Blane, 1968). Patients might seek to maintain commitment to a bad decision (a course of behavior such as smoking) by making themselves resistant to persuasion to change their beliefs about it (Festinger, 1957). By resisting therapeutic recommendations, patients may be attempting to balance the power and control in the practitioner-patient relationship. Within this framework, resistance is seen as a part of the inevitable power struggle between patient and practitioner that is the essence of medical care (Freidson, 1970; see Chapter 2 for further discussion of conflict in the therapeutic relationship, and Chapter 6 for discussion of persuasion and social influence by the practitioner).

Environmental Factors

A second variety of explanation for resistance includes the effects of the environmental aspects of patients' lives on their behavior and habits. Research suggests that barriers to compliance exist in the form of other demands made on the patient's resources (such as time, money, interest, and attention). Related to this are sociocultural explanations of patient compliance that point to the need for cultural and social supports to enhance compliant behavior and to overcome resistance (Stone, 1979). Behavioral approaches stress the need for environmental supports and reinforcements for the appropriate healthy behaviors if these behaviors are to be continued. (Environmental factors are considered in more detail in Chapter 7.)

The Practitioner-Patient Relationship

A third set of explanations for noncompliance emphasizes practitioner behavior toward the patient (an issue we examine in depth in Chapter 3). Noncompliance is sometimes explained in terms of reciprocation: the patient responds with resistance to the practitioner's control over and refusal to share information with him (Waitzkin & Stoeckle, 1972). Other approaches that focus on faulty communication between physician and patient deemphasize the intentionality of the physician's difficulties in communicating information to the patient (Svarstad, 1976). Lack of patient participation in decisions made about his or her own course of treatment has been suggested as a cause of resistance (Stone, 1979), as has the lack of caring, warmth, and understanding on the part of the practitioner (Rogers, 1957; Frank 1961). The technique-centered character of today's medical care (in contrast to earlier years) has been blamed for patient resistance because of the inevitable alienation of patients engendered by such technology (Rodin & Janis, 1979).

These three factors illustrate the diversity of theories that attempt to explain patient noncompliance. This diversity, while perhaps initially somewhat confusing, is advantageous because it helps to counteract the tendency of medical professionals to conceptualize noncompliance as a unitary phenomenon, with one specific cause, diagnosis, and treatment (Gillum & Barsky, 1974). As we demonstrate in this book, the problem of patient noncompliance with medical regimens does *not* lend itself to a single solution by a single technique (for example, only improving the communication of information, or enhancing the patient's social support). Although noncompliance can be understood in terms of a *limited number* of factors or dimensions (Cumming, Becker, & Maile, 1980), the development and maintenance of health behavior is undeniably complex. Patient compliance is embedded in an intricate web of social and psychological factors.

Understanding medical compliance in a social psychological framework, such as we are attempting to do in this book, reminds us that a patient's less than wholehearted acceptance of medical advice is not at all surprising. The giving of medical advice and the prescription of a medical regimen involves an attempt at influence on the part of the practitioner toward the patient. An influence attempt is never certain to succeed. It is possible, however, to delineate the conditions under which the suggestions of the practitioner will be manifested as behavioral change on the part of the patient. Such is our goal in this book.

OVERCOMING NONCOMPLIANCE: THE PROCESS AND CONTENT OF INFLUENCE

Cutting across the three general categories of explanation for noncompliance are two specific targets for patient noncompliance: the patient may resist the *influencer* (the practitioner) or the *advice*. These two targets of resistance suggest respectively two important themes in overcoming noncompliance: the *process* and the *content* of the influence attempts directed toward the patient. First, let us consider the targets of patient resistance to compliance with medical treatment.

A patient might *resist the influence of the provider* of care because of the provider's characteristics as a person, because of the poor quality of the therapeutic relationship, or because of the patient's rejection of the provider's position of authority. This resistance is likely to be manifested in the patient's rejection of treatment. He or she may fail to show up for appointments or may drop out of treatment and seek another health professional or alternative healer (Baekeland & Lundwall, 1975; Cobb, 1954; Hayes-Bautista, 1976). The second type of resistance involves acceptance of the provider but *rejection of the specific advice* that is given. This type of resistance is typically expressed through the patient's continued return for treatment after failure to follow the prescribed regimen or to stop an unhealthy practice proscribed by the practitioner. In this second case, the patient is assumed to be motivated to change but is apparently unable to control his or her behavior. Thus, in the first case, the patient's commitment to the practitioner's treatment is in doubt; in the second case this is not so. In this book, we examine the factors that contribute to both forms of patients' noncompliance with medical recommendations and show that these forms are in fact interrelated. Throughout, we propose and support the basic argument that acceptance of the specific health recommendations of a practitioner is very often predicated upon acceptance of the practitioner as a trusted and caring individual. Of course, the practitioner's reliability, trustworthiness, and concern for the patient as a person will depend to some degree upon the character of the recommendations he or she makes—whether they are in keeping with or far afield from the patient's belief system, and whether they are in direct opposition to the patient's cultural values and social norms. The extent to which the practitioner is willing and able to be sensitive to and deal with the psychological and social factors affecting patients' lives is likely to influence their acceptance of the practitioner as a person of influence.

Throughout this book, we likewise deal with both the process and the content of behavior change, carefully outlining the components of each and explaining their potential applications to the enhancement of patient compliance. An overview is presented below.

The Process of Practitioner Influence: Communication and Power

The verb "communicate" comes from the Latin *communis* or "common." To communicate is to attempt to establish a commonness. In anatomy, two structures in the body communicate if nothing limits the flow of a substance between them. For example, the knee's bursa and the knee joint capsule "communicate" because synovial fluid normally flows freely between them. Likewise, in terms of human social process, communication involves the unrestricted exchange of meaning between people to establish a commonness of thought, attitude, feeling, and idea. Such exchange may take place by means of words (verbal communication) or signs (nonverbal communication). For many reasons, communication is a particularly formidable problem in the medical-care setting. A common country or culture, for example, does not guarantee a sharing of language—of words and gestures as symbols—between patient and practitioner. Since illness and pain are subjective conditions (indeed, dependent not so much upon measurable physical states as upon the interpretation of them [Mechanic, 1968]), language symbols used by practitioner and patient are likely to have different meanings. Indeed, as we shall see in Chapters 2 and 3, communication is likely to be impeded when the sender and/or the receiver is anxious or emotionally upset, when there are differences between them in knowledge and power, or when disparities exist in their education and social status. Similarly, differences in priorities and purpose of information exchange as well as the use of professional "in-group" jargon severely complicate the process of communication. Pressures of time may thwart the mutual, repeated checking of interpretations necessary for an accurate exchange of meaning. Time limitations, too, may preclude the similarity of thought and congruence of feeling that are indispensable to communication. In sum, "the factors that complicate the process of shared meaning are nearly all present in doctor-patient encounters" (Barnlund, 1976, p. 721).

The following practitioner-patient exchange brings some communication issues to the forefront, defying the application of unilateral blame for problems in medical communication."

Physician: Does it hurt here?
Patient: No.
Physician: And here?
Patient: No.
Physician: Are you constipated?
Patient: No.
Physician: Do you know what constipated means?
Patient: No. [Mumford, 1977, p. 411]

Physicians seldom attempt to ascertain a patient's level of understanding, least of all for such elementary medical terms as constipation. Yet patients often do not understand the terms their practitioners normally use (Samora, Saunders, & Larson, 1961). When practitioners use these terms, most patients will not ask what they mean, preferring instead to attempt to decipher them within a given context. Thus, it is difficult, if not impossible, to assign "blame" to one or the other party, particularly when we realize that their interaction is imbedded in a social structure that imparts (or has imparted) behavioral expectations to each. Patients are expected to be cooperative and submissive (Parsons, 1958) while physicians are expected to be dominant and in control (Parsons, 1951). Such expectations, of course, influence their joint interaction, the information communicated, and its effects on patient compliance. Further, while motivation and commitment of practitioner and patient are necessary conditions for the development of effective communication, they do not automatically confer on these interactants the capacity to communicate with one another effectively. Rather, skills are needed by both practitioner and patient in order for them to translate their motives into actions.

A major aim of Chapters 2 and 3 is to delineate carefully the skills necessary for effective practitioner-patient communication. In Chapter 6 we examine the application of these skills to the practitioner's use of social power and his or her persuasion of the patient toward the goal of belief (and hence behavior) change. Throughout these chapters, we emphasize the number and complexity of factors that relate to practitioner-patient communication, and suggest that anyone who is truly serious about improving medical communication must avoid "the temptation to search for demons" (Barnlund, 1976, p. 722). No one party is to blame. Practitioners as well as patients must cope every day with anxieties, fears, and uncertainties surrounding medical treatment. Each must find "some compromise between private impulse and social expectation" (Barnlund, 1976, p. 722). Thus, the goal of our analysis of the process of influence is by no means to identify the one culprit responsible for poor communication—be it the patient, physician, hospital structure, profession of medicine, or human condition. Rather, we hope to examine precisely how each element that impinges upon the practitioner-patient relationship affects it, and what can be done to improve communication and social influence toward the goal of patient cooperation with prescribed medical treatment.

The Content of Practitioner Influence: Beliefs and Social Norms

Patients' minds are not blank tablets on which practitioners carve their prescriptions for health and well-being. Everything that a practitioner communicates to a patient about a regimen for health care must be filtered through the patient's system of beliefs about disease and about the expectations of others for his behavior. These beliefs and social norms therefore comprise the content (or substantive focus) of the practitioner's attempts to influence his or her patient's compliance.

Patients play active roles in their medical care. The beliefs and subjective norms that they construct and maintain tend to influence their health behaviors substantially. Patients make decisions regarding the necessity of treatment; they act upon the opinions they hold regarding their susceptibility to serious illness and the costs versus the benefits of receiving medical care. Partly on the basis of their beliefs, patients choose (or choose not) to seek medical advice and to follow the recommendations made to them for preventive and/or curative regimens. In addition, as members of various social networks composed of their cultural groups, families, friends, and acquaintances, patients receive medical information and advice, and learn what constitutes acceptable behavior. Patients attempt to weigh the influence of advice from medical practitioners against the advice of others who figure importantly in their lives. They try to maintain some degree of conformity with the expectations for behavior appropriate to their cultural and social identities. Therefore, psychological and social factors—patients' thoughts and others' expectations—operate in an extremely important way to influence patient compliance.

Practitioners who wish to affect their patients' health behavior must therefore clearly understand their patients' beliefs and social/cultural norms. These are the important substantive or content issues toward which the process of influence should be directed. Hence, in this book, we are compelled to deal explicitly with these issues if we are to understand compliance fully. In Chapter 4 we examine health beliefs and attitudes in detail, and consider both the Health Belief Model (Becker, 1974) and the general Value × Expectancy theory (Rotter, 1954) as valuable formats for understanding the role of psychological factors in patient compliance and health behavior. In Chapter 5 we examine the influence of the patient's cultural and social norms and expectations on compliance and preventive health action. In Chapter 7 we examine the content of barriers that hinder patients' fulfillment of their intended health behaviors. In all cases, we examine the role of the practitioner in modifying the factors that impede patients' compliance.

The Interaction of Process and Content

Our analysis of the many varied issues in the process and content of practitioner influence is not solely descriptive. Our goal is not simply to identify the factors that affect patient compliance and health protective behavior, but also to identify the influence of these factors on one another. Further, we present an implicit overall scheme. This scheme consists of a logical organization of the many factors that relate to patient compliance, and an appropriate ordering of the factors to consider in attempting behavior change. In this implicit structure (which we make explicit below), we suggest that in the development of medical compliance, certain factors are very clearly prerequisite to others. Understanding of the temporal relationships among the many factors that affect patients' health behaviors is an important step toward influencing patients' compliance.

The implicit scheme that we present suggests that a patient's behavior change (toward compliance with a prescribed regimen or toward adherence to a health-protective behavior) will not occur if barriers stand in the way of that change. In order to make alterations in their actions, patients must at least know how to monitor and control their behavior. Impediments to the new behavior (such as excessive cost) must also be removed or reduced. Certain supports for the behavior change (such as family encouragement, or skill at positive self-talk) are likely to facilitate the patient's translation of his desire to change into his enactment of the new behavior. The removal of barriers and/or the enhancement of supports will probably be effective only if the patient is committed to making the change. Otherwise, regardless of the ease of the regimen, the patient will probably not continue it for any period of time. Patient commitment to a regimen (particularly to a difficult one) is not easy for the practitioner to come by, however. Patients withhold commitment until they believe that the new health behavior is likely to be positive for them (for example, if they believe it is likely to bring positive, valued outcomes) and that they will receive social approval (or at least avoid social disapproval) for making the commitment to follow the regimen. In regard to this latter point, it is not surprising (and indeed, it is supported by empirical data) that patients will avoid treatment regimens that encourage social group (e.g., family, culture, and the like) disapproval or ostracism. If the patient's beliefs (about the regimen and about their likelihood of receiving social approval) go against the target health behavior, efforts must be exerted by the practitioner to change those beliefs and subjective norms or reduce their salience. Evidence abounds, of course, that social influence and persuasion by the practitioner demand a positive patient-practitioner relationship. Patients need to trust the practitioner before they will reveal their beliefs and subjective norms. Without trust in the practitioner, belief change is unlikely to occur. Likewise, communications from practitioner to patient must be clear and unambiguous in order for the patient to know what he is supposed to do to comply with the medical regimen, and for him to understand the appropriate change-oriented communications. Thus, each of the constructs in this scheme can be considered as a likely prerequisite to another, suggesting a logical sequence of components—from the practitioner's communication of information to the enactment and maintenance of behavior change skills. (Analyses of studies in the literature which have used single strategies, such as behavior modification, for changing behaviors have typically been undertaken *after* the prerequisites proposed here—such as rapport with the practitioner or experimenter, or commitment to the change—have been satisfied.)

We must note, of course, that our sequential "model" is supported by the many individual studies that are reviewed in the following chapters. Each study is applicable to one or two of the "links" in the sequence. No empirical research on compliance or preventive health behavior has yet tested all of these factors in a single statistical causal model or attempted to analyze causal relationships in complex experimental designs. This is an important research pursuit that could usefully apply the many operational definitions developed in this book. We feel that the organizing scheme presented here is important as a guide both for research on this topic and for clinical application (considered in more detail below). This scheme helps to organize a vast literature on patient compliance and health behavior, and suggests opportunities for more global research and practical applications than have heretofore been possible.

Practitioner as Agent of Social Influence

An important theme that will appear repeatedly in this book involves the role of the medical practitioner as an influence agent. This influence is, of course, specifically directed toward the patient regarding the health regimen. The role hosts many difficulties, for interpersonal influence requires much effort and often meets with minimal success—even in cases in which the influence is nobly initiated solely for the good of the recipient. The discipline of social psychology is largely concerned with interpersonal influence. In fact, a commonly accepted definition of social psychology illustrates the centrality of this concern: "Social psychology is the scientific field that studies the manner in which the behavior, feelings, or thoughts of one individual are influenced or determined by the behavior and/or characteristics of others" (Baron & Byrne, 1981, p. 7).

Our goal in this book is to apply social psychological principles to the practitioner's attempts to achieve patient compliance with medical recommendations. In applying these principles, we recognize that, unlike many traditional approaches to compliance (which consider noncompliance as totally irrational and hence incomprehensible, or alternately as having a single cause and treatment), a social psychological approach views the achievement of patient compliance precisely in terms of interpersonal influence. In this framework, we view interpersonal influence (as have others, e.g., Frank, 1961) as *the essential* precondition for behavior change, regardless of the particular mode of therapy employed by the practitioner. By means of a social psychological approach, we seek to delineate the precise conditions under which the wishes of one individual (the practitioner) may be translated into behavior on the part of another (the patient).

We believe that the study of patient compliance with medical regimens will be greatly enhanced by the application of a social psychological orientation. Practitioner and patient are perhaps best viewed as a "social system" (Henderson, 1935) and compliance as the outcome of a social transaction (Stone, 1979). From the initial decision to follow the treatment regimen to the elimination of barriers to the enactment of appropriate health behaviors, the context of the practitioner-patient relationship is the most appropriate setting for the solution of compliance problems. Throughout this book, then, we continually emphasize the role played by various aspects of the practitioner-patient relationship that affect the development and enhancement of patient compliance and health behavior. These include such issues as the clarity and openness of practitioner-patient communication; the fulfillment of joint expectations and desires for the conduct of the interaction; the joint understanding of practitioner's and patient's beliefs and attitudes toward themselves, each other, and the treatment regimen; their awareness of external social factors that impinge upon both the relationship and the patient's capacity to follow the regimen; and finally, the quality of the interpersonal relationship established between practitioner and patient.

The Social Psychology of the Practitioner's Role

In the social psychological approach that we emphasize, we consider the practitioner's role as central to the development and enhancement of patient compliance with medical regimens. Inherent in the practitioner's role as healer is a certain social power which, if used effectively, can be applied to change patients' beliefs regarding their treatment regimen and its efficacy. This power may also be used to change the expectations of the patient's social group regarding the regimen (perhaps by means of the practitioner's brief intervention in the family). The practitioner has enormous power to elicit from the patient a commitment to try to follow the regimen, and in demonstrating concern for the patient's difficulties, to support him or her physically and emotionally to overcome them.

The joint responsibility of practitioner and patient in achieving compliance and health behavior will be emphasized throughout. We demonstrate that both parties to the therapeutic relationship are responsible for its success—improved health status for the patient. We argue that the traditional role of the health professional as parental figure, who with reprimands and control treats patients as dependent children, is no longer acceptable to patients nor, for that matter, to many practitioners. Further, we argue that such a stance is unlikely to result in satisfactory long-term health outcomes. The goal of effective patient care requires *joint cooperation* between health professional and patient, in a mutually supportive partnership.

IMPLICATIONS FOR RESEARCH AND CLINICAL PRACTICE

Our review of the extensive research on the development and maintenance of patients' medical compliance is organized within a heuristic framework. At numerous points in our discussions of the many varied factors that influence patient compliance, we outline the important questions that deserve research attention. As we mentioned above, the scheme as a whole proposed here is also a subject for empirical analysis. Researchers might find here a valuable and important application of statistical methods for the analysis of causal models. This is made possible partly through the clear operationalization of the factors that figure prominently in the development and maintenance of compliance behavior.

This book presents not only a delineation of theory and research on compliance, but also guidelines for clinical application. The organizational scheme in this book is likely to be quite useful to clinicians in clarifying and retrieving their knowledge of various compliance-related factors that become evident as each patient's "history" unfolds. Decisions regarding the most appropriate focus for initial intervention (and the overall plan for subsequent interventions) are probably best developed with such a scheme as a guide. Thus, practitioners can base their decisions about patient care on stable research findings about compliance.

Although we believe that the approach presented here has clinical applicability, we are careful *not* to offer a cookbook, "how-to" manual. Across-the-board recommendations for practitioner action would be clearly unwise, for the best course to follow with any one patient will be determined most effectively by the practitioner's careful and intelligent use of knowledge from the compliance literature combined with knowledge of the individual patient. Of course, the organizational scheme in this book can be used to aid the practitioner in gathering information from each individual patient, and in determining the manner in which the patient conceptualizes his or her own difficulties in achieving compliance. Once these difficulties are clarified in terms of social norms, beliefs, deficiencies of behavioral and cognitive skills, and the like, they can be acted upon and changed.

The scheme presented in this book may be very useful in medical practice if it is approached by combining the statistical and the clinical understanding of health behavior. Empirical findings can suggest workable clinical interventions. This scheme can be used to teach physicians and other health professionals the cues they should watch for in their care of patients, as well as how to combine the various relevant factors to develop efficacious treatments. An analogous approach is used in the medical field in the recognition and treatment of coronary risk. Numerous studies have supported the various individual factors that relate to coronary artery disease. Partial integrative explanatory models of these factors are available. These factors include age, sex, heredity, serum cholesterol, heavy cigarette smoking, elevated systolic blood pressure, sedentary lifestyle, and the "Type A" behavior pattern. The more risk factors that are present, or the greater the severity of any one factor, the higher the patient's risk for ischemic heart disease (or a coronary event). A statistically imperfect but conceptually correct and heuristically valuable "model" links these various factors to coronary disease. This model also links the factors among themselves (Robbins & Cotran, 1979). It is used for training practitioners and employed by clinicians in medical practice. This organizational scheme identifies the important cues to which practitioners should attend in their care of individual patients, and it demonstrates how to combine those cues in recognizing coronary risk and applying interventions to reduce it. It adds to but does *not* replace, the clinician's judgment of coronary risk or existing coronary disease. It helps the clinician take into account a potentially confusing array of individual variables. Likewise, the scheme we present in this book for understanding compliance with medical regimens is intended to guide assessments of patient cooperation as well as judgments regarding interventions to improve it.

2

Practitioner-Patient Relationships: The Communication of Information

A popular stereotype of physician-patient interaction depicts the physician speaking in a hurried fashion while half running from his bedridden patient. The physician's words are garbled and mumbled. This hardly matters, however, because the medical jargon employed makes precious little sense to the patient anyway. The patient, in turn, is depicted as slow to comprehend and as reacting rather dully to the information that is conveyed. In somber interaction, the patient consistently and meekly defers when the physician interrupts. The patient seldom asserts his or her right to add yet another piece of pertinent information. The patient and the physician believe that what the patient has to say is unimportant. Rather, it is what the physician says, the questions he asks, the comments he makes, and the recommendations he gives that are of ultimate concern.

MODELS OF COMMUNICATIVE INTERCHANGE IN THE PRACTITIONER-PATIENT RELATIONSHIP

The stereotype described above (the strict enactment of which is actually a relatively rare occurrence in the everyday practice of medicine) reflects the early theories of medical sociologists such as Talcott Parsons (1951), who delineated the "proper" role of physician and patient in modern Western society. As is true of most stereotypes, however, this one (at least according to Parsons) harbors a kernel of truth. According to Parsons, the professional role of the physician demands technical competence, emotional neutrality, and a commitment to serving people. In this role as emotionally neutral healer, the physician is expected to remain detached and in control. The physician legitimizes the patient's entry into the sick role—a role that exempts the patient from many of his or her day-to-day responsibilities. In return, however, the patient is expected to seek competent medical help, to profess a desire to become well again, and to demonstrate this desire by cooperating completely with and deferring to the physician's authority.

Inherent in this relationship as described by Parsons is a disparity of power, for the physician typically occupies the superordinate, and the patient the dependent, station. The asymmetry of this relationship is based primarily upon the physician's expert command of an esoteric body of knowledge and, of course, upon his resources and skills in applying that knowledge. Parsons (1975) labeled this information differential the "competence gap." He suggested that this competence gap ultimately justifies the physician's social position as legitimate authority and professional, as well as the patient's obligation to trust in and comply with the physician's clinical prescription.

Parsons argued the existence of these roles from a functionalist perspective. He reported on what he observed, and argued that this state of affairs existed because it was functional. We should note that the Parsonian formulation remains rather pervasive in the present-day study of practitioner-patient interaction. Many empirical researchers who have studied communicative interchange have employed methodologies and interpreted findings with an eye toward supporting or toppling Parsons' seminal conceptualization of the sick role (see for example, Wolinsky & Wolinsky, 1981).

Medical sociologist Eliot Freidson (1970) has persuasively challenged Parsons' analysis of the sick role. Freidson criticized Parsons for presenting too unrealistic and narrow a view of physician-patient interaction. Freidson asserted that Parsons derived his definition of the sick role from a single and quite limited perspective—that of the physician. Freidson criticized Parsons for ignoring the patient's unique perspective, and for giving short shrift to what *actually happens* in the medical encounter while emphasizing mere expectations instead. According to Freidson, Parsons' sick-role analysis describes how both physician and patient *should* behave in medical interaction. As such, "it serves as a fixed standard by which we may measure the variable deviation of reality. However, it cannot really explain reality. It can only say what reality should be and note exceptions: it can note that the patient should submit to professional authority but, in fact, does not" (Freidson, 1961, p. 190). Parsons, therefore, labored to describe what should happen, whereas Freidson strove to depict what actually does happen.

What happens, according to Freidson, is conflict. In fact, Freidson argued that we cannot ignore the *necessity* of conflict in the physician-patient encounter. He argued this contention by noting that "the professional expects patients to accept what he recommends on his terms; patients seek services on their own terms. In that each seeks to gain his own terms, there is conflict" (Freidson, 1961, p. 171). While Parsons portrayed the physician-patient relationship in terms of the strict enactment of patterned sequences of behavior (albeit within the laudable framework of a mutually defined goal—the patient's eventual return to productive social functioning), Freidson presented a more situational perspective. He did not deny the existence of patterned social expectations, but he questioned the weight of their influence in relation to more direct interpersonal determinants of behavior.

Information exchange, in Freidson's approach, becomes a somewhat complicated proposition. Patients are not lowly or childlike in their perspective, nor do they adhere to a strict pattern of expectations because of limitations in knowledge and expertise. Patients' expectations are quite different from those of the physician. These expectations derive from the patient's position in a social network. According to Freidson, interpersonal influence and the weight of expectations derive precisely from the social position of the participant in the interpersonal relationship. Thus, for many patients the authority of the physician is far from absolute. For example, the patient's degree of education or the support he or she receives from family and friends may indirectly affect the information exchange between physician and patient.

The interpersonal context of the interaction between physician and patient is also brought to the fore in Freidson's analysis. Freidson suggests that in order to resolve the conflict that inevitably arises between the physician and patient in medical interaction, a kind of reality negotiation must occur:

> Interaction in treatment should be seen as a kind of negotiation as well as a kind of conflict. This point is suggested in Balint's psychiatric sense that the patient is using his symptoms to establish a relationship with the physician (Balint, 1957) but more particularly in the sense of negotiation of separate conditions and of separate perspectives and understandings. The patient is likely to want more information than the doctor is willing to give him—more precise prognoses, for example, and more precise instructions. As Roth's study indicated, just as the doctor struggles to find ways of withholding some kinds of information, so will the patient be struggling to find ways of gaining access to, or inferring, such information (Roth, 1963). [Freidson, 1970, p. 322]

Parsons (1951, 1975), then, argued that the therapeutic relationship contains, of necessity, an asymmetry of power. He proposed that in order for the therapeutic encounter to be a success, the practitioner must maintain his position of institutionalized authority. Freidson (1970), on the other hand, took a less rigid stance. Like Parsons, he granted the physician the status of technical expert, but did not insist upon the need for professional dominance.

Thomas Szasz and Marc Hollender (1956) have similarly taken issue with Parsons' requirement for physician dominance. They suggested that differences in interaction style can be successfully evidenced in the physician-patient relationship in accord with the nature of the patient's particular illness. Szasz and Hollender proposed three distinct types of physician-patient interaction: (1) the active-passive model; (2) the guidance-cooperation model; and (3) the mutual participation model. The active-passive model is typified by an emergency situation (coma or severe injury) in which the physician is necessarily active and the patient passive. The guidance-cooperation model is employed when the patient has an acute illness (such as an infection or a sprain). In this case, the patient seeks advice and the physician provides direction and technique. The mutual participation model, on the other hand, is used in managing long-term or chronic illness conditions. Here, the physician occasionally meets with the patient but the success of the intervention requires a high degree of patient responsibility and action directed primarily toward caring for him- or herself. The Szasz and Hollender conceptualization provides us with a fair degree of latitude in approaching the communicative interchange between physician and patient. Szasz and Hollender noted that no one model is better than the others, but rather that "each . . . is entirely appropriate under certain circumstances and each inappropriate under others" (Szasz & Hollender, 1956, p. 591). The circumstances, as we have noted, stem from the nature of the patient's organic symptoms.

Freidson also took Szasz and Hollender to terms for failing to extend their analysis to its logical limits. In order to be complete, Freidson contended, Szasz and Hollender should have included the situation in which the physician assumes a passive role in the practitioner-patient relationship:

> [W]hile the existence of situations where the practitioner more or less does what the patient asks him to do may not be denied, such situations are rejected out of hand as intolerably nonprofessional, nontherapeutic, and nondignified to be conceded for mere logic and dignified by the recognition of inclusion. This lack of concern for being logically consistent and systematic is characteristic of virtually all writing about the doctor-patient relationship by medical men . . . so long as medical writers persist in crippling their logic by normative considerations, they cannot expect serious intellectual consideration. [Freidson, 1970, p. 317]

Freidson suggested two situations in which such relationships might occur. The first (which we label the cooperation-guidance model) portrays the patient guiding and the physician cooperating, for example, when the patient designs his or her own therapeutic regimen (see Cousins, 1979) and the physician follows along, providing some input. The other (which we designate the passive-active model) portrays the physician as passive and the patient as active, such as when the patient demands and gets a specific prescription (see Freidson, 1961).

An important related issue is the role of the patient as an active participant in his or her own medical care. Over the last decade and a half, medicine has witnessed the birth of the patient-as-consumer movement. Haug and Lavin (1981) have discussed the implications of this orientation: "A consumerist stance clearly constitutes a challenge to physician authority. It focuses on purchasers' (patients') rights and sellers' (physicians') obligations, rather than on physicians' rights (to direct) and patients' obligations (to follow directions). *Caveat emptor*, 'let the buyer beware,' rather than trust in the seller's goodwill, characterizes the transaction" (p. 213). The consumer movement is firmly based upon a wish to narrow the "competence gap" between patient and practitioner. Indeed, the average level of education has steadily risen in Western society over the last few decades and the public is better informed now than ever before about health matters. Most medical knowledge is, however, of a highly technical nature. As a result, many have argued and it is widely believed that because of the highly technical nature of medical knowledge, only medical professionals are capable of judging the quality of medical work (Freidson, 1970). The consumerist orientation disagrees, however, and argues that for many reasons the patient is qualified to make such judgments, and indeed should feel free to decide whether the physician is performing his or her job appropriately (Lebow, 1974). While some data do indicate a high degree of congruence between the judgments of physicians and patients regarding the quality of the technical and interpersonal care delivered (DiMatteo & DiNicola, 1981), there is still insufficient evidence to suggest that consumers can make such judgments, and that a consumerist orientation may be effective in closing the competence gap. Certainly patients should be encouraged to assess various aspects of the quality of their medical care, and when they have done so, possess the freedom to seek services elsewhere if necessary (Freidson, 1961). That patients will ever close the competence gap is actually quite unlikely. This limitation, without doubt, has important implications for the practitioner-patient relationship.

This is *not* to say that patients are destined to remain passive and dependent in their medical care. Their control and expertise lie in their capacity to formulate their own private beliefs on the basis of the information they receive, to reconcile their beliefs with those of important persons in their lives, to make commitments to perform various health actions, and to take control over the many factors that shape their behavior. These are realms over which the practitioner, in fact, has little control. Here we are simply arguing that patient and physician possess *different forms of expertise and different potentials for control*. In later chapters of this book we will carefully examine how medical treatment can be greatly enhanced by the judicious joint application of both these forms of expertise and control.

Analysis of the consumer orientation brings to light the process of negotiation which has been said to characterize practitioner-patient interaction. Negotiation is consistent with Szasz and Hollender's (1956) mutual participation model, and with Freidson's (1970) theory of conflict in the therapeutic relationship. It is, however, strictly at odds with Parsons' (1951) conceptualization of the sick role. Negotiation is thus a construct used by some theorists to describe and further explore the process of practitioner-patient interaction. Because we see it as a dominant theme, we continue to explore it in this chapter as we examine information exchange in the therapeutic relationship. Although thus far we have cursorily examined a few major theories that directly concern information exchange in the practitioner-patient relationship, others exist which we have not considered at all. Some examples are theories of the physician-patient relationship proposed by Freud (1924), Balint (1957), Bloom (1963), and Henderson (1935). Thus, while the theme of negotiation in information exchange is important, it is by no means the only framework within which one might examine practitioner-patient interchange. The extent to which the practitioner-patient relationship can be characterized *empirically* as an interplay of disparate perspectives (of doctor and patient) regarding highly valued medical information is another matter.

Precisely how much information is actually negotiated and exchanged in practitioner-patient relationships is an important question for research. This empirical gap exists despite an abundance of research that describes various individual components of the practitioners' and patients' behavior. What the literature presently lacks is research on the *interaction* between practitioner and patient. Very few studies have examined the behavior of one participant as a direct function of (or in response to) the behavior of the other. In addition, while many have theorized about the potential consequences of information negotiation in the practitioner-patient relationship (for example, that negotiation might destroy the various "nonspecific" factors in the healing process [see Chapter 3]), for the most part empirical information regarding the precise effects of various aspects of information exchange has been limited. It is rather important, however, to identify the effects of information exchange on outcomes of the practitioner-patient relationship such as patient satisfaction, the physical outcome of treatment, and (of special concern in this book) patient compliance with the prescribed treatment regimen.

Recent research on practitioner-patient interchanges has described individual responses of the participants to the interaction (although it has largely overlooked the precise effects each participant has on the other in the interaction). Our goal in this chapter is to review much of the current research and to describe the typical behavior of each participant in the interchange. Our approach remains social-psychological throughout, and so we focus on the social interaction between people. We do not confront outright the broader sociological, political, and economic issues that inevitably arise in considerations of the medical practitioner-patient relationship.These broader issues are dealt with elsewhere in some detail from a number of different perspectives by various experts (see Gallagher, 1978; Illich, 1976; Zola, 1975; Jeffreys, 1970; Waitzkin & Waterman, 1974).

In the following sections, we examine the empirical research on the practitioner-patient relationship in terms of the specific details of interaction—behaviors such as finishing a thought, getting a word in edgewise, ascertaining that the other person is listening, asking questions, and making sure that questions are answered. We must consider such details in order to begin to understand information sharing in medical encounters. As a result, such questions as the following also become important: Who talks most in the practitioner (physician)-patient relationship? Who interrupts whom? Who listens, how often, and how well? Is information actually communicated? Does the transmission of information result in any demonstrable effects? Recognizing that some major questions remain to be answered (and indeed, pointing these out), we consider the empirical research that has sought to answer them. Thus, in the following pages, we seek to describe the practitioner-patient relationship not as it *should* be but as it *is*.

THE EDUCATION OF PATIENTS

Health professionals very often rely on sources other than themselves to communicate health knowledge to their patients. Physicians all too often assume that their patients have been exposed to and influenced by messages from mass-media health information programs (Surgeon General, 1979). Two important questions remain unanswered, although their answers are critically important to decisions regarding the manner in which patients should be given health education: (1) Are patients typically exposed to and receptive of mass-media health messages? and, (2) Is mass-media health education more or less effective than health education from a medical practitioner?

In a review of the literature on the effects of mass-media health campaigns, Kelley (1979) has noted that indeed they are valuable as sources of public-health information. Their limitations as catalysts to behavior change, however, have led some researchers to conclude that health education (toward the goal of healthy behavior) is best accomplished by health practitioners directly (Hingson, Scotch, Sorenson, & Swazey, 1981). Let us consider the evidence. People vary in the extent to which they are exposed to health messages and in the extent to which they learn anything of value from them. Feldman (1966) for example, demonstrated that variations in health knowledge are closely related to an individual's educational attainment, age (older people have less health knowledge than younger people), and sex (men have less health knowledge than women). Differences in health knowledge both reflect and influence receptiveness to health information. Media information of all kinds generally reaches and is assimilated by those who are initially most interested in the particular topic. Information campaigns typically bypass groups of persons who have the least interest in them (Klapper, 1960). In the case of health information, then, education campaigns bypass those in the greatest need of the information. Further, the persuasiveness of mass communication is considered rather low in comparison to individualized persuasion efforts (Zimbardo, Ebbesen, & Maslach, 1977). Mass-media messages usually have an impact only when they attempt to reinforce the existing behavioral predispositions of the audience, and usually work only when social norms and ties, personal influences, and other mediating factors do not contradict the message (De Fleur, 1966).

In a related manner, school programs in health education have the potential to teach preventive health behavior on a wide scale to a captive audience. These programs, however, are for the most part ineffective (Hingson, Scotch, Sorenson, & Swazey, 1981, p. 40). Priorities in this area are usually low and resources are often limited. In addition, most health education programs in the schools put heavy emphasis on moralism and considerably less on health knowledge. Therefore, the credibility of the messages is often called into question. When the representation of hazards from such substances as marijuana is exaggerated, students may mistrust the more accurate messages, such as the warnings about the dangers of cigarette smoking or heroin use. Thus, while mass-media and school health education programs are potentially valuable in promoting preventive health care, their current manifestations have severe limitations, particularly in contrast with direct communication from practitioners to their patients.

Face-to-face communications between practitioners and their patients are more compelling than other forms of health education (Hingson et al., 1981). Radio, television, and newspaper messages are easily ignored, but it is probably more difficult to ignore a message given directly by a knowledgeable, caring health professional in face-to-face interaction. The face-to-face encounter also provides an opportunity for practitioner and patient to recognize and correct misconceptions and inaccurately perceived messages. The individual patient's health knowledge can be assessed and the communication program geared appropriately to it. In face-to-face encounters with practitioners (as opposed to media campaigns), the patient's social ties and ability to engage in self-control can also be readily assessed. Finally, persuasive messages can be developed specifically for the individual, and consequently, the effectiveness of persuasion can be greatly enhanced. While in later chapters we consider these issues, such as persuasion (Chapter 6), social norms and ties (Chapter 5), health beliefs (Chapter 4), and supports for self-control (Chapter 7) in much greater detail, we allude to them here in order to emphasize how important the one-to-one practitioner-patient encounter is for effective health education.

Evidence suggests that opportunities for health education by practitioners do become available. In any given year, three-fourths of all Americans have some contact with a physician. The average person has nearly five contacts per year (Hingson et al., 1981, p. 102). Furthermore, patients surveyed from all economic classes tend to report that most of their health information comes from physicians (David & Boldt, 1980). Yet, practitioner-patient encounters are by no means wholly successful in changing patients' health behaviors and in enhancing their compliance with medical recommendations. The influence that practitioners actually enjoy over their patients typically falls rather short of its potential. A number of problems and limitations in practitioner-patient communication attenuate its effects, and a complete understanding of these is necessary if efforts are to be made to overcome them.

Limitations in the Practitioner's Communication to Patients

Misinformed Patients. A surprising number of patients leave their doctor's office with little idea of what they are supposed to do to follow their treatment regimen. A number of important empirical studies have demonstrated this point very clearly, using methodologies that range from interviews to clinic and pharmacy records to observations of actual practitioner-patient encounters. In one of these studies, Svarstad (1974, 1976) found that 50 percent of patients could not correctly report how long they were supposed to continue taking their medication. As we will see below, an important reason for this was their physicians' negligence in informing them. Seventeen percent of patients could not correctly report how often they were supposed to take their medication, and 23 percent could not identify the purpose of the drugs they were taking. Other research identified similar problems. Brant and Kutner (1957), for example, conducted interviews with 50 hospitalized surgical patients, nearly all of whom were found frequently to experience anxious uncertainty. Although they reported their findings in qualitative terms, the authors noted that patients rarely knew in advance about the normal, predictable postoperative events they would experience. Often patients did not even know why they were having surgery. In yet another study, Kane and Deuschle (1967) conducted interviews with medical patients who had been discharged (up to 13 months previously) from a university medical center in Kentucky. Among patients who were taking medication, 72 percent could not accurately identify their medicines, 26 percent had no idea why they were taking the medicines, and 37 percent "could not be counted upon to know when or how much of a prescribed medicine to take" (p. 263).

Many important issues are relevant to informative communication with patients. Even after flawless communication from practitioners, patients are prone to forget what they have been told. Typically, however, communication from the practitioner is far from flawless. Thus, in the grand scheme of things, problems in practitioner-patient communication cannot be appropriately considered the fault of one or another party. For every physician who offers no explanation, there is a patient who does not press for one. For every patient who makes an interpretive error or misunderstands directions, there is a physician who did not check to see if the patient understood what he or she said. The assignment of culpability seldom advances our knowledge and understanding of how to improve practitioner-patient communication. Instead, we must approach the therapeutic relationship with at least some degree of detachment, and with an empirical orientation to the analysis of practitioner-patient interaction.

Physician as Teacher. The word "doctor" is derived from the Latin *docere* which means "to teach" (Eisenberg, 1977). The *American Heritage Dictionary* describes this meaning (of doctor as teacher) as "obsolete." The obsolete status of "doctor" in the English language stands as a metaphor, since in modern times the role of the doctor as teacher seems indeed to be almost totally outmoded. One major reason why patients misunderstand their treatment regimens involves their physicians' negligence in explaining those regimens to them.

Empirical research supports this explanation. Pratt, Seligmann, and Reader (1957), in a study of physician-patient interactions in a clinic, noted that particularly when a patient initially seemed poorly informed, physicians avoided taking the time necessary to translate medical explanations into terms the patient could understand. (It is interesting to note that physicians tend to grossly underestimate the comprehension level of their patients [Segall & Roberts, 1980]). Instead, the physicians allowed these patients to remain confused and uninformed. Similar findings were more recently reviewed by Duff and Hollingshead (1968), Cartwright (1964), and Taylor (1979). In the hospital, explanations were found to be particularly difficult to obtain. Brant and Kutner (1957) and Golden and Johnston (1970) found that physicians in hospitals rarely met with their patients in unhurried conference or stayed to talk with them after explaining something in order to be sure they understood it. Cartwright (1964) found that physicians did not even introduce themselves to the hospitalized patient in a significant number of cases.

Whether or not practitioners in general give explanations and information to patients, and the conditions under which the medical practitioner's role as teacher might be enhanced are important subjects for future, in-depth empirical examination. Although empirical research on this issue is still relatively sparse, a few provocative studies do exist. These studies give us a fairly detailed look at practitioner-patient communication. Waitzkin and Stoeckle

(1976), for example, reported the results of a pilot study involving the direct recording and analysis of physician-patient communications. During the medical visit (which lasted, on the average, 20 minutes) the physician was found to spend less than one minute communicating information to the patient or informing the patient about some aspect of his or her illness or treatment. Waitzkin and Stoeckle reported that those same physicians estimated that they spent 10 to 15 minutes (that is, 50 to 75 percent of their interaction time) giving information to their patients. These results are supported with similar data from Freemon, Negrete, Davis, and Korsch (1971), and Davis (1971). The former study demonstrated that physicians gave information or instructions to mothers of pediatric patients during only about 8 percent of the interaction time, and the latter study found that physicians "gave suggestions" to patients during only about 10 percent of the interaction time. Bain (1976) reported that "giving instructions" occurred somewhat more frequently—during 16 percent of the interaction time. Finally, when the category "patient education" was widened to include "those planned attempts to facilitate behavioral change that contributes to the improvement or maintenance of health" (Bartlett, 1980, p. 863), estimates of time spent by primary-care physicians in patient education was increased. Bartlett (1980) reviewed four studies (other than those considered above) and found a weighted average of 27.5 percent of the medical visit spent in broadly defined patient education. It is important to remember, however, that patient education was defined more broadly in these studies than in the former studies. It did not represent the mere transmission of information, but included all activities related to facilitating behavioral changes.

The question of how much time medical practitioners devote to patient education is likely to be explored more completely and effectively in years to come, as methodologies for analyzing practitioner-patient interactions become more highly developed. Research by Stiles, Putnam, Wolf, and James (1979a) has demonstrated the importance of developing precise methods for categorizing practitioner utterances. They noted that without very specific categories, communications that differ greatly in character are likely to be labeled in the same manner. Stiles and coworkers found, for example, that the category that represented physicians' utterances to their patients actually contained many kinds of communications. Two-thirds of physicians' utterances to patients were acknowledgments (such as, "yes, I see"), questions, reflections, or interpretations, and only one-third were advisements (or instructions). This latter category contained commands of immediate relevance (such as, "Please sit up," and "Let me look at your foot") as well as instructions about the treatment regimen. Thus, even Stiles et al.'s complex coding scheme did not measure the very specific behavior of giving information about the treatment regimen. Another important contribution of their work was Stiles et al.'s division of the medical visit into three parts: history, examination, and conclusion. They found that the percentage of time in each devoted to "advisements" from the physician was respectively 2 percent, 23 percent, and 9 percent, with an overall average of 10 percent. Since the conclusion of the medical visit is likely to be the part during which the practitioner explains medical regimens and prescribes treatments, this research suggests that the physician spends only 9 percent or less of the time instructing the patient.

An important study by Svarstad (1976) demonstrated that regardless of the amount of time spent by physicians in talking to their patients, physicians may still be ineffective communicators. Svarstad recorded the specific verbal instructions given to patients during their medical visits and compared these instructions with those attached to the patients' medication containers. She found that the physician often did not even discuss his intention to prescribe medication with the patient. Of the 347 drugs prescribed to the patients in this study, 60 were never discussed during the observed visit. In 90 percent of the drug-prescribing incidents, physicians gave their patients no specific verbal advice on how to use the medication. The observer concluded that the physicians usually inferred that their patients could easily figure out the dosage required, and when and how the medication was to be taken. An additional problem occurred in the prescribing of medication. Often, physicians verbally changed the dosage of a drug that the patient had at home, but gave the patient no written record of the change. Physicians assumed that their patients understood the change and would remember it. In addition, instructions to be written on prescription drug containers almost never included the length of time that the drug should be taken. Ninety-seven of the 347 drugs were dispensed to be used for symptomatic relief, but only 42 of these were dispensed with labels indicating such. A patient's misunderstanding of the purpose of the medication, in fact, might have led him or her to take the medication regularly. In 20 percent of the prescription cases, the pharmacist incorrectly specified some condition of the administration of the medication. (This may or may not have resulted from the physician's illegible handwriting.) Finally, in 29 percent of the cases of drug prescription, the physician did not give the patient the name of the drug, or any information about its purpose.

Is the Doctor Listening? Sir William Osler (1899), noted physician-educator, once told young doctors to listen to the patient for the patient will tell the diagnosis. Indeed, listening can be a critically important aspect of patient care. A patient has the opportunity to gather many clues about his own condition, such as details of the character and timing of symptoms. The physician may in fact miss an important key to differential diagnosis by restricting the patient's description of his problem. Much may be lost by insisting that patients respond to questions with one-word answers. Listening fully to all the patient has to say may help the physician avoid the tendency of many in medical diagnosis to formulate a hypothesis too quickly and then fit the empirical evidence to that hypothesis (Elstein, 1976). Listening also suggests the physician's respect for the patient, and his or her willingness to share the power in the relationship (Stone, 1979). Listening to the patient tell his story in his own words is a lesson which is repeatedly emphasized in medical training (Engel & Morgan, 1973).

In four major empirical studies, physician-patient verbal communication has been analyzed in detail. In these studies the various forms of verbal communication emitted by patient and by physician were tallied from tape recordings of the actual medical visit (Freemon et al., 1971; Davis, 1971; Bain, 1976; Stiles et al., 1979a). In all four studies, similar patterns of verbal interaction were found despite differences in population and setting. In the history-taking portion of the medical visit, Stiles et al. (1979a) found that the patient talked 54 percent of the time and the physician 46 percent. This was the only study of the four in which (in only one part of the visit) the patient talked more than the physician. In the other three studies, and in the other two portions of the medical visit in the Stiles et al. study, the physician talked significantly more than the patient. Since a major goal of the physician is to collect information from (indeed to listen to) the patient, this statistic is somewhat surprising. Physicians tend to verbalize quite extensively, although their utterances tend *not* to be explanations or communications of information. Rather, about two-thirds of what physicians say are acknowledgments, questions, reflections, and clarifications (which are, of course, necessary components of communication if used judiciously). Freemon et al. (1971), however, noted that physicians are not even aware of this latter aspect of their communications. According to these reseachers, most physicians believe they spend much more time listening to their patients than talking to them.

A final study which is relevant to the physician's listening was conducted by Dangott, Thornton, and Page (1978). These researchers interviewed various health professionals including dentists, physicians, nurses, and medical technologists. The purpose of the study was to investigate how health professionals communicate with their patients about pain. It was found that health professionals were very prone to use disconfirming messages, which did not allow the patient an opportunity for response. For example, practitioners tended to emphasize the importance of "mental attitude" and insisted that they did not inflict "pain" on their patients. In fact, they often denied the existence of pain. For example, practitioners often said, "This might pinch a little" and subsequently did not allow their patients to disagree, and say that it actually hurt. That practitioners sometimes flatly ignore or contradict a patient's communication—particularly about such an important issue as pain—suggests that the degree to which practitioners typically listen to their patients may be somewhat less than optimal.

The Practitioner and Medical Jargon. "You have essential hypertension," said the physician to his patient. "I'd like you to take hydrochlorothiazide b.i.d. to eliminate fluid retention. You should also reduce your sodium intake." "Thank you," said the patient. Although he had no idea what the physician was talking about, the patient was impressed.

Many patients are impressed by incomprehensible medical jargon (Korsch, Gozzi, & Francis, 1968). The physician's use of medical terminology is sometimes taken by the patient as a compliment to his intelligence. Jargon may signal that the patient can relax into the submissive, but safe, sick role. By using jargon, the practitioner stays in control (Shapiro, 1978). It is a long-standing habit:

> They make a great display of Hippocrates and Galen, utter unknown words, apply their aphorisms to everything, and stuff men's minds with unheard-of names, leaving them full of meaningless sound.
>
> —John of Salisbury, *Metalogicus*
> 1250 A.D. [cited in Strauss, 1968]

The use of medical jargon may impress some patients but it communicates very little useful information to them. As a result, many patients become distressed and rebellious. For example, in a survey of health care and its relationship to social class, Koos (1954) found that much of his respondents' dissatisfaction with medical care was the result of poor communication with their physicians. One respondent noted that "maybe things would be better if the doc understood us, and if we always knew what the hell he was driving at—and not in big words either" (Koos, 1954, pg. 77).

Medical terminology, of course, is necessary to facilitate communication among medical professionals. Sometimes, however, as Christy (1979) has pointed out, jargon even obscures communication within the discipline of medicine. However, according to some critics, that is not so important, for medical jargon is high sounding, formal, and frightening, and it serves the purpose of elevating the physician's status with respect to the patient (Shapiro, 1978). Indeed, according to Barnlund (1976), jargon makes practitioner-patient communication an exercise in the mystification of meaning.

Physician-patient communication cannot be maintained if the patient does not know the relevant medical vocabulary (Becker & Maiman, 1980). Korsch, Gozzi, and Francis (1968), for example, found that pediatricians in a clinic used many vocabulary words that parents simply did not understand. Words such as "incubation period" and "workup"—common terms in medical settings—confused and perplexed the parents to whom they were spoken. After the visit, parents were left with no better idea of what was wrong with their babies than they had before it. The chance of noncompliance in the care of their children was, as a result, quite high. Mazullo, Lasagna, and Griner (1974) found similar use of medical vocabulary among physicians and comparable confusion among patients. Many patients in this study, for example, thought the phrase "as needed for water retention" meant that their diuretic pills should be taken to cause water retention. Some patients reported that they would take the pill at night before going to bed so that they would be able to sleep through the night without needing to urinate. They probably experienced a rude awakening!

A major systematic study of patients' knowledge of medical vocabulary was carried out by Samora, Saunders, and Larson (1961). This study involved a heterogeneous population of patients. A list of 50 words, judged by practitioners as appropriate for use in conversation with patients, was constructed. Each word was then embedded in a context sentence. One hundred and twenty-five patients (largely lower class) were asked to define each word. That definition was then scored according to the patient's apparent degree of understanding. The least number of words that any patient could define adequately for communication in the hospital was 11. The most any patient knew was 47. The average number of words defined was 29 (the median was also 29). Twenty-five percent of the respondents knew 40 or more of the words, and 25 percent knew 20 or fewer words. The most commonly missed words were "malignant," "secretions," "cardiac," "respiratory," "tendon," "terminal," and "nerve." On the other hand, "appointment," "vomit," "relieve," and "constipated" were known by more than 90 percent of the respondents. A more recent follow-up was conducted by Segall and Roberts (1980), who used a format similar to that of the Samora et al. (1961) study, with three major modifications. Respondents filled out their questionnaires at home (presumably with access to a dictionary), respondents were of higher socioeconomic class, and the vocabulary definition task required recognition instead of recall. It was found that the medical vocabulary words missed by subjects in the Samora et al. study were much more often correctly understood by patients in the Segall and Roberts study. Of course, it was likely that the conditions of the latter study made the task quite a bit easier than it was in the former. It is also possible, however, that patients have become more knowledgeable about medical vocabulary than they were in the past.

Patient Fallibility

So far, we have focused on the practitioner's role in the often confusing and unsatisfying communication between practitioner and patient. This approach has been too limited, of course, for a patient's lack of knowledge about his or her therapeutic regimen is not solely the fault of the practitioner. Patients forget what they have been told, they make interpretive errors, and when they do not understand what they have been told, they neglect to say so. Unassertiveness and passivity on the part of the patient contribute as much to problems in communication as does the practitioner's deficiency in explanation. Shapiro (1978) noted, however, that patients often express their confusion through communication channels (primarily nonverbal) that are different from the ones that physicians are accustomed to reading (primarily verbal) (also see Friedman, 1979). Thus, patients tend to signal their distress and confusion to practitioners but they typically do so only through the less overt channels of facial expressions, body movements, and tone of voice. Later in this book, we will return to the role of nonverbal communication in the practitioner-patient relationship, and we will examine some of the reasons for patients' reluctance to assert their wishes to their physicians. Here, we examine some of the other factors involved in patients' contributions to communication problems in the practitioner-patient relationship.

A Failure of Memory and a Failure of Judgment. In order for effective communication to take place—communication which results in patient cooperation with a treatment regimen—the recipient of a message must remember what he or she has been told. An investigation by Ley and Spelman (1965) demonstrated, however, that shortly after their consultation with the practitioner, clinic outpatients forgot about one-third of what was told to them during the medical visit. For example, 20 percent of the prognoses of a condition were forgotten by patients; 56 percent of the instructions were forgotten; 48 percent of the statements about treatment were forgotten. Other research has shown that patients make interpretive errors. In one study, Mazullo, Lasagna, and Griner (1974) examined patients' responses to typed instructions for ten commonly prescribed medications. Sixty-seven patients were interviewed and asked to read the label on each of ten pill bottles. They were then asked to describe how they would take the drug. There was not one instance in which a label was interpreted the same way by all patients. The responses indicated marked variability in patients' interpretations of what most physicians would consider straightforward instructions. Even when the instructions were not at all ambiguous, the frequency of interpretive errors ranged from 9 to 64 percent. Pilot research by Hellmuth, Johannsen, and Sorauf (1966) similarly demonstrated significant distortion of physician recommendations by cardiac patients in a study that measured patient distortion reliably, and examined the factors to which distortion was related. In this research, patient defensiveness was found to be significantly related to their distortion of information. Finally, Snyder, Lynch, and Gruss (1976) found that patients' misunderstanding and failure to listen to instructions were positively related to the degree of trust they placed in the physician. This latter finding suggests a possible negative outcome of trust in the therapeutic relationship (see Chapter 3), and points to the importance of future research on the effects of trust on patient responsibility for their care.

Cassata (1978) has summed up the communication research as it relates to patient distortion and patient forgetting of medical recommendations. These are the major findings:

1) Patients forget much of what the doctor tells them.
2) Instructions and advice are more likely to be forgotten than other information.
3) The more a patient is told, the greater the proportion he or she will forget.
4) Patients will remember: a) what they are told first; b) what they consider most important.
5) Intelligent patients do not remember more than less intelligent patients.
6) Older patients remember just as much as younger ones.
7) Moderately anxious patients recall more of what they are told than highly anxious patients or patients who are not anxious.
8) The more medical knowledge a patient has, the more he or she will recall.
9) If the patient writes down what the doctor says, he or she will remember it just as well as if he or she merely hears it. [Cassata, 1978; p. 498]

Passive, Unassertive Patients. A few studies have demonstrated that patients typically know more about medical issues (conceptual issues, *not* medical jargon) than their physicians anticipate is the case (Pratt, Seligmann, & Reader, 1957; Kane & Deuschle, 1967). Unfortunately, the physician's underestimation of the patient's knowledge is likely to be detrimental to their communication. Pratt, Seligmann, and Reader (1957) found that when physicians underestimated patients' knowledge, they were then less likely to discuss illness at length with the patient. The practitioner assumed that the patient would not understand what was being discussed and consequently the explanation would require a prohibitive amount of time. The physicians decided not to bother. This problem is compounded, of course, when the patient, who knows relatively little, is afraid to ask for more information. He or she may then simply let the physician decide what information to convey. Patients rarely attempt to inform their physicians when they do not understand, or when they would like further explanation. Instead, they nod their heads knowingly at explanations they do not comprehend, and refrain from asking questions when given the opportunity. Objective analyses of verbal communication in physician-patient encounters supports this hypothesis overwhelmingly. Stiles et al. (1979), for example, found that in analyses of verbal response modes in 52 clinic visits, patients asked questions of the doctor only 7 percent of the time. In the Freemon et al. (1971) study, less than 5 percent of the time in the average visit was taken up with the mother's request for information or instructions, or with her disagreement with the physician. Similarly, in the Bain (1976) study, patients' problem-related expressions ("I am worried about my job") and questions ("How long will I be out of work?") each took up less than 7 percent of the interaction time. Thus, as Coe (1970) has noted, patients are reluctant to ask the physician any questions during the interview for fear of demonstrating ignorance or incomplete trust in the physician. Consequently, questions are not asked and dissatisfactions are not voiced. The participants in a critically important interchange actually communicate very little.

Some Unanswered Questions

It is important always to keep in mind that problems in practitioner-patient communication stem from both patient and practitioner variables—from practitioners' "failure" to explain as well as from patients' "failure" to comprehend. These variables have heretofore been examined separately—a practice which represents a significant flaw in the research to date. Precisely how practitioners' behaviors affect patients' behaviors and vice versa has yet to be carefully examined. The nature of practitioner-patient *interaction* has yet to be explored.

The literature on physician-patient interactions, despite about 25 years of (albeit sporadic) research, is filled with some serious gaps. The editorial writings abound with prescriptions for how things *should* be. There is, however (particularly in the work from the 1950s and 1960s), a paucity of methodologically sound studies that examine the phenomenon in objective fashion and reflect how things really are.

Research on verbal communication in physician-patient interactions has been furthered tremendously in the past decade by the application of formats for the analysis of interaction process. Most notable among them is the verbal response modes analysis of Stiles, Putnam, Wolf, and James (1979a). This taxonomy of verbal response modes is particularly noteworthy because it was developed specifically for the study of medical interactions. This taxonomy is based on categories developed from conceptual principles of the practitioner-patient relationship, and it has demonstrated intercoder reliability. Nevertheless, research with this coding scheme is time-consuming, complicated, and tedious. It may be much too unwieldy for many researchers. The work done by its developers is herculean, and one wonders how often such extensive studies will be done in the future. While it may be very difficult to preserve the methodological excellence of the Stiles et al. approach, perhaps a less cumbersome measurement method that would preserve some of its qualities can be developed. This should be a high priority for researchers in the field. Subjective measures, such as those used in the early days of the research reviewed here, will never again be adequate.

INFLUENCES ON PRACTITIONER-PATIENT INTERCHANGE

Earlier in this chapter we considered various individual components of communicative interchange between practitioners and patients in the health-care setting. We have seen that physicians, for the most part, do not consistently explain illness and treatment to their patients. In a complementary fashion, patients misunderstand or forget what is explained to them. Patients rarely ask questions of their practitioners. Such facts have been unearthed through detailed analyses of physician-patient interactions and by means of examination of the perceptions of professionals and patients about one another. These facts, however, do not explain the *cause* of communication problems and do not point to the source of these limitations. Why might it be that physicians do not explain? Why do patients misunderstand and forget? Why don't patients ask questions?

The answers to these questions lie partly in the interrelationships that exist among the various components of problematic communication in the practitioner-patient relationship. As facets of an interactive process, each problematic component of communication has the potential to elicit a problematic response. This notion is supported by the studies of interaction process considered so far (Freemon et al., 1971; Davis, 1971; Bain, 1976; Stiles et al., 1979). In these studies, the various components of communication were correlated with, rather than treated as independent of, one another. For example, since interaction time was usually limited, the more a physician talked, the less a patient was able to talk. Similarly, when patients asked fewer questions, physicians provided fewer explanations. As Pratt, Seligmann, and Reader (1957) pointed out, physicians who expect that their patients already know little about their medical care refrain from providing any information at all lest they be forced to spend a great deal of time and effort filling in the gaps. If the patient indeed knows little or nothing about the medical problem or treatment, or if he or she does have knowledge but fails to display it, a conflict may ensue. The patient may assume that the practitioner refuses to tell him or her anything, and is withholding information. In such situations, patients may abandon their attempts to find out what they would like to know, and they may even become quite angry. Practitioners may assume that these patients have relinquished control over themselves and their health. Thus, the mutual influence of these communication factors is pervasive, and their reciprocal operation is the essence of "interaction."

Practitioner-patient interactions do not occur in a vacuum. They are influenced by many factors that are not obvious components of the two-person interaction. The constraints on behavior of practitioner and patient are determined, in part, by the wider social context. The structure of the society and of the medical-care delivery system in which the interaction takes place determine, in part, its course. This context exerts influence on the day-to-day workings of the seeking and providing of medical care. Thus, we are sometimes forced to look beyond the immediate practitioner-patient interaction in order to make sense of the problems that occur in it.

In this section we briefly examine some of the more broadly conceived factors that are hypothesized to limit practitioner-patient communication. We note, however, that no one explanation independently or fully accounts for the phenomena we observe. There is no one cause for the problems that exist in information exchange, and the tendency of some researchers and theorists to focus on, and argue for, a singular explanation limits understanding rather than enhancing it. As Barnlund (1976) pointed out, *nearly all* of the barriers to effective communication that have been identified in general communication research can be found in the practitioner-patient relationship. Further, these limiting factors can occur simultaneously and influence one another.

Anxiety, Distress, and the Patient's Role

As we noted earlier in this chapter, a sick person occuppies a social role, the entry to which is governed by physicians. Physicians are the "gatekeepers"of the sick role in American society (Parsons, 1958). They take charge of the person who is ill, dispensing (for the society as a whole) privileges (e.g., absence from work) in exchange for obligations (e.g., cooperation and the expression of a desire to get well). Because of the importance that is typically placed on hospital and health-care-center routine, the patient faces another obligation as well—the obligation to be unswervingly cooperative and compliant with every detail of care and to submit totally to the authority of the practitioner. Many have noted that patients are often quite willing to accept the role of passive participants in their care (King, 1962; Lederer, 1952; Skipper & Leonard, 1965). Patients are often anxious and fearful, and when they are sick, many wish simply to be cared for.

It has been suggested that one important reason why patients do not ask questions of their practitioners is that they have relinquished responsibility for their medical care. The source of this abandonment of self-control is, however, debated. The patient's passive acceptance of all that is dealt him (and all that is hidden from him, such as information) has been attributed to his regression to a childlike state in response to illness (Lederer, 1952). Others (Taylor, 1979; Lorber, 1975) have argued that a passive role is forced on patients because those who do ask questions and demand answers are labeled "bad patients" by practitioners and hospital staff. Bad patients are often ignored, prematurely medicated, or referred to psychiatrists (Lorber, 1975; Katz et al., 1970). For whatever reason, illness behavior usually carries with it some degree of dependency. This dependency is unfortunately likely to interfere with patient participation in the communication process.

Barnlund (1976) has pointed out that the anxiety and ego involvement that tend to accompany physical incapacity, illness, and disease can easily interfere with effective communication. People rarely comprehend information clearly when they are emotionally upset. Learning and information processing take place most effectively when the individual is experiencing an intermediate level of anxiety. High anxiety, such as may accompany illness and dealings with the medical-care system, might also trigger defense mechanisms such as denial and repression. For many reasons, the patient may become distracted from what he or she is being told. Thus, explanations given to patients might do little to change their state of knowledge about their condition or their treatment *unless* their anxiety level is also reduced. Of course, a frustrating search for information or the absence of it altogether may precipitate enormous anxiety in the patient, which the provision of information might significantly reduce (Langer, Janis, & Wolfer, 1975; Vernon, 1971). Thus, anxiety may be the cause and the effect of the patient's poor state of knowledge. There is, without doubt, an intimate relationship between anxiety and information but the precise character of that relationship cannot yet be specified. It is critical to understand this relationship in attempting to clarify and enhance practitioner-patient communication in medical care. It is clear that further research on this question should have high priority.

Poor communication between patients and practitioners might be a reflection of patient resistance to influence by the health professional. A patient's reluctance to ask questions and to provide clarifying information may represent his attempt to keep the practitioner uncertain of his beliefs, feelings, and behaviors. The patient may be able to "resist" without openly asserting his desires or confronting the practitioner with opposition to the treatment or regimen prescribed. If the patient does not comprehend the instructions, he cannot be held responsible for noncompliance. This method of engineering his noncompliance may be appealing to the patient who wishes to gain control in the therapeutic relationship (Hayes-Bautista, 1976a,b).

The notion that patients may sabotage communication with their practitioners in order to gain control through noncompliance is not new (Haley, 1963; 1973). It suggests that patients value control (although they may use inappropriate means to achieve it). Patients' attempted rebellion against control by their practitioners might even suggest that patients are willing to take control over their own lives, and wish to avoid dependencies on their health professionals (Blane, 1968). A theme that will appear again and again throughout this book is the importance of patient control and responsibility in the development and maintenance of patient commitment to the therapeutic regimen. We will consider various constructive means available to patients for expressing their desire for control, and various ways in which health professionals may help to enhance patients' feelings of control and self-determination. It is important to note here, however, that the above considerations represent another example of the reciprocal relationship between information exchange and an outcome variable such as compliance. It is not possible to state unequivocally that deficient communication between practitioner and patient causes noncompliance. Indeed, the causal link may go in the opposite direction. Here again, further research is necessary.

The Practitioner's Role

As we have noted, ineffective communication between practitioners and their patients has been attributed to the practitioner's incorrect expectations of the patient's state of knowledge and capacity to learn (Pratt, Seligmann, & Reader, 1957; Kane & Deuschle, 1967). It has also been suggested that practitioners assume that patients' knowledge is considerably higher than it really is and so they fail to offer crucial information about the treatment (for example, precisely what constitutes a low-fat or low-sodium diet), or that practitioners simply have no idea of their patients' state of knowledge (Golden & Johnston, 1970; Segall & Roberts, 1980). Most researchers and theorists have assumed, however, that practitioners are oriented, by and large, to the benefit of the patient and that they try to act in accord with that orientation.

The possibility that practitioners' behaviors may be self-serving has been suggested, although empirical support has rarely been offered. Since the formulation of effective explanations and the communication of clear and unambiguous information may require a great deal of effort (Martin, 1978), some practitioners are likely to dispense with the goal of patient education simply because they are unwilling or unable to expend the necessary effort. Similarly, some practitioners may wish to maintain a high degree of emotional detachment from their patients (Daniels, 1960; Lief & Fox, 1963). This detachment may serve as a means of self-protection, although it is rationalized as necessary for the proper conduct of medical care. Practitioners may keep their patients unaware of their condition or of relevant information about their case in order to prevent patients from arguing from a knowledgeable position. Practitioners may simply want to prevent their patients from causing them "trouble" (Lorber, 1975; McIntosh, 1974), bringing malpractice litigation against them (Thurlow, 1969), or exhibiting unmanageable emotional reactions (Skipper, Tagliacozzo, & Mauksch, 1964).

Barnlund (1976) has hypothesized the interesting notion that "mystification" helps *both* practitioners and patients to escape from the anxiety, embarrassment, and frustration that accompany the uncertainties inherent in medical care. Although it is an appealing notion, it is challenged by such empirical studies as Davis' (1960) research on practitioners and parents of children with polio. Long after the children's prognoses were established with a fairly high degree of certainty (for example, whether or not they would walk again), health professionals (such as physicians and nurses) told the parents that the prognoses were still quite uncertain. Davis' investigation demonstrated that the withholding of information from the parents served to delay (and sometimes to eliminate altogether) the physician's obligation to counsel or comfort them. Under the guise of concern for the child and his family, the practitioners apparently served their own needs.

In order to understand practitioners' motives and behaviors fully, one must look to the broader societal context. Parsons' (1951) analysis of the role of the physician characterizes it as one of high status and control vis à vis the patient. The disparity in power and control carves an emotional chasm between physician and patient—a chasm that is bridged only by the physician's altruism and orientation to serving people. The physician assumes control and power in the patient's best interest. They are necessary for the practitioner to perform his healing function. Freidson (1970) and Waitzkin (Waitzkin & Stoeckle, 1972; Waitzkin & Waterman, 1974) advocate a different viewpoint. They have interpreted the physician's custody of power with much less emphasis on the physician's altruistic motives. In their view, the physician maintains control not because it promotes the interests of the patient, but rather because it maintains the institutional authority of the physician. Practitioners are believed to withhold information in order to maintain patients' dependency. The practitioner's competence, expertise, and legitimized status as a healer bring with them social and political power, which physicians as a group strive to maintain. The goal of maintaining institutional authority and power is emphasized and reinforced throughout medical training (Shapiro, 1978). New members of the profession learn the ideology that supports practitioner power and dominance. According to these reseachers (particularly Waitzkin & Stoeckle, 1972), the practitioner's dominance is manifested in the practitioner-patient interaction through subtle behaviors. These behaviors include not only the withholding of information but also less obvious but perhaps more perverse interpersonal behaviors such as interrupting the patient's speech as an expression of dominance and power in the conversation (West, 1981). While the research is, as yet, sparse, the microanalyses of verbal and nonverbal interactions have begun to show promise as a very useful methodology for analyzing therapeutic communications.

Practitioner and Patient: Differing Backgrounds and Perspectives

Surveys of the occupational status of various jobs and professions in American society have placed the physician second only to Supreme Court Justice

(Duncan, 1961). Other health professions are also high in occupational status. They all demand a relatively high level of education. Thus, the chances are good that most patients will have had less formal education and will enjoy lower occupational status than the practitioners they encounter. Health professionals are experts and their status derives from their special knowledge as well as from their income and education. For many patients, medical practitioners also represent authority. As Barnlund (1976) has noted, the presence of higher-status individuals often provokes fear and tension in the patient, which may interfere with his or her processing of information. As demonstrated by White (1953) and by Seeman and Evans (1962), any emphasis on status distinctions between practitioner and patient will affect their personal interchange. Status hierarchies are likely to promote patient avoidance of contact with the professional, withholding of information, and even distortion of the information that is conveyed.

Differences in social status, in family background (a large percentage of health professionals come from professional families), in education, and in income represent still other discrepancies between practitioners and their patients. The value of health and the willingness to engage in preventive health practices is likely to be at variance for the two groups (Larson & Sutker, 1966) and may easily cause problems in communication. Health practitioners also tend to have a better developed sense of the future than their patients have (Mumford, 1977). Practitioners typically deal every day with health statistics (such as the chance of stroke from uncontrolled hypertension), and treat patients who have not beaten the odds. Further, their long postponement of immediate goals in favor of education tends to reflect their belief in and commitment to the future. Few patients will have as strong a commitment, even where their own future health is concerned.

Finally, miscommunication and misunderstanding may result from practitioners' and patients' differing perceptions of medical care, and their differing concerns regarding it. To a practitioner, the sick person represents a job. No matter how concerned and caring the practitioner may be in his or her approach, each patient is one of many who must be cared for. To the patient, the illness is a very significant life event and may be accompanied by pain, discomfort, and anxiety. Anderson and Helm (1977) have noted that physician-patient interaction actually involves a process of negotiation about how the medical problem will be perceived. In fact, if concordance in perceptions is not achieved, difficulties in the interaction are likely to ensue, and the patient is likely to be unsatisfied and uncooperative (Taylor, Burdette, Camp, & Edwards, 1980; Jellinek, 1978). Differences in concerns may become obvious to the interactants, such as in the study by Freemon et al. (1971). There, mothers of pediatric patients openly expressed significantly more emotion (generally negative, such as tension) than did the physicians, "suggesting that a medical visit with a sick child generally is a more emotionally charged experience for a mother than for her doctor" (p. 308). Considering the many ways in which practitioners and patients differ in their perspectives, it is not at all surprising that communication difficulties would arise between them.

In the Context of Medical Care

Time is a critically important issue in practitioner-patient interaction. Physicians often claim that they are limited by time in how well they can care for and educate each patient in their practice (Seligmann, McGrath, & Pratt, 1957). Patients cite the physician's apparent lack of time for them as one of the most important factors in their decision to change doctors (Gray & Cartwright, 1953). Detailed analyses of practitioner-patient interactions have focused attention on this issue of time. Lorber (1975), for example, noted that in the hospital, patients who took up too much time (usually by asking for information) were labeled by the staff as "bad patients." Skipper (1965) noted that hospital patients often refrained from asking questions precisely because they expected that the staff had no time to answer them. Thus, it seems that increased interaction time should improve practitioner-patient communication.

This is not the case, however. Studies of the effects of time (measured objectively) on patient satisfaction and patient cooperation with treatment paint an unexpected picture. Freemon et al. (1971), for example, found that the length of the physician-patient interaction was not correlated with patient satisfaction. (This was also reported by Korsch, Gozzi, & Francis, 1968.) The length of the interaction did correlate with patient compliance with treatment, but surprisingly, the shorter interactions were associated with higher compliance, and the longer interactions were associated with lower compliance. Qualitative analyses of these longer interactions between pediatricians and mothers demonstrated that the physicians often wasted time, particularly by letting themselves be trapped into petty quarrels with the parent. Korsch, Gozzi, Francis (1968) offered an example. A mother described what she called "vomiting" by her baby. The physician corrected her, referring to the baby's reaction as "regurgitation." Each countered the other's statement with insistence on the term he or she had chosen. The physician never acknowledged the mother's use of her own language to describe what she thought was wrong with her child. The physician continually repeated the information he wanted to convey, but never sought to reassure her or demonstrate that he understood what the mother was trying to say. The mother felt that the physician never understood that the child was vomiting, and as a result she ignored his prescription for treatment.

The National Ambulatory Medical Care Survey (Feller, 1979) indicated that the average time spent in face-to-face contact between office-based internists and their patients (in the late 1970s) was 18 minutes. The average time across all specialities was 15 minutes. Korsch et al. (1968) suggested that if no time is wasted in unproductive miscommunication, practitioner-patient encounters can be satisfactory and effective in as little as five minutes. By 1990, it is estimated that the present health manpower shortage will be eased substantially. It is expected that an adequate number of physicians will be available for 94 percent of the United States population (Feller, 1979). Nurses, nurse practitioners, and other health personnel should become more plentiful as well. Perhaps soon, lack of time will not be considered an acceptable reason for ineffective communication with patients. While less obviously true, it is not an acceptable reason now.

Finally, the structure of medical care may affect practitioner-patient communication in the following, rather subtle way. Health-care settings, particularly hospitals, operate as "total institutions" (Goffman, 1961). They govern every aspect of the patient's life—his daily routine, his hygiene, his eating schedule, his clothing, his spending of free time, his contact with his social network, etc. Clinics operate in similar ways, although the patient's time under their jurisdiction is limited. For the sake of efficiency, hospitals and clinics strip patients of their identities along with their clothing. Patients are examined, prodded, percussed, and palpated by their practitioners. They become medical cases. Individual variations among patients in their physical conditions (their electrolyte balance, their SGOT and BUN tests, their blood gasses) tend to capture and maintain the interest of health professionals much more easily than do individual variations in patients' comprehension of information, their personality, and their style of coping. Depersonalization is common in the health-care system and it is considered necessary for the smooth functioning of the medical system and the efficient delivery of health care. It is easy to see, of course, that an enormous potential exists for misunderstanding and poor communication between patients and their health-care practitioners.

THE POSITIVE EFFECTS OF COMMUNICATING INFORMATION

We began this chapter with the assumption that patients must first understand the behaviors required of them if they are to fulfill their medical regimens. In this section, we review the supporting evidence for this assumption. We consider the measurable results of effective communication between practitioners and their patients. We also provide evidence that practitioner-patient communication is amenable to modification, and we examine various methods for enhancing communication between practitioners and their patients. In reviewing the empirical literature, we describe the effects of providing information on various health-care outcomes, including patient compliance with treatment, patient satisfaction, and the results or outcome of care.

Information and Patient Cooperation with Treatment

Patients must know specifically what to do to fulfill their required regimens. This is one important reason why information is important to compliance. A number of important questions then arise. What kind of information best improves cooperation with treatment? To whom, and how should it be delivered? It is likely, we might guess, that if patients understand their regimens *and* the rationale for them, they can answer various questions that may arise in the course of treatment for themselves. Some patients might wonder, for example, if a course of antibiotics should be discontinued as soon as the symptoms (usually pain) of a urinary tract infection disappear. Knowledge of the purpose of a full ten-day course of the medication would be extremely important in preventing premature discontinuance of an important treatment. In other cases, patients' full understanding of their regimens may be required in order that they may explain the details of treatment to their family members, who in turn may help to provide support and reminders. Further, the communication of information, including the careful explanation of the treatment regimen, is likely to indicate to the patient that the practitioner is concerned with and mindful of his welfare. For these and other reasons, effective communication is a critical prerequisite to patient cooperation.

An excellent review of factors affecting "drop-out" from treatment (both medical and psychotherapeutic) has been presented by Baekeland and Lundwall (1975). Their review documents drop-out from treatment as a very troublesome feature of long-term medical care for chronic conditions. Patient drop-out from treatment for such chronic conditions as hypertension and diabetes has been found to result from poor instruction concerning the problematic consequences of avoiding adequate treatment. Patients were more likely to discontinue treatment if they were not aware of the potential health dangers of their medical problems and the necessity of remaining under close medical supervision. Interestingly, a similar phenomenon occurs in psychotherapy. Studies of patient drop-out from psychotherapy suggest that patient-initiated termination of treatment is often the result of the patient's lack of information about and understanding of the treatment rationale. In fact, it was found that when various options were explained to patients, they were more likely to remain in treatment.

Other correlational research has documented a positive relationship between the practitioner's offer of information to the patient and the patient's cooperation with treatment. Francis, Korsch, and Morris (1969), for example, reported that in their study of 800 tape-recorded visits to a pediatric outpatient clinic with follow-up interviews measuring compliance, a key factor in noncompliance was the parent's failure to receive an explanation of the diagnosis and cause of the child's illness. In a similar study using tape recordings, Freemon et al. (1971) found a trend toward high compliance in cases where the pediatrician focused discussion with the parent specifically on the diagnosis of the child's problem. Interestingly, and perhaps contrary to expectations, the quantity of discussion about treatment did not relate to compliance. Thus, in both studies, discussion of etiology and meaning of the child's symptoms seems to have been very important to parents' cooperation with the recommended treatment. Simple explanations, free of jargon, were particularly important in helping mothers to understand the medical problem and hence the importance of cooperation with the treatment. Of course, the treatment had to be clearly presented and the patient aware of precisely what he or she was supposed to do in order for compliance to ensue.

Compliance with long-term regimens for chronic illness, however, seems to require quite a bit of understanding on the part of the patient regarding details and potential variations of the course of treatment, if errors are to be avoided. Hulka, Cassel, Kupper, and Burdette (1976) investigated the actual amount of information transmitted from physician to patient and how that affected patient cooperation with treatment. The research involved 357 chronically ill patients with diabetes and congestive heart failure. They were the patients of 46 primary-care physicians in solo and group practice. All patients were visited in their homes by a nurse interviewer who asked them to describe the current medications used in their treatment, the function of each medication, and its recommended scheduling. The medication prescribed and the specific dosage and timing recommendations were determined by checking patients' medical charts and, when necessary, pharmacy records. Physicians were asked a series of pertinent questions about the information they had conveyed to each patient. They were asked whether the patient had been instructed or informed in each area of concern, including when to take the medication, for how long, and under what conditions (e.g., on an empty or a full stomach). Patients were asked corresponding questions about the information transmitted to them by their physicians. The researchers sought to measure whether the patients did, in fact, understand and remember correctly what had been told them by their physicians. (In this research, of course, a lack of correspondence between physician and patient report did not necessarily reflect the patient's memory failure or misunderstanding. It could reflect, instead, that the physician's report was in error and that the physician believed that he or she had communicated some piece of information, which in fact he or she had not.) Any discrepancy between the information believed by the physician to have been given to the patient (and thus important for treatment) and that received or processed by the patient could be expected to result in noncompliance if information is indeed important to compliance. Hulka et al. (1976) therefore devised a communication score that reflected the amount of information which had been successfully transmitted from physician to patient.

In this research, the dependent variable was patient compliance. The nurse-interviewer who visited each patient at home asked him or her to describe precisely the manner in which the patient was taking the drug. Drug error rates were then determined by the discrepancy between the patient's behavior and what was prescribed for him or her. In this research, four kinds of "noncompliance" measures were generated which were particularly useful in determining the effects of information on patient medication taking: *omission rate*, the proportion of the drugs the patient was *not* taking of those prescribed by the physician; *commission rate*, the proportion of the drugs the patient *was* taking which the physician *had not* prescribed; *scheduling misconception rate*, the proportion of prescribed drugs taken by the patient for which the patient *did not know* the correct schedule; and *scheduling noncompliance rate*, the proportion of prescribed drugs taken by the patient for which the patient *knew* what was prescribed but *did not take* the medication according to the correct schedule. These separate measures represented a valuable addition to the empirical research on compliance because they allowed a meaningful distinction to be made between intentional and unintentional noncompliance (the former representing a kind of rebellion on the part of the patient, and the latter representing an error for which the patient is not directly responsible).

In this research, Hulka and her colleagues found that when all types of medication errors were combined, the average patient's medication error rate was 58 percent. On the average, omissions occurred in 18 to 19 percent of the drugs prescribed and commissions in 19 to 20 percent of the drugs prescribed. Scheduling errors occurred in the use of about 17 percent of the drugs prescribed. Interestingly, the average scheduling (intentional) noncompliance rate was only 3 percent, indicating that patients only rarely failed to follow a regimen that they understood. The scheduling noncompliance rate was so low and had such low variability that it was eliminated in further analyses. The correlation between the other three medication error measures and the information conveyed from physician to patient demonstrated that communication was very important and accounted for significant differences in drug omission rates and commission rates. There was also a trend indicating a relationship between misconceptions and physician-patient communication. The less information communicated (that is, the lower the communication score), the lower the patient's accuracy in taking the prescribed medication.

In regard to the general issue of information and its relationship to compliance, Davis (1968) noted that "while there is not complete agreement on exactly how the doctor-patient relationship affects compliance, most investigators do recognize the importance of communication and explanation" (p. 287). Davis reviewed 20 studies in which this relationship was demonstrated.

An experimental study by Roter (1977) has provided some compelling evidence for the role of information in patients' commitment to treatment. This study is especially important because it used the random assignment of subjects to treatment groups, and involved an experimental intervention that was designed to increase the information obtained by patients by motivating them to ask questions of their physicians. In this research, experimental group patients, prior to their visit with a physician, were assisted by a health counselor to formulate questions they would like to ask their physicians. These questions (about diagnosis, etiology, treatment, and prognosis) were written down in order to help the patient to remember. Control-group patients were given some general information but no special help or encouragement to ask questions for their physicians. The results showed that experimental-group patients (given the special intervention) asked more direct questions of their physicians than did control-group patients. This was determined through analysis of tape recordings of the medical visit. Experimental group patients also demonstrated significantly higher appointment-keeping ratios than did control patients. Subsequent analyses of these data (Roter, 1981, prepub. ms.) showed that among experimental (activated) patients, the earlier in the interaction the first question was asked by the patient, the more questions were asked during the entire medical visit, the shorter time the visit took, and the higher appointment-keeping (compliance) rate was demonstrated by the patient. Thus, patient-initiated requests for information resulted in improved compliance, as well as in a less time-consuming visit.

Information and Patient Satisfaction with Treatment

Perhaps not surprisingly, popular notions that patients who are informed by their practitioners are more satisfied with the medical care they receive are supported by empirical research. Many correlational studies have found a positive relationship between patient satisfaction and the practitioner's provision of information about diagnosis, treatment, and prognosis. Korsch, Gozzi, and Francis (1968) studied the expectations of mothers who brought their children to an emergency clinic. Tape recordings of the physician-mother interaction were made and later analyzed in conjunction with the results of chart review, postvisit interview, and a follow-up interview with the mother. A striking finding of the research was each mother's intense concern with and need for information and explanation of her child's disease and its cause. Mothers especially wanted to be reassured that they were not to blame for their children's illnesses. Failure to fulfill a mother's need for an explanation of the diagnosis and etiology often resulted in significant dissatisfaction on the part of the mother. Other correlational research (using interviews, questionnaires, and chart reviews) has also linked the provision of information to patient satisfaction. Houston and Pasanen (1972) found that patients' satisfaction with their care was directly related to the amount of information they received. Liptak, Hulka, and Cassel (1977) found that pediatricians' awareness of maternal concerns, and their communication to the mother were correlated with the mothers' satisfaction with medical care.

In their objective analyses of patterns of interaction exchange in the physician-patient relationship, Stiles, Putnam, Wolf, and James (1979b) found that patient satisfaction, as expressed in a postvisit questionnaire, was related to the physician's transmission of information in "feedback" exchanges during the concluding segment of the visit. During feedback exchanges, physicians gave their patients information about illness and treatment, and patients were allowed to ask clarifying questions. In a previous study of direct observation of interaction (Freemon, Negrete, Davis, & Korsch, 1971), researchers had failed to find an association between physicians' offering of information and patient satisfaction. Stiles et al. (1979b) attributed this null result to limitations in the widely used coding systems of the early 1970s, which failed to distinguish the direct communication of information from other common physician responses (such as acknowledgments).

In another study, behaviors of physicians and patients were coded from videotaped interviews (Smith, Polis, & Hadac, 1981). The importance of information to patient satisfaction was again supported. In this study, the verbal (and in some cases nonverbal) behaviors of physicians and patients were coded from 29 videotaped practitioner-patient encounters. Postvisit interviews were conducted with patients to determine their degree of satisfaction with the visit, and their understanding of what was told them by the physician. Statistically significant (and substantial) correlations were found between two sets of variables: the proportion of time in the interview spent by the physicians giving information, and the patient's satisfaction with the visit and understanding of what had been communicated. In addition, satisfaction and understanding were respectively correlated with time spent discussing prevention, and time spent (by the doctor) located within three feet of the patient (proximal distancing—a nonverbal cue). Significant negative correlations were found between the proportion of time the physician spent during the visit reading the patient's chart and both satisfaction and understanding. Interestingly, the sheer length of time of the visit was significantly positively correlated with patient satisfaction, although not with patient understanding of the information communicated.

Two experimental studies have addressed the relationship between the communication of information and patient satisfaction. In one study in a family-practice clinic, Bertakis (1977) tape-recorded physician-patient visits to determine the amount of information conveyed by the physician to the patient regarding diagnosis and etiology of the illness, further investigations such as laboratory tests, and treatment regimen required. In the intervention group, patients were asked to recall exactly what had been told them immediately after the visit. Patients were, overall, more satisfied with physicians who gave them information. In addition, patients who retained more of all forms of information about their illness were more satisfied. The experimental group patients were also asked to restate what they had been told immediately after the visit and were given feedback. After their treatment for the illness was completed, experimental patients retained 83.5 percent of what they had much earlier been told compared with only 60.8 percent of the information retained by control patients who were not asked to recall what they had been told. Patients in the experimental group were also more satisfied with treatment than were patients in the control group. Thus, a focus on patient recall of information given by the physician increased its salience and hence its retention, and also increased patient satisfaction.

In the experimental study by Roter (1977) described above, experimental-group patients were "activated" by an intervention that helped them to ask questions of their physicians. Measures of resultant patient satisfaction showed some surprising results. Although patients in the experimental group asked more direct questions of their physicians, they were less satisfied than control-group patients who were not encouraged to express to the physician their desire for information. Experimental-group patients also displayed greater negative affect toward their physicians during the visit. Indeed, it is possible that when patients must assert to the physician their desire for information about their care, they experience distress and anger at the physician.

The relationship between the provision of information and patient satisfaction needs further study, since many questions still remain unanswered. For example, is patient satisfaction enhanced only when information is given freely to the patient by the physician, and not as a result of the patient's request for information? Such a conclusion might be teased out of the findings considered so far, but a direct test of this question is mandatory before a final conclusion can be drawn. Similarly, do patients who ask their physicians to share information with them come to resent their practitioners? Do patients dislike having to take an active role in their treatment?

The question of whether patient satisfaction is a worthy goal in itself is, of course, relevant to the examination of the relationship between information giving and patient satisfaction. Whatever its other value, satisfaction does seem to be related to compliance, at least in preliminary work on this issue. Ware, Davies-Avery, and Stewart (1978) reviewed the literature on patient satisfaction with treatment and noted that it is indeed an important aspect of medical care. Patient satisfaction can be reliably measured and it has validity in terms of health-care outcomes. Satisfaction is related to patient cooperation with treatment (Korsch et al., 1968), to patient commitment to medical (versus nonmedical) treatment (Cobb, 1954), and to patient commitment to a particular physician (DiMatteo, Prince, & Taranta, 1979). Because of the weakness of simple correlation in deciding direction of causality, Roghmann, Hengst, and Zastowny (1979) used multiple-regression techniques to predict patient utilization of medical-care services from their satisfaction, and vice versa. The results showed that, indeed, satisfaction influences utilization, not the other way around.

Information and the Outcome of Treatment

Outpatient Treatment. In the care of both acute and chronic illness, the treatment of patients as passive recipients of care may not be in their best interest. Particularly when regimens require long-term medical involvement, an active patient orientation may be necessary in order both to improve patient cooperation and to enhance the physical and psychological well-being of the patient. In a study by Schulman (1979), a systematic attempt was made to vary patients' active orientation toward medical care—an orientation that enhanced their knowledge of the regimen and their participation in it. The participants were 99 hypertension patients whose direct involvement in their care was considered in relation to their treatment outcome. Patients' active orientation was induced by various methods of treatment but was measured as a quantitative variable using a self-report measuring scale. Additional oral and written questionnaires were given to patients, asking about their cognitive, behavioral, and physical outcomes. Blood-pressure measurements were also recorded. Patients with a highly active orientation to their care were significantly more likely to have their blood pressure under control and were less likely to report side effects of their medications. They also adhered more closely to their treatment recommendations and were more likely to engage in health-enhancing behaviors (such as stopping smoking, relaxing more, reducing their salt intake, and consuming no alcohol). On a cognitive level, patients with a highly active orientation also expressed greater feelings of self-efficacy, greater confidence in their professionals' expertise, and a greater belief in the benefit of treatment over the cost.

Stressful Medical Examinations and Procedures. Research has demonstrated an overwhelming amount of evidence to support the assertion that pain is a psychological phenomenon. Pain perception is complex and is subject to cognitive and emotional factors (Melzack, 1974). Pain experiences are modified by thoughts regarding the "meaning" of the situation to the patient, by the person's anxiety about the source of pain, and by attentional factors (to what extent the person is focusing thoughts on the pain) (Beecher, 1959). Studies of various experimental interventions (for example, Kaplan, 1982) have shown that the provision of information to the patient can have a significant impact on his or her ability to cope with an unpleasant or painful medical examination or treatment procedure.

Folklore suggests that when one faces a stressful event that is likely to cause pain, it may be best "not to think about it." Studies of avoidant thinking, however, suggest that this is not an effective coping mechanism for most people who face medical procedures. In a study of patients waiting to receive electric shocks, Houston and Holmes (1974) found that the provision of distracting material designed to produce avoidant thinking actually resulted in more intense psychophysiological reactions among subjects than did the opportunity to assess the seriousness of the threat. In the face of expected pain or discomfort, the opportunity to think about the details of what one is about to experience actually reduces the distress of experiencing it. Information is one of the best treatments for the stress attendant on facing a difficult medical procedure.

Numerous intervention studies have examined this issue in naturalistic settings with patients who are facing these stressful procedures. In one experiment, Johnson and Leventhal (1974) studied 48 patients who were about to undergo an endoscopy examination (which requires that a tube as thick as a thumb be passed down the throat into the gastrointestinal tract, while the patient is fully awake). Patients were given either one of two types of preparatory information, both types of information, or no information at all. One type of information concerned the sensations that would be experienced (what would be seen, heard, felt, tasted), while the other instructions told patients what they would be asked to do during the examination (make swallowing motions). The results showed that the instructions that gave a complete description of the sensory experiences reduced patients' emotional distress most effectively. The information concerning what the patient was expected to do was only effective when it was used in combination with the sensory information.

Similar findings have come from studies of other medical procedures such as pelvic examinations (Fuller, Endress, & Johnson, 1978), blood donation (Mills & Krantz, 1979), and a sigmoidoscopy (Kaplan, 1982). The provision of sensory information (what would be experienced by the patient, the specific sensations, feelings, sounds, tastes, smells, etc.) had a profound effect on reducing self-reported anxiety and its behavioral concomitants (such as agitation, muscle tension, amount of analgesic or tranquilizer required, etc.), many of which might interfere with the medical procedure itself. Shipley et al. (1978) found that the repetition of explicit information about the process of an endoscopy examination was most effective in reducing distress during the examination.

There is preliminary evidence that some personality factors might mediate the effects of information on the patient's ability to cope with noxious procedures. Kaplan (1982) has reported that in some laboratory research, as well as in a study on reactions to dental surgery, the provision of very specific information is only effective for patients who have an internal locus of control (that is, those who believe that what happens to them is a function of their own behavior, not of external factors). In some cases, it has been noted that individuals with an extreme external locus of control react better when they are not given any specific information about what will happen to them. This is not a well-established finding, however, and the role of personality factors in patients' coping with information and medical examinations requires considerably more research. At this point it appears that information has an overall positive effect on patients' coping, and the provision of information to patients along with their treatment recommendations is a well-advised approach to patient care.

Surgery. Studies of the effects of providing surgical patients with preliminary information about their surgical experience have been carried out over the past two decades, stimulated initially by the work of the psychologist Irving Janis (1958). Janis examined the phenomenon of the "work of worrying" on patients' adaptation to the stressful events that surround surgery. In the early 1960s, researchers in the anesthesiology department of the Massachusetts General Hospital began to explore the results of providing information to patients. They used as their outcome criteria various physical and psychological variables, including patients' anxiety level before surgery, their calmness, their need for pain-killing medication, and their postoperative course (including the total number of days of hospitalization). Egbert, Battit, Turndorf, and Beecher (1963) found that information provided to patients in a supportive visit by the anesthetist prior to surgery had a more positive effect upon their drowsiness and calmness before surgery than did the tranquilizing drug pentobarbitol. When the drug was combined with the informative visit, the most positive effect was achieved. A further investigation of this phenomenon (Egbert, Battit, Welch, & Bartlett, 1964) showed a positive effect of a supportive visit by the anesthetist, a visit in which sensory information and instruction in a method of relaxing spasmodic abdominal muscles after surgery was provided. Patients in the experimental group required less pain medication for the five postoperative days than did control-group patients. They were judged to be more comfortable and in better physical and emotional condition, and were discharged from the hospital an average of 2.7 days earlier than control-group patients. All of the dependent measures in these studies were gathered by individuals who were blind to the experimental conditions of the patients. It is important to note that in this study, the information about the future pre- and postoperative experiences was not the only information given to patients. They were also told what specific coping techniques to use in their adjustment to the surgical pain. Thus, it is not clear whether the positive effects achieved were the result of information in general, or of the specific instructions (such as for muscle relaxation) provided.

Whether sensory information alone is enough to ease the difficulties of surgery has been the topic of a good deal of research. Langer, Janis, and Wolfer (1975), for example, provided various forms of preoperative preparatory information to 60 adult surgical patients. One of the interventions involved instruction in a cognitive coping device that included calming self-talk, a reappraisal of anxiety-provoking events, and cognitive control. For example, patients were taught ways to reinterpret problem events so that these events would not seem so bad, and ways in which to talk to themselves in order to achieve calm and better enable themselves to deal with problems that arise. The intervention with which it was compared consisted only of information about what the patient would experience during the pre- and postoperative phases of care. One group of patients (the control group) received no intervention, another group received both interventions, a third group received the cognitive coping intervention alone, and a fourth group received the information intervention alone. The amount of pain relief medication and sedatives requested by patients served as the dependent measures. Interestingly, the most favorable outcomes occurred in the cognitive coping condition, with no preparatory information. Other studies (such as Newton & Reading, 1977; and Schmitt & Wooldridge, 1973), however, have suggested that the most positive effects for surgical and nonsurgical preparation result from a combination of information and coping techniques presented to patients. Relatedly, in an extensive and thoughtful review of the literature on the short-term effects of psychological preparation for surgery, Reading (1979) examined all the studies to date on this topic and concluded that optimum patient care probably requires a combination of information and coping techniques, with an emphasis on the latter.

Finally, research has shown that information and support presented to the person who is significant to the patient (such as a family member) may have important effects on the patient's reaction to surgery. Skipper and Leonard (1968) presented experimental data indicating that social interaction with hospital personnel who provided information and emotional support reduced a mother's stress and changed her perception of the threatening nature of her child's hospitalization. In turn, her child's stress was reduced, and in turn the child's social, psychological, and physical reactions to hospitalization and surgery were influenced profoundly.

Mediating Mechanisms. Precisely *how* information (and suggestions for specific coping) operate to enhance the outcomes of patient care is still not clear. Reading (1979) has overviewed the various theories and has offered the following explanations: (1) information reduces patient anxiety (sensory information may cause the least reduction in anxiety, information about practical details more reduction, and coping instructions the greatest reduction in anxiety); (2) information enhances feelings of personal control (resulting in greater stress tolerance and the capacity to reduce feelings of hopelessness); (3) information can improve the patient's attitude toward the procedure (focusing on the positive rather than the negative effects of the experience); and (4) the provision of instructions utilizing established techniques for coping with pain helps to reduce the pain experienced by the patient. Now that information has been well established as important to the outcome of treatment, it is time to orient research efforts toward understanding the precise mechanisms that bring about these beneficial effects. Only then will researchers and practitioners be able to decide the optimum preparatory format for many different patients under many varying conditions.

A Final Note. Nearly all of the studies to date of the relationship of information to patient satisfaction and cooperation in ambulatory care settings have been correlational. On the other hand, studies of the relationship of information to the outcome of surgery or stressful medical procedures have been, for the most part, experimental. The divergence in methodologies between these two topics is hardly coincidental. It seems to reflect a divergence in characteristics of those settings. While in outpatient care there tends to be a natural variance in the degree of information provided to patients (and this variance in information is then correlated with factors such as satisfaction and compliance), in surgical and procedural treatment settings, the typical course of events provides a natural "control group" of the experimental design. The control group receives no information. The experimental intervention—the provision of information to patients who are about to undergo surgery or a stressful medical procedure—is a new endeavor. It is a deviation from normality, and an experiment. As this situation changes, and modern medical care sees the provision of information to patients becoming a routine component of care, it is likely that naturalistic studies will be done in inpatient settings. The incorporation of experimental intervention studies in outpatient settings is very important as well. Both naturalistic and intervention studies must be combined in order that mediating and attenuating factors in the link between information and health-related outcome may be carefully examined.

CONCLUSION

Throughout this chapter, the communication of information within the context of the practitioner-patient relationship has been examined. A picture of the typical therapeutic interaction has been sketched—with the patient asking few questions and the practitioner volunteering little information. The communication problems typically encountered in practitioner-patient interactions have been examined, as have the many barriers to the provision of information to patients. The benefits of explanation and education (in enhancing patient satisfaction, compliance, and the outcome of treatment) have also been considered.

For many years, health educators have extolled the virtues of providing information to patients. This is in fact the primary goal of the field of health education. Health education programs are designed to reach large numbers of individuals and to convey relevant health information to them within the constraints of their social, economic, and cultural contexts (Green, 1979). Although for many years health educators have been far removed from physicians, nurses, and nurse practitioners, lately they have become more actively involved with primary-health-care providers. The explicit goal of health education within the primary-care context is client self-sufficiency (Roter, 1977) and the promotion of the practitioner-patient relationship as a partnership (Stone, 1979; Currie & Renner, 1979). It is interesting, and perhaps a bit distressing as well, to note that in at least one major study (Roter, 1977), patients' own active orientation to their care (enhanced by a health educator's prompting to ask questions of their physician) caused patients to experience emotional discomfort. The reasons for this are not at all clear, and so this issue presents an important topic for research—particularly before the concept of the practitioner-patient partnership crumbles under unrealistic expectations.

Another major issue related to information giving in the physician-patient relationship is in need of future research. This is the controversy regarding the practitioner's sharing of the medical record with the patient. The few studies on this topic show mixed results. Stevens, Stagg, and Mackay (1977), for example, reported that giving hospitalized patients access to their medical records had little or no effect on any of the process or outcome variables they measured. Although patients were given free access to their hospital charts, few actively sought and studied their records. Most did elect to look at them when the charts were available as part of routine ward rounds. There was no measurable difference, however, between experimental (free-access) and control patients in their ability to list diagnoses or medications, their self-assessment of depression, anxiety, or contentment, or their attitudes toward various aspects of the health-care system. Access to records was found partially to facilitate practitioners' communication with patients. Fischbach et al. (1980) did find a positive effect of having patient and practitioner co-author the medical record. They noted, however, that the success of their approach may have come precisely from the *coauthorship*, which by its very nature required communication and an open-ended dialogue. Fishbach et al. warned that simply issuing a copy of the record to the patient without explanation or support may promote no positive effects on the practitioner-patient relationship, and might, in fact, be harmful and have negative effects (such as arousing fear in response to record entries which the patient does not understand). Studies of patients' desire for paticipation in their treatment suggest that the majority of patients wish not to assume full responsibility for decisions about care, but rather wish to share it with the physician and rely on his or her expertise (Vertinsky et al., 1974).

Even aside from the question of the appropriateness of a patient-practitioner partnership, we find that the therapeutic communication is a very complex issue. While the accurate transmittal of information is necessary for patient compliance, the transfer of facts by means of patient education is neither the only component of communication nor the only factor that affects compliance (Sackett et al., 1975). As Green (1979) has noted, communication in the practitioner-patient relationship demands attention to the manner of expression, to the rapport that exists in the therapeutic relationship, and to the psychological and social situation of the patient. Educating patients also demands an understanding of what they know, and what they are willing to learn and capable of learning. In this sense, our entire book is about communication in the practitioner-patient relationship.

The complexity of these issues is great, and careful examination is necessary. In the following chapter we consider another crucial factor in communication—interpersonal rapport—which relates in some very important ways to compliance.

3

Practitioner-Patient Relationships: Rapport and the Art of Medicine

The meeting of practitioner and patient in the medical setting sometimes results in a dispassioned enactment of their stereotypic social roles, as was demonstrated at the beginning of Chapter 2. The practitioner approaches the patient as a nonjudgmental healer who is affectively neutral, portrays little emotion, and maintains an air of objective professional concern. The practitioner always appears confident in his or her medicotechnical skills. The patient, on the other hand, enacts the complementary role of passive recipient, prepared to cooperate fully with the practitioner's technical ministrations, expecting nothing more than the practitioner's total dedication to the eradication of their common enemy, the disease. As many have noted, however, empirical research and theoretical analyses of actual medical encounters have characterized the practitioner-patient relationship as significantly more complicated than the simple enactment of these social roles.

The social roles of practitioner and patient were initially proposed because, in theory, they are functional. They insure that practitioner and patient will behave "appropriately" toward one another—particularly that, despite the competence gap between them and the superior knowledge and expertise of the practitioner, the patient will not be exploited (Parsons, 1951, 1958). These roles facilitate the development of an important component of the practitioner-patient relationship—the factor of trust. Since practitioner and patient cannot be counted on to follow the role requirements first set out by

Parsons, however, other factors must be called into play to enhance the development of trust.

It is interesting that although many other interpersonal factors have been found to promote trust in the practitioner-patient relationship, the contention that the classical roles of physician and patient operate to enhance trust has never been empirically demonstrated. (In fact, some research has suggested that the strict enactment of these social roles of active practitioner and passive patient may result in patient distress and unsuccessful medical treatment [Taylor, 1979; Lorber, 1975].) In this chapter, we review those other interpersonal factors, and examine how they might operate to establish the patient's confidence in the benevolence of the practitioner. We also examine the importance of trust to patient compliance and other outcomes. In our analysis, we maintain the orientation that patients generally desire much more from their medical practitioners than the classical role of the practitioner has to offer (Reader, Pratt, & Mudd, 1957). Patients want understanding, caring, and concern for themselves as people (Freidson, 1970; Eisenberg, 1977). Very often they desire information as well (as examined in detail in Chapter 2), and are becoming increasingly demanding of respect as thinking, feeling human beings (Eisenberg, 1977; Engel, 1977a). Practitioners, in turn, desire that their patients exert some control over their own behavior and accept some responsibility for their health (Knowles, 1977). The eradication of the disease also demands more from practitioner and patient than they have classically been expected to give. The current emphasis on nonspecific factors in healing (Beecher, 1959; Frank, 1977), on the mind-body relationship (Pelletier, 1979), and on the role of interpersonal relationships in patient care (Friedman & DiMatteo, 1982; DiMatteo & Friedman, 1979, 1982) points to a newly demonstrated, scientifically valid effect of the practitioner-patient relationship on the enhancement of healing. There seems to be little doubt that the outcome of even an apparently purely technical medical procedure can be profoundly affected by the rapport and interpersonal quality of the practitioner-patient relationship. One important reason is the significant contribution of these interpersonal factors to patient cooperation with the treatment process. Interpersonal issues in the therapeutic relationship influence the patient's beliefs in the efficacy of the treatment, and his or her expectations for its positive outcome (DiMatteo, 1979). These issues, thus, affect the patient's willingness and ability to overcome resistance and to participate in the prescribed health-care regimen.

In this chapter, we examine the interpersonal factors in the therapeutic relationship that contribute to patient compliance with medical treatments and recommended health behaviors. We examine these factors as they influence compliance both directly (in their influence on health behavior), and indirectly (as they operate in the development of trust). We argue that trust is necessary if the patient is to share with the health practitioner the beliefs, values, attitudes, and social normative influences that affect his compliance. Entrusting these to the practitioner places the patient in a vulnerable position and renders the patient likely to be persuaded and influenced. Throughout this entire chapter, we present the therapeutic relationship as a setting for the inevitable negotiation that must take place between individuals with profoundly disparate goals and points of view, whose mutual interdependency places a premium on their cooperation and trust.

PRACTITIONER, PATIENT, AND ILLNESS

The relationship between a patient and his or her medical practitioner is limited in time compared with most other relationships in the patient's life. Nevertheless, this relationship often assumes paramount personal importance. People usually remember much about the emotional and interpersonal tone of their encounters with health professionals (Korsch, Gozzi, & Francis, 1968; Francis, Korsch, & Morris, 1969). In general, people tend to view their medical practitioners as very important figures (King, 1962). It is easy to see why this is true. Physicians and other health practitioners are present at most emotionally momentous occasions in people's lives—such as determinations of pregnancies, births, surgeries, pronouncements of terminal illness, and deaths of loved ones. These practitioners are typically approached under conditions of high anxiety and deep concern. Patients tend to be very sensitive to the interpersonal treatment they receive from their medical practitioners because of the emotional uncertainty they feel when they are faced with unfamiliar scientific jargon and procedures, novel surroundings, and separation from the comfort and support of loved ones (Friedman, 1979a). Patients are often completely at the mercy of their practitioners, whom they have initially sought out because of their high level of hope and confidence in the ability of these healers to relieve their distress. In addition, very few physical or emotional boundaries separate practitioners from their patients. Health professionals are privy to all parts of the patient's body and to the most intimate details of the patient's life. Mixed emotions usually accompany the presence of the practitioner—a reduction in anxiety as well as an increase in it, the experience of fear as well as the experience of hope, and sometimes feelings of profound attachment.

Regression in Illness

Among medical practitioners, it is commonly reported that when people are sick or highly anxious, they tend to "regress"—that is, to assume a childlike, dependent role that is characteristic of an earlier stage of their development

(Nemiah, 1961; Lederer, 1952). Regression is noted to be a common phenomenon in the hospital, where it tends to be supported by a certain degree of infantilization imposed on the patient by the medical-care process (Lorber, 1975; Taylor, 1979). Health professionals care for patients when the latter are most vulnerable, emotionally as well as physically (Lederer, 1952). In part because of this vulnerability, patients tend to experience ambivalent emotions toward their health professionals. They are highly sensitive to their practitioners' demonstrations of protection and caring for them. They are also highly sensitive to their practitioners' negative behaviors and are quick to become angry and rebel against them.

Transference. Psychodynamic explanations of patients' reactions to illness invoke the concept of transference. It is important to consider transference here because so many health practitioners embrace it as an explanation for their patients' behaviors toward them. Transference, broadly defined, refers to patients' manifested attitudes and behaviors which reflect their previous relationships with authority figures (typically their parents, but sometimes previous practitioners as well). Transference is associated with regression, and as such is believed to reflect patients' "infantile" concerns. Thus, transference if often brushed off by busy health practitioners as inappropriate "acting out" on the part of the patient of some long forgotten conflict, memory, or feeling. Most health professionals feel that, as they have neither the expertise nor the time, they are in no position to deal with a patient's deep-seated "unconscious" processes (particularly if these involve negative feelings toward the practitioner). They therefore ignore the patient's needs. Sometimes, however, the patient's negative expressions of anger or rebellion (whether due to some degree of transference or not) represent predictable responses to disrespectful, discourteous, or condescending behavior on the part of the practitioner. While the patient's negative reaction may be reminiscent of his or her childhood rebellion against authoritative parents, the patient's assertion of freedom and attempts at counter-control may actually be quite adaptive. They may help to prevent the development of helplessness and depression, and aid the patient to attain what he or she needs from the medical-care system. The practitioners' discounting of the patient's behavior as "unconscious acting out" reduces the legitimacy of the patient's requests. Such a label fosters the feeling among practitioners that patients' complaints are not worthy of notice. Because of this tendency, we feel that while psychodynamic notions of regression and transference may provide excellent explanations for the character of patient behavior during illness, they tend to reduce the importance of the patient's legitimate requests. In this chapter, therefore, we take a somewhat different approach and view the patient as an equal partner with the practitioner in a process of negotiation.

The Practitioner's Conduct

Unquestionably, emotions run deep in the medical encounter. The stakes are high and the issues weighty. Patients are highly sensitized to the subtleties of the situation and of the behavior of the practitioner. This sensitivity invariably affects patients' perceptions of the medical care that is rendered to them. As Doyle and Ware (1977) have noted, the physician's conduct is the most important factor in the patient's evaluation of his or her health services. Thus, the practitioner's behavior toward the patient is an important part of the patient's care. As we shall see in this chapter, the potential for good as well as for harm is quite profound in the practitioner-patient relationship.

SELF-PRESENTATION, NEGOTIATION, AND EXPECTATIONS IN PRACTITIONER-PATIENT ENCOUNTERS

In a small-scale but intensive study of general practice in Wales, two sociologists, Stimson and Webb (1975) analyzed the face-to-face encounters between practitioners and patients in terms of two guiding themes: self-presentational strategies and negotiation. They conceptualized practitioner and patient as actors, much in the fashion that the symbolic interactionists propose that, through interaction, people create reality (Hewitt, 1979). Their approach was similar to that of Goffman's (1959) dramaturgical analysis of social interaction, in which he argued that all the world is a stage and that people are actors who present themselves in ways they see fit (see Chapter 5 for a more detailed discussion of symbolic interaction and its relevance to health care issues). According to Stimson and Webb, practitioner and patient are likewise engaged in a process of effective self-presentation. The patient does *not* relinquish control and decision-making power to the physician; rather, he or she maintains control through self-determination and through contact with outside social and lay referral networks (which, as we see in Chapter 5, are comprised of individuals who either directly or by means of social norms influence the patient's behavior at least as much as the physician does). The patient, however, uses the illusion of dependency on the practitioner as a self-presentation strategy in order to manipulate the practitioner's sentiments and behaviors. The patient's goal is to direct the consultation along his or her own desired lines, and to persuade the physician to view the problem from the perspective of the patient. Stimson and Webb viewed the consultation in terms of each actor's attempt to influence the other. They conceived of the interaction in terms of the second theme—a process of negotiation.

Stimson and Webb argued that negotiation is indeed a *process*, the outcome of which is the result of mutual influence which takes place during the medical consultation. This process does not guarantee the achievement of a compromise that will be acceptable to both parties. Whether or not this compromise is reached will depend heavily upon the interpersonal skills of the practitioner and the patient. These researchers also suggested that the consultation does not take place in a vacuum but that it is influenced by its social context, and that the negotiating parties have some initial information or expectations about one another. These may have been derived from their prior knowledge of one another as persons (if they have met before) or from their stereotypes of one another (what the patient thinks about medical practitioners, and what the practitioner thinks about patients). Their expectations for one another's behavior are therefore likely to influence, in part, their negotiation process.

Expectations and Requests

Some studies have claimed to demonstrate a correlation between the "fulfillment of expectations" during the medical encounter and patients' satisfaction and compliance with treatment (Korsch, Gozzi, & Francis, 1968; Francis, Korsch, & Morris, 1969). In the patient-care literature (according to Lazare, Eisenthal, Frank, & Stoeckle, 1978), the meaning of expectations is confusing. The term can appropriately refer to different issues, but these meanings have been confused in the research. The same term has been used to apply to what patients anticipate will happen (expectation) and what they want to happen (requests). These researchers have shown that the two concepts are not identical (Lazare, Eisenthal, & Wasserman, 1975). A patient may expect that a practitioner will deliver a certain form of care (e.g., be efficient, and technically sophisticated) but may not desire that form of treatment at all. The fulfillment of expectations (in the sense of anticipation) is likely to correlate with positive outcomes of care such as satisfaction and, perhaps as a result, compliance. Social psychological research has demonstrated the positive effects of predictability and has shown that people are comfortable with and evaluate positively both events and other people that they feel are predictable. Thus, predictability itself may be a reason for positive evaluation.

The fulfillment of patients' *desires* for their care have been explored in a number of medical contexts. Careful examination of the meaning of expectations in the studies by Korsch (Korsch, Gozzi, & Francis, 1968; Francis, Korsch, & Morris, 1969) reveals that the fulfillment of mothers' implicit requests for the visit with the practitioner predicted their satisfaction and compliance with care. Research by Lazare, Eisenthal, Frank, and Stoeckle (1978) found that patients were in fact able to state in detail the nature of their request regarding the practitioner's action during the clinic visit. In the psychiatric-clinic setting, where this research took place, requests were of many different types. They included administrative and community triage, control (e.g., "keep me from killing myself"), reality contact, ventilation, succorance, psychodynamic insight, and social intervention (e.g., "tell my wife not to leave me").

According to Lazare and colleagues (1978), patients' requests have been largely ignored in the literature on practitioner-patient interactions. While a few studies, such as those cited above, have examined this potentially important determinant of patient compliance and satisfaction, for the most part the issue has received little careful scrutiny. This deficiency in the literature probably partly reflects practitioners' beliefs that patients desire to receive a satisfaction of their unconscious needs (such as transference) from the therapeutic interaction. In this view, asking the patient what he or she wants would involve turning control of the interaction over to the patient. Practitioners may also feel that eliciting the patient's request would be like opening a Pandora's box of insatiable demands. Still other practitioners probably feel that patients do not know what they want anyway. On the other hand, the paucity of research may reflect the maintenance of the status quo in which patients fail to state a request because they believe it is not their role to do so, or because they fear exposing their desires and experiencing humiliation by the clinician. Whether or not these assumptions about the practitioner-patient relationship are in fact valid remains to be seen after empirical examination.

Negotiation

The concepts of requests and expectations have also led to a view of the practitioner-patient relationship as a process of negotiation. Lazare et al. (1978) hypothesized, on the basis of their investigations of patients' requests, that conflict between physician and patient is often present. Sometimes this conflict is explicit, such as when the patient wants a prescription and the clinician is unwilling to give it, or when the patient expresses a desire for treatment of a specific problem (e.g., a prescription or device to deal with the patient-defined problem) but the clinician focuses on a different problem (which the patient sees as irrelevant). This type of explicit conflict was examined in the Korsch et al. research noted above. In the analyses of unsatisfactory clinic visits, the pediatricians and mothers under study tended to define the baby's problems in totally discrepant ways. Mothers who were interviewed after the visit were able to describe the precise nature of their disagreements with the physicians. In other cases, however, the conflict and negotiation may be much more subtle and may remain unstated. The differences between practitioner and patient may center in such issues as the definition of the problem, the cause of the illness, the goals of treatment, and the priorities of treatment, but these differences may be unknown or unacknowledged by practitioner or patient. An excellent example of the operation of this difference in perspectives is the interaction in the emergency room between a physician and a patient who is complaining of abdominal pain. Until the diagnosis is made, the practitioner must withhold pain-relieving medication in order to chart the course of the pain. The patient does not know this (and the practitioner does not explain it). The patient believes that the physician is withholding medication out of cruelty, and is withholding communication (of diagnosis and prognosis) out of secretiveness. Neither practitioner nor patient recognizes that they differ in their definitions of the medical problem. It is also important to recognize that conflict and negotiation may take place, as Stimson and Webb (1975) noted, over completely intangible issues such as self-esteem, honor, and saving face.

Indeed, there are many issues that might give rise to conflict in the practitioner-patient relationship, and therefore a high probability exists that at least one issue will result in some conflict. Many theorists therefore hold that conflict is inherent in the practitioner-patient relationship, and that conflict resolution through the process of negotiation is a critical part of any helping relationship (see Freidson, 1970; Balint, 1957). The process of negotiation refers to a coming together or conferring over a source of conflict with the purpose of achieving some agreement. It is a process whereby each of two or more parties attempts to determine what each will give or take or perform in a transaction between them (Rubin & Brown, 1975). An important general goal of each party to the practitioner-patient negotiation process is this: the practitioner seeks to feel that he has done what he believes to be professionally appropriate while the patient wishes to receive what he feels is in his own best physical and psychological interest. Compromises are acceptable as long as they still provide enough satisfaction to make the relationship worthwhile for the patient and will not breach the clinician's professional standards.

What happens when the negotiation does not result in a compromise that is acceptable to both parties? Usually, practitioner and/or patient attempt one of the following: coercion (exertion of power by the practitioner), sabotage of the regimen (by the patient), rejection of the other by one or both parties, or lying (the presentation of pseudomutuality whereby the patient, for whatever other reasons he might have, continues to see the practitioner but does not admit that he is not following the advice or regimen; the practitioner avoids any confrontation that might reveal noncompliance). In the patient-practitioner relationship, the failure to resolve or negotiate the issue successfully is a serious problem. It "may be followed on the patient's part with dissatisfaction, noncompliance with treatment recommendations, changing physicians, and/or litigation. On the clinician's part, failure to negotiate may be followed by referral elsewhere or by the withholding of goodwill and support that would otherwise be offered" (Lazare et al., 1978, p. 127).

The process of negotiation has been proposed as central to the practitioner-patient relationship—so central that it may embody *all* of the most important components of practitioner-patient communication. Lazare et al. (1978) argued this very point:

> We believe that the most sensitive and sought-after clinicians are the most effective negotiators. They sense the patient's worries, misconceptions about the illness, and hesitations about treatment. They create an atmosphere which encourages patients to present their perspective, on the one hand, and encourages them to hear the clinician's perspective, on the other hand. These clinicians know how to be forceful but they have also learned how to compromise without losing their professional integrity. [Lazare et al., 1978, p. 129]

Lazare and colleagues have argued on the basis of the empirical literature (and sound theoretical development as well) that the practitioners who best manage their relationships with patients—those who are most effective interpersonally—are sensitive to each patient's feelings, are warm and empathic, genuine and self-disclosing, and use their social influence to find solutions that satisfy the patient and fulfill the requirements of the role of professional healer. Interpersonally effective practitioners go beyond the patient's medical diagnosis to consider the patient's emotional reactions to the disease, and his or her needs in relation to it. These practitioners do *not*, however, simply give in to those needs at all costs. They maintain control and professional integrity, ever aware of the technical requirements of the care they deliver.

Indeed, research on patients' evaluations of the care delivered by their physicians suggests that patients evaluate as interpersonally most effective those physicians whom they also rate as technnically most effective (DiMatteo & DiNicola, 1981). One problem in the reconciliation of research findings arises, however, when we consider that in the DiMatteo and DiNicola (1981) research, those physicians who were rated as technically (and interpersonally) most competent by patients were *not* the same physicians who were rated as technically (and interpersonally) most competent by other physicians. In fact, the correlation between supervising physicians' ratings of resident physicians' technical skill and patients' ratings of that skill was only .16. The correlation between supervising physicians' ratings of residents' technical skill and patients' ratings of the residents' interpersonal skill was only .02. The equivocal nature of these data in relationship to the theory and empirical research cited above suggests the need for more methodologically sound, theoretically well conceived research on the evaluation of practitioners' technical and interpersonal care of their patients.

Self-Presentation

The usual practitioner-patient relationship is characterized by the withholding of information. As we noted in Chapter 2, practitioners are habitually very selective about the information they give to their patients, for they fear the latter will not fully understand the information, that communication will require an extensive time commitment, and/or that the patients will exhibit unmanageable reactions. Patients also withhold information from their practitioners. Stimson and Webb (1975) have noted that this is often done in an effort to "manage the impression" (in a symbolic interaction sense) shown to the practitioner in the interactions. By withholding information, patients try to avoid placing themselves in a disadvantaged position with respect to the practitioner.

By means of information control, patients attempt to influence the practitioner. (This attempt at influence is not necessarily a conscious one on the part of the patient.) Open conflict between practitioner and patient is rare. Formality and restraint are typically exercised by both parties in order to prevent an openly hostile encounter. As we will examine in more detail below (when we consider nonverbal communication), practitioners and patients are usually very subtle in their communications of distress or dissatisfaction with the other's behavior, which necessitates a high degree of sensitivity from the other interactant. When the conflict nears the surface, one or both parties is likely to back down or withdraw—the practitioner into detached unconcern and the patient into noncompliance.

The patient's noncompliance is of particular concern to us in this book. As we noted in Chapter 1, practitioners often have a great deal of difficulty recognizing noncompliance among their patients. This is partly the result of each patient's self-presentation. As we saw in Chapter 2, patients whose desires for information are frustrated by their practitioners usually do not press further for answers. Instead, they withdraw into apparent acquiescence. Patients suppress their dissatisfaction with the interpersonal behavior of the practitioner in like manner. This self-presentational strategy is then maintained throughout the interaction, only to give rise to resistance to the regimen after the clinical visit. Thus, regardless of what the practitioner observes, the patient maintains control (beneath the facade of acquiescence) by withholding his or her thoughts, feelings, and beliefs about the interaction (and his or her desires for it), about issues relevant to the diagnosis and treatment, and about his or her intentions to cooperate with the required regimen.

The process of negotiation between practitioner and patient involves expression of their desires for the conduct of the interpersonal interaction between them and for the resultant outcome. We examine in particular detail later in this chapter the behaviors required of the practitioner for effective negotiation with the patient. As noted by Lazare et al. (1978, p.129, quoted above), these include the practitioner's empathy and genuineness in the relationship, his or her sensitivity, expressiveness, and self-disclosure, and the capacity to communicate warmth to the patient while maintaining the necessary level of social power. There we note the relationship between these factors and the broader global issue of trust as a basic element in the practitioner-patient relationship and hence in patient cooperation with treatment.

It is important to remember that negotiation involves content as well as process. One critical aspect of this content consists of the patient's and practitioner's (usually divergent) beliefs about both the disease and the treatment regimen. These beliefs involve such issues as whether or not the disease (or potential disease, in the case of a preventive regimen) is worth the attention it requires—how serious it is, and how likely it is to be visited upon the patient. Patient and practitioner typically also hold (usually divergent) beliefs regarding the efficacy and cost of treatment. The differences in their perceptions are particularly likely to emerge because of patients' and practitioners' differing perspectives on the meaning of symptoms and disease, and their potential danger. Patient and practitioner view the cost versus benefit of the treatment differently, too, because of the differences in what is required of them. The practitioner simply prescibes the regimen while the patient must alter his or her own behavior in order to follow it (Stone, 1979). Therefore, as we consider the process of negotiation in this chapter, we must remain aware that the *content* of the negotiation will depend heavily upon each patient's entire set of beliefs regarding health care and illness. Taking this argument a step further to the origin of the content, we find that the patient's family and social network are also relevant because they determine, at least in part, the patient's contribution to the negotiation. The practitioner-patient negotiation takes place within the context of a social network that consists of friends and family. As we will see in Chapter 5, such social influences are very important to the content of the negotiation between practitioner and patient.

In the following sections of this chapter, we consider important factors in the negotiation between practitioner and patient—particularly the practitioner's interpersonal behavior toward the patient. Before we do this, however, let us examine some general issues (primarily social and historical) as they reflect patients' desires for their practitioners' behavior.

PATIENTS' VIEWS OF MEDICAL PRACTICE

It is curious that dissatisfaction with medicine in America is at its most vociferous just at a time when doctors have at their disposal the most powerful medical

> technology the world has yet seen. The "old fashioned" general practitioner, with few drugs that really worked and not much surgery to recommend, is for some reason looking good to many people—in retrospect, at least. . . . Present-day disenchantment with physicians, at a time when they can do more than ever in history to halt and repair the ravages of serious illness, probably reflects the perception by people that they are not being cared for. . . . The patient wants time, sympathetic attention, and concern for himself as a person. [Eisenberg, 1977, pp. 235, 238]

In today's modern technical medicine, patients report that they feel they are treated like *cases* by their physicians (Skipper & Leonard, 1965). Care is also often fragmented and episodic, and as a result patients are often bewildered and angry (Koos, 1955; Freidson, 1961; Poole & Sanson-Fisher, 1979). Surveys of patients' evaluations of their medical care suggest that the interpersonal aspects of care, as opposed to the technical, are the most important to them and that patients feel they are not receiving the quality of care that they desire (Koos, 1955; Friedson, 1961; Caplan & Sussman, 1966; Reader, Pratt, & Mudd, 1957; Poole & Sanson-Fisher, 1979).

In response to these perceptions, the popular press is sometimes relentless in its punishment of the medical-care system. Popular authors (for example, Lear, 1980; and Ryan & Ryan, 1979) berate practitioners for insensitivities that had a profound personal effect on them. Practitioners are characterized by these authors (and by many in the popular media) as cold, excessively brisk, brusk, inaccessible, and unfeeling. On the whole, the medical system is portrayed in these writings as immensely impersonal. The impact of this popular, emotional writing, while it refers to isolated practitioners and isolated medical care settings, has contributed to branding the entire profession, criticizing its handling of the practitioner-patient relationship, and emphasizing the apparent lack of communication and understanding afforded to patients. The public concurs. (Interestingly, as Brown [1980] has noted, patients characteristically describe *physicians in general* in quite negative terms, while at the same time they rate *their own physicians* positively, and as "exceptions to the rule.")

The goal of medical practice encompasses both the delivery of effective treatment for existing disease and the prevention of future disease (Isselbacher et al., 1980). Billions of dollars are spent every year in the United States on research and training programs designed to find better ways to cure disease and prolong life. In fact, medical care is one of America's largest industries, accounting for approximately 10 percent of the gross national product. Despite its stated commitment and expansive budget, medicine often fails to accomplish its goals because many patients are dissatisfied with the care provided to them. This dissatisfaction may strongly influence the efficacy of medicine.

As we shall examine in further detail in the later pages of this chapter, patients' compliance with medical treatment is often predicated upon their satisfaction with the medical-care encounter. Many patients who have curable or preventable conditions become or remain ill as a result of their dissatisfaction with the interpersonal manner in which they are treated by practitioners. Besides failing to follow their treatment regimens, they often fail to seek medical care in the first place, and/or turn to nonmedical healers (often quacks and charlatans) in the hope of obtaining both a caring attitude and a cure (Cobb, 1954). Patients may recriminate through malpractice litigation (Vaccarino, 1977; Blum, 1957, 1960; Mechanic, 1977), thereby causing their practitioners to become even more detached and inaccessible than before (Thurlow, 1969). Patient commitment to the practitioner is highly influenced by interpersonal factors as well (DiMatteo, Prince, & Taranta, 1979; DiMatteo & Hays, 1980). While patients rarely change physicians because they think they are technically incompetent, they often do so because of what they consider inadequate personal treatment and attention (Gray & Cartwright, 1953; Kasteler et al., 1976). Thus, since medicine's powerful technology is effective only if that technology is used, the interpersonal aspects of medical care that influence its use are critically important to the fulfillment of the promise of medicine.

THE ART OF MEDICINE: A BRIEF HISTORY

During the fourth century B.C., Hippocrates posited a series of critical arguments in support of the importance of the "art of medicine." He defined the art of medicine as the *manner* in which a practitioner provides care to a patient. In the *Corpus Hippocraticum*, Hippocrates described the power of the art of medicine in this way: "The patient, though conscious that his condition is perilous, may recover his health simply through his contentment with the goodness of the physician."

The art of medicine has figured prominently throughout the history of medicine. As we noted earlier, the practitioner's manner of caring for the patient has been posited as the explanation for medicine's success as a healing profession (Shapiro, 1960; Frank, 1977). Prior to the twentieth century, most medical remedies had absolutely no demonstrably therapeutic effects. Often, they were rather dangerous (such as the widely prescribed strychnine and arsenic tonics) (Shapiro, 1960; Houston, 1935). Until the advent of technological medicine, the art of medicine was by far the most critical aspect of the care of the patient.

During the early part of the twentieth century, effective medical treatments began to be developed. Antibiotics became available and their therapeutic effects began to be understood. The developments of many scientific disciplines were applied to the care of patients and medicine became a composite of many academic scientific disciplines. In 1910, the Flexner report to the Carnegie Commission (Flexner, 1910) argued for an end to the purely clinical teaching of the proprietary (privately owned, profit-motivated) medical schools of the day. Flexner deemed mere clinical instruction inadequate. Instead, only university-based, basic science-oriented medical schools were allowed to grant medical degrees. New, stringent licensing laws led to the close of the proprietary schools, giving rise to a model of medical education that was firmly grounded in the basic sciences such as anatomy, physiology, microbiology, pathology, pharmacology, and neurology. These were taught as separate disciplines, and instruction in medicine centered in a definition of disease as negatively altered biology instead of as signs and symptoms present in a human being (Ebert, 1977). Particularly during the 1940s and 1950s, more and more discoveries of the basic sciences were applied to medical practice. The sheer volume of relevant scientific material forced a significant rift between the technological aspects of medicine and the care of the patient. The new technology of medicine was seen as powerful and effective while the art of medicine lost its prominent place and was typically viewed as superfluous, and even as a waste of time.

As medicine's scientific side grew in importance, physician-educators began to recognize the potential seriousness of a growing gap between the science of medicine and its actual practice. Shattuck (1907), for example, warned that the disease is one thing, but the diseased person is quite another. He proposed that the gap between the science of medicine and the care of the patient could be bridged by the art of medicine. Shattuck warned that the scientific aspects of medicine should not replace compassion, cheerfulness, and gentleness. The *care of the patient*, not scientific research, should remain the ultimate goal of medicine. Similarly, in 1904 another prominent medical educator and physician, Sir William Osler, told medical students, "The practice of medicine is an art, not a trade; a calling, not a business; a calling in which your heart will be exercised equally with your head" (Osler, 1904). Despite the emphasis on traditional scientific medicine, however, a few notable medical educators throughout the twentieth century kept alive an interest in the art of medicine and stressed its importance. Among them were Henderson (1935), Engel (1977a, 1977b), and Eichna (1980).

While not a research topic of overwhelming popularity, the practitioner's interpersonal treatment of the patient (the art of medicine) and its antecedents and consequences have received some theoretical and empirical attention, particularly from the perspective of social science and public health. Recent reviews of this literature are available (see DiMatteo & DiNicola, 1982; DiMatteo & Friedman, 1982). Practitioner-patient relationships are by no means simple in character; health-care settings are normally quite anxiety provoking and emotionally trying for both patients and practitioners (Taylor, 1979; DiMatteo & Friedman, 1982, chap. 10). Some important findings are available, however, to guide further research, as are applications in the clinical practice of medicine. We review these findings briefly, synthesizing them in a new and we hope more valuable manner in order to understand the practitioner-patient relationship as it affects patient cooperation with medical treatment.

MUTUALITY AND PRACTITIONER-PATIENT RAPPORT

Practitioners who value the art of medicine speak of the central importance of "rapport" with their patients (Osler, 1904; Engel, 1977a). The *American Heritage Dictionary* defines "rapport" as a relationship of mutual trust, caring, understanding, or emotional affinity. This definition suggests that rapport is not one-sided, and that it may *not* be solely under the practitioner's control.

Mutuality, in the sense in which this word is used in the definition of rapport, implies equity or reciprocity. It suggests that each participant must contribute something to the relationship in which rapport is established. The precise nature of the contribution of practitioner and patient to their relationship varies somewhat according to the theoretical framework in which the practitioner-patient relationship is viewed. Freidson (1970), for example, described the basis of rapport as a mutuality of hope: "The primary characteristic of the situation we find when a patient seeking help interacts with a physician trying to give help is mutual hope. The patient would not be likely to seek help if he did not believe a physician could help him, and the practicing physician would not undertake help if he did not feel he could do something effective" (p. 263). Cassell (1976), on the other hand, viewed rapport as firmly rooted in a mutual sharing of values between physician and patient:

> At the time of the first visit . . . the patient somehow manages to convey to the physician his or her beliefs about the body, life, fate, sickness, and death, probably without ever discussing those topics; and the doctor . . . responds in kind. The first visit often establishes whether or not the doctor and patient share similar values. (If not, the patient rarely returns.) More important, perhaps, the first visit also establishes whether or not the doctor understands the patient. [p. 94]

Parsons (1951), as we have noted earlier, viewed rapport in the practitioner-patient relationship as a mutuality of goals. Practitioner and patient seek to eliminate the illness and restore the patient to a healthy state. Their mutual role definition and validation (practitioner as technically competent, emotionally neutral, selfless healer; patient as compliant occupant of the sick role) brings about rapport. Finally, rapport has been conceptualized as interpersonal warmth, trust, and caring in the practitioner-patient relationship (see DiMatteo & DiNicola, 1982).

Despite the existence of definitions and theoretical orientations that emphasize the reciprocity and mutuality of rapport in the practitioner-patient relationship, little empirical research has addressed this orientation. While some researchers (e.g., Korsch, Gozzi, & Francis, 1968) have examined the mutuality of practitioner and patient expectations as important to the success of their interaction, for the most part the role of the patient in the establishment of rapport has been bypassed. This is especially true of approaches to rapport that focus on mutuality of caring, interpersonal warmth, and trust. Evidence suggests, however, that a focus on such reciprocity and mutuality of caring, trust, and warmth may be important for practitioners as well as for patients. The development of mutually close interpersonal relationships with their patients has been cited by physicians as the most important factor determining their contentment with and personal fulfillment in medical practice (Ort, Ford, & Liske, 1964).

Regardless of the focus of the mutuality (whether of hope, values, roles, or affective behavior), the establishment and maintenance of rapport requires some sustained effort on the part of both practitioner and patient. Unfortunately, however, because of circumstances of their encounter (such as the patient's confusion, discomfort, fear, pain, or anxiety), the responsibility for establishing rapport is likely to fall most squarely upon the shoulders of the practitioner. Thus, nearly all of the existing research on the art of medicine or rapport in the practitioner-patient relationship has focused exclusively on the behavior of the practitioner and the perceptions of the patient. The research we review in the following discussion reflects this bias toward the practitioner's behavior. Nevertheless, we should not forget that both persons determine the character of the "relationship." Thus, the patient's hopes, expectations, values and demonstrations (toward the practitioner) of caring, warmth, trust, and concern must also be caught in the investigator's net if he or she is to claim that their relationship has been studied. Since it is likely (theoretically speaking, at this time) that the practitioner's behavior will be elicited in response to the behaviors of the patient, the *interaction* between them is an important goal for any research that attempts to understand the art of medicine. Such a goal appears particularly important in the light of findings (reviewed later in this chapter; see Hall, Roter, & Rand, 1981) that suggest that patients' requests for information from their physicians are often delivered with negative affect. The influence of patient's negative affect on practitioners' responses is likely to be an important issue for exploration in future research that considers the practitioner-patient relationship as a *reciprocal interaction.*

TRUST

Earlier in this chapter, we considered theories and empirical research that have supported a view of the practitioner-patient relationship as a process of self-presentation and negotiation. Such an approach holds that the patient is motivated to withhold from the practitioner information that may be relevant to his or her care. An openness of communication that facilitates the patient's discussion of his or her problems and feelings, as well as the willingness to be influenced by the practitioner, will depend upon the building and maintenance of trust in the therapeutic relationship (Johnson, 1980; Johnson & Matross, 1975). Trust is often defined as the belief that one can rely on the support and affection of other people. Trust is likely to vary from person to person (since, for some, trust will be easy to attain while for others it will be elusive). Beyond individual differences, trust is a characteristic of a relationship between people. As such, trust can vary as the relationship varies and changes.

Despite the potential importance of trust in helping relationships, Johnson (1980) has noted that very little research has been devoted to the basic features of trust or to the manner in which trust develops. This is surprisingly true, even concerning research on the psychotherapeutic relationship in which we would expect trust to be extremely important as a facilitator of personal disclosure by patient or client. Likewise, trust in the physician-patient relationship has received little empirical attention. Part of the reason for this lies in the enormous complexity of the construct.

Achieving Trust

Johnson and colleagues (Johnson, 1980; Johnson, 1972; Johnson & Johnson, 1975; Johnson & Noonan, 1972) have sought to clarify this construct of trust. They have developed what they called an operational model, and have begun to support each component of it with empirical research (which they have either generated or reviewed). This model specifies the process of building and maintaining trust in a helping relationship: (1) the client takes risks by disclosing problems, feelings, attitudes, beliefs, and behaviors (this usually takes place during the medical interview and history); (2) the helper responds with warmth, accurate understanding, and an expression of cooperative intentions (the first two defined as necessary for therapeutic change [Rogers, 1957]); and (3) the helper reciprocates to some exent the client's self-disclosures by disclosing some information (such as perceptions of and feelings about the client, reactions to what is taking place in the helping encounter, and relevant appropriate personal information) (this is the third factor proposed by Rogers, 1957).

A key element in trust is self-disclosure. In the psychotherapeutic relationship, for example, the client must disclose relevant information about his or her attitudes and concerns in order to receive help from the therapist (Johnson, 1980). Likewise, a medical patient must disclose health beliefs, attitudes, and subjective feelings of normative pressure in order for the physician or other health-care practitioner to assess accurately the forces that support or inhibit health behavior and to decide how most effectively to influence and change these factors in order to achieve cooperation. Such disclosures, of course, render the patient vulnerable to possible rejection, scorn, ridicule, shame or exploitation by the health professional. For example, the patient's understanding of health issues may be minimal and his beliefs about disease and its cure quite crude and characterized by superstition. The patient may be aware of his own ignorance about health matters, and fear exploitation as well. An enormous degree of trust in the practitioner may therefore be required for the patient to disclose these beliefs. Thus (theoretically speaking, at least), trust is likely to be a key component in the enhancement of the initial steps toward compliance in the therapeutic relationship.

In order for trust to be developed, a patient's disclosures must be greeted by the practitioner with acceptance and understanding. Trust is damaged when the client (or patient) feels rejected or feels that the helper uses his power for harm and exploitation (Johnson & Noonan, 1972). Warmth, empathy, and the expression of cooperative intentions (reassurance) instead are necessary in response to patient's disclosures in order for trust to be enhanced. Johnson and Noonan (1972) and Johnson, McCarty, and Allen (1976) have noted that trust does not require a conflict-free relationship. Trust can still be enhanced in relationships in which unresolved conflicts exist between the participants. Thus, the trust that is necessary for continued self-disclosure by the patient can be built even in the midst of the conflict and negotiation that are naturally present in the practitioner-patient relationship.

In regard to the issue of trust, it is important to note that some patients are likely to be unwilling to trust implicitly in either the expertise or the ethical values of practitioners. They may therefore be unwilling to accept the practitioners' authority (Haug, 1978). Patients may try to obtain as much medical information as they possibly can, and to engage in various approaches to self-care. It is highly unlikely, however, that the "competence gap" will ever be closed between the practitioner (particularly physician) and the patient with regard to medical care. (We do not doubt that a patient may know more than the practitioner about one or a few isolated facts regarding the patient's care, particularly if the patient is well read on the topic. For the most part, however, the physician's overall knowledge of the patient's illness and treatment well outweigh that of the patient.) While the patient may reject the practitioner's authority and/or advice, he may not be better off for having done so. We argue that a partnership should be oriented toward effective control of the medical problem as well as toward patient cooperation with treatment. Such a partnership requires trust—particularly that trust which is based on the caring, concern, warmth, and interest expressed by the practitioner. The patient needs to be assured that compliance can be safely granted (Haug, 1978). The establishment of trust can do much to help the practitioner forestall the "revolt" of the patient against his or her authority.

Trust as a Condition for Change

Some theorists and researchers have suggested that trust is central to the practitioner-patient relationship and that as such it is one of the most important factors in *any* approach to helping people change. All psychotherapies and treatments that are oriented to medically relevant behavior change have as their common basis the relationship between practitioner and patient (Gillis, 1974; Frank, 1973, Goldstein, 1971). Central to therapy is the practitioner's achievement and maintenance of power on the basis of his or her expertise. That power is then used to persuade patients that they should adopt new ways of viewing themselves, and new ways of thinking (believing) and behaving. Strupp (1973) and Strong (1968) have proposed that a helper's power base [or influence base] with the helpee is achieved through the latter's perception of the expertness and trustworthiness of the former. The application of this power to the process of persuasion and social influence is examined in Chapter 6. The specific therapeutic techniques that are applied (e.g., insight, reflection of feelings, behavioral reinforcement) are important only insofar as they provide a vehicle for establishing and delivering the healing message. Trust is effective in enhancing the therapeutic relationship, and hence the therapy, because it insures the patient's "expectant faith" (Frank, 1973, 1977). Scientific practitioners covertly "manipulate" the patient's positive expectations (for example, by means of the reputation of the therapeutic technique). With trust in the practitioner, the patient's faith can be maintained, and healing (in this case, behavior change) can be achieved.

The Components of Trust

The question of precisely what constitutes trust (and practitioner behaviors that instill trust) has not yet been adequately answered. The "nonspecific" aspect of the practitioner-patient relationship has been the subject of theory for many years, but trust in the medical-therapeutic relationship remains a topic in need of empirical attention. Some answers are available and may suggest some useful directions for empirical research.

Caterinicchio (1979) endeavored to study the interpersonal circumstances under which patients' trust in the practitioner is developed and maintained.

In his review of the literature on trust, Caterinicchio proposed the existence of at least two theoretical dimensions of trust: (1) the perceptions of gains and losses associated with the choice of an ambiguous path involving a desired outcome contingent upon another's behavior; and (2) the experience of anxiety associated with the probability of the occurrence of an undesired or unpleasant outcome. Caterinicchio found in recursive path analysis that among outpatients, past successful treatment interactions with the physician (successful in terms of positive emotional and physical outcomes) were critical prerequisites to the development of trust in the physician. This research suggested that once the interpersonal trust has been established through past successful treatment sessions, and the physician is considered a reliable source of instrumental and socioemotional care, the perception of trust in the practitioner will be a powerful determinant of the patient's positive assessment of the value of continued or future medical treatment. According to Caterinicchio, patients who report a high degree of trust in their physicians will comply with a regimen even if compliance demands considerable personal cost in terms of time and resources. This is true because past experiences of trusting in the physician have led to positive outcomes. This researcher also found that trust did not require continuity of treatment; that is, while a high degree of treatment continuity may be required for the incremental development of interpersonal trust in one particular practitioner, the mere frequency of primary-care contact was not a necessary condition for trust in practitioners in general to develop. Patients reported a high degre of trust even when they had received medical treatment from many different physicians over a given period. When each of those encounters was successful, clients expressed feelings of trust in the clinic, viewing it as a collection of physicians, all of whom were trustworthy.

In the next section of this chapter where we consider five important factors in the practitioner-patient relationship, we will return to the issues of trust, rapport, warmth, empathy, and interpersonal genuineness, particularly as they affect patient cooperation with medical treatment. Before we do, however, we consider one last definition of trust—a provocative one that may help to clarify some of the issues that color and complicate patients' perceptions of their care and the practitioners who deliver it.

Trust: No Other Choice

Bidwell (1970) has proposed that two factors are likely to influence the level of patients' trust in the therapeutic relationship: (1) the patient's technical familiarity with the professional service (primarily his ability to assess the skillfulness of performance); and (2) the patient's need for professional service (how urgent he perceives the situation is). The less technical knowledge he has and the more compelled he is to obtain the medical-care service, the more absolute his trust must be. Bidwell suggested that under conditions of low knowledge and high urgency, the patient has no choice but to trust in the practitioner. Such an approach to trust as the only option available suggests one possible reason for patients' sometimes ambivalent feelings about their medical practitioners—their simultaneous belief in the goodness and supportiveness of the practitioner, and rebellion against the practitioner's authority and control.

Trust and Cooperation with Treatment

According to social psychologist Morton Deutsch (1962), trust is a central requirement for cooperation between people in any social interaction, just as it is important to the practitioner-patient relationship. Trust is the attitude that one can rely upon the support and the affection of other people and as such it is a requirement for successful and prolonged cooperation with them. As we noted earlier, trust is required for any individual to allow himself or herself to be vulnerable to others. Thus, one view of the relationship between patient trust and compliance posits that control resides within the practitioner, and the patient's submissive trust of him or her facilitates cooperation with the medical prescription.

A different theoretical approach has been proposed by Waterman (1981), who viewed trust as related to self-determination. Easterbrook (1978) has proposed that when important life outcomes are perceived as beyond one's personal control and are determined by the actions of others, apprehension and mistrust are felt. The mistrust is highest when the dependency is involuntary, and when the persons depended upon are not personally known. Waterman (1981) derived from Easterbrook's notions several hypotheses regarding trust. He also presented a unique approach to the concept of trust. Waterman proposed that trust is most likely to emerge in the presence of feelings of competence and confidence, for when an individual has high self-esteem, others are not a threat. Low self-esteem leads to feelings of vulnerability and fear of exploitation. When a person decides voluntarily to participate in a given activity and he or she feels free of constraints (not a pawn of fate), trust is facilitated. According to Waterman, trust is most readily established when the person has been allowed personal input into the selection of the individuals on whom he must depend in a joint effort, or when the person has a sense of personal control over the behaviors that he must enact. Although not tested directly, these hypotheses have potential importance for the practitioner-patient relationship. Waterman's notions about trust suggest that this important component of the practitioner-patient relationship may be best enhanced by the practitioner's emphasis on developing within the patient a sense of competence, self-control, and personal responsibility. Trust, and the means by which it is achieved, are likely, in turn, to enhance patient compliance with treatment.

Many of the issues such as trust and rapport that we have considered so far have been concerned with theoretical aspects of the art of medicine. We turn now to the empirical literature in an effort to summarize the findings to date (organized within five factors) regarding the interpersonal aspects of medical treatment (including trust and rapport in the practitioner-patient relationship). Further, we examine the effects of these factors on patient cooperation with medical regimens.

THE INTERPERSONAL ASPECTS OF TREATMENT: EMPIRICAL FINDINGS

Factor 1: The Practitioner's Affective Communication

The interpersonal behavior of a medical practitioner is typically scrutinized rather closely by his or her patients. Particularly when verbal communications toward the patient are limited and little information is dispensed (as is often true in the setting of medical care), patients attempt to gain information about their care and clues to the assessment of their own and their practitioners' performance by means of affective or emotional cues. For example, patients often focus on their practitioners' distressed expressions (which may be brought about by fatigue or confusion) as evidence for their practitioners' dislike of them, disapproval of their behavior, or grave concern about their threatening medical condition (Friedman, 1979). They rarely try to clarify their perceptions by asking questions. Since patients usually know relatively little about the purely technical aspects of the medical care they receive, they often judge the quality of their care on the basis of their own responses to the affective behavior of their practitioners (Freidson, 1970).

Research supports the theoretical suggestions that patients evaluate the overall performance of their practitioners on the basis of the practitioners' interpersonal, affective behavior (Mechanic, 1968; Ben-Sira, 1976, 1980). (It is important to note here again that there is evidence that technical and interpersonal performance of physicians is highly correlated, not only among the ratings made by patients but also among those made by physicians. Thus, interpersonal and technical performance of physicians may in reality be highly correlated, as one may demand the other for the effective practice of medicine [DiMatteo & DiNicola, 1981].) In fact, patients' evaluations of the affective behavior of their practitioners has been found to have a somewhat stronger relationship to their overall commitment to care from those practitioners than did their evaluations of the technical performance of the practitioners. In a questionnaire survey of over 200 patients, Segall and Burnett (1980) found that patients were more satisfied with physicians who conformed to their ideas of how physicians should behave interpersonally. Physician conformity to patients' expectations for their affective behavior was reported to be considerably more important to patients' overall evaluation of care than was physician conformity to procedural or administrative expectations. Acording to Segall and Burnett (1980), patients' expectations "transcend the desire for instrumental competence, since patients expect social and psychological, as well as physical, relief from their encounters with their physicians" (p. 277). Similarly, DiMatteo, Prince, and Taranta (1979) found that among medical-clinic patients, the intention to return to a particular physician was more dependent upon the patient's perceptions of that physician's affective behavior than upon perceptions of that physician's technical performance. More general surveys have also found that patients place interpersonal factors higher in importance than technical factors in their statements of what they wish to have from their medical care (Koos, 1955; Freidson, 1961; Reader, Pratt, & Mudd, 1957). It is likely, of course, that patients simply expect that all medical practitioners possess an adequate level of technical competence, and as a result they tend to focus more readily on interpersonal variables that they have often found lacking in the health care they have received.

The importance of the practitioner's affective behavior has been noted by Ben-Sira (1976) who argued that the communication of positive affect from physician to patient is essential for the development of a patient's confidence in the physician. This idea is not new. In the fourth century, B.C., Hippocrates suggested the physician must "bear in mind [his] manner of sitting, reserve, arrangement of dress, decisive utterance, brevity of speech, composure, bedside manners, care, replies to objections, calm self-control. . . . His manner must be serious and humane; without stooping to be jocular or failing to be just, he must avoid excessive austerity; he must always be in control of himself" (Hippocrates, *On Decorum*).

Research in counseling has shown that nonverbal cues (such as facial expressions, body movements, and voice-tone expressions of emotion) are extremely important in the communication of empathy, warmth, and caring. They may be even more important than verbal cues in many cases (Haase & Tepper, 1972). This phenomenon holds true in medical settings as well (Friedman, 1979, 1982). The practitioner's nonverbal cues of affect figure prominently for a number of reasons. Patients and practitioners often experience uncertainty in the medical arena. Patients typically know little about what constitutes a serious medical development, or in precisely what manner a procedure is going to affect them physically and emotionally. For example, "a lower G.I. series" is an unusual experience for most patients. They do not know what to expect or how to react to the sensations that accompany the procedure. Consequently, patients will look to the subtle nonverbal cues of their health professionals for some indication of what is going to happen to them. They often need to know whether their own interpretation of the situation is appropriate. Moreover, patients seldom understand the content of the verbal communications between practitioners about their illnesses. They attempt to infer meaning from the emotional context of the medical jargon which is used by the health professionals who are overheard discussing the patient's medical case. Dependence on the emotional context of the message is also likely when the patient fails to decipher the technical language with which practitioners typically provide explanations to their patients. Hence, patients look to the nonverbal cues of their health professionals in order to deduce information about their conditions. The facial expressions of the physician who discloses to a patient his diagnosis of multiple myeloma may have a greater impact on the patient's perception of his prognosis than would any verbal description of the likely course of the disease. In addition, patients look to the nonverbal cues of their health professionals for indications of acceptance and caring. Although the health professional's primary interest or focus during the interaction is upon content such as information relevant to a diagnosis, the patient's priorities tend to fall more along the affective dimension. Patients desire indications of positive interpersonal reactions from their practitioners and they look to the practitioners' nonverbal expressions for those reactions. Thus, they may depend to an inordinate extent upon nonverbal cues for information about how much their health professionals care about them.

In the following discussion, we consider a number of aspects of nonverbal communication between health professionals and patients, and the theory and research that support their importance. We also suggest some implications for patient care. We point to ways in which health professionals might utilize their own nonverbal communications to enhance their development of rapport with patients, and through the enhancement of trust bolster their positions as agents of social influence toward the goal of patient compliance.

Touch. One extremely important component of nonverbal communication as it affects the establishment of rapport with patients is touch. Tactile stimulation can be extremely soothing to ill patients as well as to human beings in general, and it can serve to communicate reassurance, comfort, value, and caring. Social scientists have found that touch may serve a tension-reducing function and that it is central to healthy social development (Montagu, 1978). Touch often enhances the therapeutic abilities of the health professional (Blondis & Jackson, 1977).

The effects of touch are likely to depend upon both the emotional context in which the touching takes place and the interpersonal meaning attached to it. A gentle touch of the patient's head may be perceived by the patient as a reflection of the health practitioner's caring, understanding, and concern. This touch might just as easily signify the practitioner's control, however, because touch denotes power (Henley, 1977). Health professionals regularly touch patients, but patients rarely purposely touch their health professionals. Thus, the practitioner's touch on the patient's head might be interpreted as condescending and as representing the health professional's power and complete access to the patient's body.

The potential for a negative effect of touching is illustrated in a study by Larsen and Smith (1981). These researchers videotaped 34 first-time physician-patient visits (the interview/conversation portion only) at a family-practice center. These videotapes were scored by trained judges according to the specific nonverbal behaviors exhibited by the physicians. After the visit, patients completed a questionnaire that was designed to evaluate their satisfaction with the visit and their understanding of the information given to them by their physicians. Among other findings, it was determined that the more the physicians touched their patients during the conversation, the less satisfied those patients were with the doctor and with the visit. The authors suggested that touching may have been interpreted by patients as aggressive, since this was their first visit with the physician. More touching was also associated with less understanding on the part of the patient—a finding that suggests that the physician's touch during conversation may have been distracting to patients. As we will examine in more detail below, the meaning of the nonverbal cue may be clarified by a comforting verbal communication (e.g., "You'll be better soon. Try to bear with the pain a little longer"). In this way, the comforting intent of the touch may be understood.

Gaze. Gaze is another significant nonverbal cue which researchers have found to be extremely powerful (see Ellsworth, 1975). People are usually aware of being stared at, and staring is likely to evoke a noticeable response. Eye contact, for example, intensifies the emotion (positive or negative) in a particular situation. A pleasant situation (such as a counselor or health professional communicating positive feedback and exhibiting warmth and understanding) may be experienced as even more positive in the presence of eye contact (La Crosse, 1975). An arousing, upsetting, or threatening situation, on the other hand, may become even more negative when accompanied by eye contact (Ellsworth, Friedman, Perlick, & Hoyt, 1978). Thus, eye contact may be used judiciously by a sympathetic, encouraging, supportive health professional to enhance rapport and trust in the therapeutic relationship. Failure to maintain eye contact, on the other hand, might arouse feelings of suspicion in the patient, or suggest the practitioner's interpersonal deviance or secretiveness.

Friedman (1979) has pointed out that excessive staring at a patient will most likely have a negative interpersonal effect. Indeed, Larsen and Smith (1981), in the videotape study of first-time family-practice clinic visits described above, found that greater use of "observation" (which consisted of the physician looking directly at the face of the patient) was associated with lower patient satisfaction. It is possible (following Ellsworth et al., 1978) that the anxiety felt by patients during their visit with the physician was intensified by the physician's (possibly excessive) eye contact to produce an overall negative evaluation of the physician.

Finally, eye contact might be maintained in an effort to avoid staring at a patient's physical deformity (a common reaction under such interpersonal stress; Kleck, 1968). This is particularly true because patients usually expect that health professionals will visually assess their physical problems without apparent distress or disgust (Blondis & Jackson, 1977). Overt discomfort, expressed through the practitioner's inappropriate use of gaze, is likely to affect practitioner-patient rapport, although precisely how the effects of gaze will be manifested under various circumstances is open to empirical research. As we have seen, however, preliminary evidence suggests that gaze is likely to be a very powerful nonverbal cue in the medical-care setting.

Facial Expressions and Voice Tone. Psychologists who have studied nonverbal communication have found that much detailed information about emotional states can be determined from facial expressions (Izard, 1977). It is usually easy to determine from a person's facial expression his or her fatigue, confusion, or distress. Facial expressions are important in the communication of pain and related negative emotions such as fear, sadness, distress, disgust, and anger. A health professional's feelings and reactions to a patient can be readily communicated through facial expressions (Friedman, 1979, 1982).

Voice tone can likewise communicate emotion. Variations in pitch, loudness, emphasis, and the temporal spacing of words are independent of the verbal content of the message and can convey, usually quite clearly, such emotions as anger, sadness, and happiness. Health practitioners' anger can be perceived in their tone of voice as well, and may have a significant effect on patients. For example, in a study by Milmoe, Rosenthal, Blane, Chafetz, and Wolf (1967), the amount of anger judged to be present in a doctor's voice when he was talking about alcoholics was correlated significantly with the resistance demonstrated by his alcoholic patients to enrolling in a detoxification treatment program.

Research on the nonverbal expressiveness of medical practitioners has examined both facial expressions and voice-tone cues in relation to the practitioner-patient interaction. DiMatteo, Taranta, Friedman, and Prince (1980) reported two studies that directly measured the nonverbal expressiveness of medical house officers and examined the relationship of this communication ability to the satisfaction with care expressed by their patients. With audiotapes and films, the expressions of 47 medical house officers were recorded as they attempted to express three different verbally neutral sentences in four different emotions or affects: happiness, sadness, anger, and surprise. The films were then displayed to college-student judges who guessed which emotion was being communicated. The degree of accuracy of the college-student judges at labeling the emotions served as a measure of the physician's ability to communicate messages of affect through facial expressions and voice tone. Patients' ratings of satisfaction with the interpersonal behavior of these physicians were also collected. Patient satisfaction was found to be positively and significantly correlated with the physicians' skills at sending (or deliberately expressing) specific emotions.

Body Postures and Movements. Finally, the enactment of certain bodily cues and gestures can cause a person to be perceived as either warm or cold, empathic or nonempathic. Certain affiliative nonverbal behaviors on the part of the practitioner such as smiles, head nods, gestures with the hands, and a 20-degree foward lean, for example, have been found to increase perceptions by clients of their counselor's attractiveness and warmth (LaCrosse, 1975). Closed arm positions seem to indicate coldness, rejection, and inaccessibility, while moderately open arm positions tend to indicate warmth and acceptance (Spiegel & Machotka, 1974; Smith-Hanen, 1977). In the study of physician-patient interactions in a family-practice center, higher patient satisfaction was associated with physicians' forward lean and bodily orientation toward the patient (Larsen & Smith, 1981). Backward lean and "neck relaxation" with chin elevated (possibly implying the communication of superiority) were correlated with patient dissatisfaction.

Nonverbal Cues in Context. Nonverbal cues are, of course, only meaningful and interpretable within a situational context. This context may be the particular environment of the individual interaction and/or the verbal context of the communication. Nonverbal behaviors can be observed against the backdrop of the environmental context or they can interact with the environment—particularly the verbal communication that occurs.

When used alone, nonverbal cues can serve a regulating function. For example, by nodding or by breaking eye contact, an individual may signal that he is yielding the turn to speak to another person (Duncan, 1972). Nonverbal communication is also used to inform others of whether or not their messages are being received. Eye contact, facial expressions, and head movements can provide feedback that the listener is attending to the speaker. Nodding may indicate understanding. Nonverbal communication might also function as a substitute for verbal behavior. The nonverbal message might actually replace the verbal one. For example, a physician might frown at a patient who talks at length during the physical examination, which disturbs the physician's concentration and makes it difficult for the physician to ask questions. The negative facial expression may indicate to the patient that his behavior is inappropriate. The nonverbal communication of the physician serves as a substitute for a verbal admonishment.

Nonverbal cues also interact with verbal ones. First, a nonverbal message may serve to accent a verbal statement that has already been made. For example, a health professional might nod his head while saying, "You really are doing well taking your medication. Your blood pressure is nearly under control." Nonverbal messages may complement verbal messages and add to them. For example, the physician might touch the patient's hand and say, "I think I understand how you feel." The nonverbal communication enhances the verbal and vice versa. Voice tone, for example, may be used to emphasize a particular point made to a patient about his treatment regimen. Finally, nonverbal cues can contradict verbal cues (or can at least *appear* to contradict them). If inconsistent verbal and nonverbal messages are conveyed to the patient, the likely result will be the patient's doubt concerning what is conveyed, or the patient's diminished trust in the practitioner (Friedman, 1979a, 1982).

It is therefore critically important to understand the role of verbal-nonverbal cue combinations. They are likely to affect many aspects of the practitioner-patient relationship. Research on these cue combinations suggests that together they convey a special message, different from the message conveyed by either cue alone. For example, Friedman (1979b) combined affective cues from photographs of the facial expressions of "teachers" with written scripts of statements purportedly "spoken" by those teachers in the photographs. Positive facial expressions that were combined with negative verbal cues (statements) were perceived by high-school-student judges as "sarcasm." Negative facial expressions combined with positive statements were seen as insincere and dominant. Consistent combinations were, in general, judged as more sincere and easier to understand. Consistent combinations were more likely to produce consistent ratings by the observers. Woolfolk (1978) studied actual voice tone, words, and facial pleasantness communicated by teachers and found a similar effect of combining positive verbal with negative nonverbal cues. This combination was seen as assertive, businesslike, serious, and most effective for high performance among sixth-grade students. These studies demonstrate that in settings in which interpersonal influence is a primary goal (as it is in the practitioner-patient relationship when the goal is compliance), the nature of verbal/nonverbal cue combinations is likely to influence the message received.

In the only study presently available on the role of verbal/nonverbal cue combinations in physician-patient interaction, Hall, Roter, and Rand (1981) analyzed 50 tape-recorded physician-patient interactions that occurred during routine visits for chronic disease. The tape-recorded interactions were rated by judges on anger, anxiety, dominance, sympathy, assertiveness, and businesslike manner. The judgments were made of electronically content-filtered speech (voice tone), original speech (voice and words), and transcripts (words only). Patient contentment with the medical visit, and patient return for appointments (compliance) were correlated with the ratings of the communication in the physician-patient interaction. The results showed that patient contentment and compliance were associated with the simultaneous combination of *positive verbal* and *negative nonverbal* communication from the physician. Such communications were judged as businesslike and serious—appropriate for the role of the physician. This finding is similar to that of the research on physician-patient interactions by Davis (1968) which examined patterns of communication and their relationship to compliance. Patient noncompliance was found to occur when the physician was permissive with an active patient, and when the physician was verbally antagonistic. Similarly, Davis and Eichhorn (1963) found that a businesslike orientation (in which the physician was kind, but firm and serious) was most effective in bringing about patient compliance.

As Hall, Roter, and Rand (1981) noted: "Interaction takes place in more than one communication channel, and it appears that the constellation of effective physician attributes such as sincerity, concern, task orientation, and perhaps assertiveness may best be transmitted through the combination of positive words and negative voice tone" (p. 28). This issue requires much further study before clinical applications and interventions can be proposed. It is likely that the next decade of research on the practitioner-patient relationship will use the newly developed technology and will explore the role of verbal and nonverbal cues, as well as their interaction, in the determination of patient satisfaction and compliance with medical treatment.

Factor 2: The Practitioner's Sensitivity

In the course of medical treatment, patients experience a wide range of emotions—from security and relief to profound fear and rage. As a result, a critical factor in the practitioner-patient relationship is likely to be the practitioner's sensitivity to patients' emotions. The value of this sensitivity will be predicated, of course, upon the practitioner's willingness to accept and to deal effectively with the emotions that patients communicate.

Verbal Communication. From the viewpoint of the practitioner, a major goal of the practitioner-patient interaction is to obtain specific medically related information. While this information is usually sought throughout the entire medical encounter (for example, during the examination the practitioner asks, "Does it hurt here?"), it is sought perhaps most intensively during the interview/medical-history portion of the visit. Questions asked by practitioners typically require simple responses, usually of the multiple-choice kind ("yes" or "no") (Bernstein & Bernstein, 1980). Similarly, practitioners tend to focus on specific events and tangible data such as the location and timing of symptoms. They are usually unconcerned with details, impatient with elaborations, and insensitive to emotions. Yet, sometimes these very pieces of information may be the most useful ones the practitioner receives (DeGowin & DeGowin, 1976).

Medical educator, Sir George Pickering (1978) noted that "Hearing the patient's message is the *sine qua non* of a great physician. . . . I become daily convinced that the chief cause of bad medicine . . . is the failure of young doctors to understand what the patient is trying to tell him" (pp. 554-555). Sir William Osler (1899) also emphasized that the physician should listen to his patient because the patient will reveal many clues to the diagnosis. Listening is likely to enhance the technical aspects of medical care. It is one issue that brings together the art and the science of medicine. Patients usually know quite a bit about their medical condition, and with some help from the practitioner in articulating that information, can provide many important clues concerning their state of health. Listening fully to all the patient has to say and only then attempting to consolidate the information may help to prevent the all too common problem among practitioners of formulating a theory about the diagnosis and then fitting the data to support that theory (Elstein, 1976). This can result in an inaccurate diagnosis. Thus, listening can enhance the technical aspects of medical care.

Listening to the patient is also important to the art of medicine because listening can enhance the practitioner's understanding of how disease affects the patient as a person. Listening communicates respect to the patient and indicates the practitioner's willingness to share power and control in the interview (Stone, 1979). Empirical research suggests that it is extremely important to attend to the patient's own version of his history as well as to his expression of emotion. Baekeland and Lundwall (1975), for example, reviewed many studies that not surprisingly suggest that patients' willingness to continue in psychotherapy treatment is related to the opportunity they have to express themselves in the therapeutic relationship. The findings are equally striking in the research on medical practitioners. Linn and Wilson (1980) developed an instrument to measure a physician's ability to facilitate and clarify patients' communications and to be responsive to patients' thoughts and feelings. This instrument, the Facilitating Response Inventory (FRI), was administered to 71 residents in internal medicine and proved very reliable. Among internal-medicine residents whose specialty was primary care, the FRI was found to predict positively the physicians' appointment-keeping rate in the general medical clinic. In this research, then, patients were more highly committed to physicians who were willing and able to facilitate patients' verbal communications. Interestingly, the FRI also correlated positively with the ratings of the residents' clinical competence (ratings made by their attending physicians in the residency program). Thus, physicians' open-ended, nonauthoritarian responsiveness played an important role in their technical care of patients as well. Physicians' acceptance of patients' communications has also been found to be related to patient satisfaction with care (as determined from analyses of tape-recorded interactions between physicians and patients (Stiles et al., 1979). Patients in this research were more satisfied with the care they received when they were allowed to tell their story in their own words at the opening of the medical interview.

Words carry tremendous weight in the health-care arena, for they usually symbolize issues that are of central concern to patient and practitioner. Issues of life and death, of health and illness can be very complex. The words used by patients in health-care interactions normally reflect their understanding of these issues, and the meaning each issue holds for them. Therefore, it can be very important for health practitioners to facilitate patients' expression of their feelings through verbal communication. There exist methods for the verbal facilitation of patients' expressions, and these methods are stressed in the training of counselors and psychotherapists. Such skills represent an important component of the training of psychotherapists, and are delineated in detail in Ivey's (1977) work on "microcounseling" skills, and in Brammer's (1979) overview of counseling methods, as elsewhere. Our purpose here is not to review those skills, since complete descriptions of them may be readily obtained. While their successful application to medical training and practice as yet requires careful empirical documentation, it is likely that verbal facilitation methods used in psychotherapy will find important application in medical practice as well.

Nonverbal Communication. Raymond Birdwhistell (1970), noted anthropologist and expert on nonverbal communication has noted that a human being should not be viewed as a "black box" that emits something called "communication"—the content of which is informative but colorless. In fact, the manner or process by which a person expresses ideas and communicates information is critically important to an understanding of that person and his or her message. Communication has a *nonverbal* component that appears in everything that people do and say. Nonverbal communication is especially important in the therapeutic relationship, as Sigmund Freud (1912) noted in the early part of this century.

The art of medicine and practitioner-patient rapport demand the practitioner's ability to receive, interpret, and accept patients' *nonverbal* communications. These nonverbal communications appear in all forms other than the written or spoken word. They involve facial expressions, body movements, body postures, voice tone (e.g., frequency and pacing of speech), extralinguistic cues (e.g., groans, grunts), touch, and the distance between persons in the interaction. For many reasons, the practitioner's ability to "decode" these messages from patients may be critically important to the practitioner-patient relationship.

Rapport and the Art of Medicine

In the health-care setting, patients typically experience a number of emotions that may be more easily recognized by attending to their nonverbal cues than to what they say. Since patients have little experience hiding or controlling emotions (such as fear and pain) in the medical setting, these emotions are often readily apparent in their nonverbal behaviors. A health professional who is sensitive to patients' nonverbal communications will be provided with important insight into the patient's feelings and will be afforded a valuable opportunity to understand the patient. It is important, too, to note that many patients are hesitant to express their feelings regarding certain matters (for example, embarrassing disabilities, their discomfort in the medical setting, or dissatisfaction with treatment). In attending to the patient's facial expressions, body postures and movements, voice tone, and other nonverbal cues, the health professional may be alerted to the possibility that something is wrong, or that a particular issue should be further explored.

The art of medicine involves understanding the patient's nonverbal communication in the medical interaction. Nonverbal cues are subtle and they add information to verbal messages (such as how the patient feels about what he has said). They may also provide independent messages, and express feelings that are not subject to the communicator's conscious control. This is especially true of body movement and posture cues, in which feelings are more likely to become apparent than in any other channel (Ekman & Friesen, 1969, 1974). By recognizing cues of dissatisfaction and negative affect in the body language of patients, the practitioner can, for example, become aware of the patient's distress, and deal with it before the patient terminates the relationship, attenuates treatment effects by noncompliance, or retaliates with malpractice litigation. By accurately reading the nonverbal cues of the patient that accompany his or her verbal expression of understanding of a treatment regimen, the practitioner may be able to identify signs of confusion or discomfort that indicate the patient's lack of understanding or possible unwillingness to follow the prescription.

Recent studies by Rosenthal, Hall, DiMatteo, Rogers, and Archer (1979) have produced evidence supporting these suggestions in one kind of therapeutic relationship. These investigations measured nonverbal sensitivity with the PONS test. The PONS is a 45-minute, 16 mm film test with 220 items. It yields quantitative measures of the test taker's sensitivity to various channels of nonverbal communication by measuring the number of situational-emotional communications of a woman in the film that the test taker can describe accurately. This test measures the respondent's abilities to decode accurately the nonverbal communication of affect in another person's facial expressions, body movements and postures, and voice tone. The studies involved counselors and psychotherapists and persons in training for those professions. Within each of six samples, there was a tendency for individuals rated high (by their supervisors) in therapeutic skills and effectiveness to be more sensitive to nonverbal information, particularly body movement and postural cues to emotion.

Nonverbal sensitivity has been linked significantly to patient satisfaction with care from the physician. DiMatteo, Friedman, and Taranta (1980), for example, reported two studies involving 64 medical house officers and hundreds of patients at an urban community teaching hospital. The nonverbal sensitivity of the physicians was measured with the PONS. An average of six of each house officer's patients were interviewed about their satisfaction with the physician's interpersonal treatment of them. In both studies, ratings of the physicians by their patients were significantly correlated with the physicians' PONS-measured accuracy at decoding emotion expressed through body posture and movement. This was not surprising, since, as noted earlier, studies by Ekman and Friesen (1969, 1974) have implicated the body channel as the one from which unintended cues to emotion are most likely to leak. These studies, therefore, provide some important evidence that a practitioner's ability to decode nonverbal cues may be an important factor in his or her ability to provide the understanding required for the effective care of patients.

By understanding the patient's nonverbal cues alone or as they accompany verbal cues, the practitioner may enhance his or her ability to identify important signs of confusion and discontent in patients (Friedman, 1979a). As an example, consider the physician's characteristic inquiry of the patient: "Do you have any questions?" Usually, the physician leaves the patient's presence promptly after hearing the patient's unconvincing "I don't think so." Yet many times patients provide clues to their confusion or distress with their nonverbal behavior, especially their body movements and postures. They may appear to sit down tensely, cast their gaze downward shyly, and/or wring their hands nervously. Practitioners who are sensitive to these cues are likely to wait, and to probe the issue a bit further. The manner in which this brief, exiting question is dealt with by the practitioner—whether the patient's distress and confusion are recognized or ignored—can mean the difference between the patient's understanding and implementation of the medical regimen and his or her misunderstanding or resistance to it.

It is important to mention that this component of the art of medicine—sensitivity to and understanding of patients' expressions of emotion (on both verbal and nonverbal dimensions)—closely resembles one of the necessary conditions for therapeutic change defined by Carl Rogers (1957). That condition is *empathy*, and it involves the capacity of the practitioner to understand (and perhaps even to feel) the patient's experiences, needs, sorrows, joys, anxieties, and hurts as if they were his own. Truax and Carkhuff (1967) have suggested that nonverbal decoding skills (and encoding skills which we examined earlier) comprise part of a general ability to relate empathically to people in a therapeutic relationship. The empirical research to date suggests that the art of medicine, and rapport in the practitioner-patient relationship, depend partly upon the practitioner's ability to understand the patient's nonverbal cues of affect, and to communicate that understanding by means of his or her nonverbal expressiveness.

Factor 3: Practitioner Warmth and Friendliness

Some of the earliest descriptions of the art of medicine, as they appear in the writings of such prominent early physicians as Hippocrates (1932 translation), Sir William Osler (1899), and Frederick Shattuck (1907), stress that the practitioner's warmth and friendliness toward the patient are central to the therapeutic encounter. Theoretical writings in medicine and psychotherapy have focused on warmth, friendliness, politeness, and positive regard (or favorable disposition toward the patient) as embodying the essence of the practitioner's role. It has been argued that in order to facilitate interaction with the patient, the practitioner must exude these qualities—the expression of which will bring about the patient's feelings of acceptance, positive self-value, and security in being cared for. Such characteristics help the patient feel "at home," whether in the practitioner's office or in the hallways of the hospital (Mayerson, 1976).

Warmth, friendliness, positive regard, acceptance, and politeness are very similar in character. In fact, in the *American Heritage Dictionary* most of them are used reciprocally to define one another. Indeed, Carl Rogers (1957) used these characteristics interchangeably to describe a general factor that he has referred to as "unconditional warmth and positive regard." This factor was proposed as one among three necessary and sufficient conditions for positive therapeutic change. Social-psychological research has demonstrated that people tend to infer a host of personality characteristics to accompany their perception of a person's warmth (Asch, 1946). An individual perceived as warm is also described as generous, happy, good-natured, humorous, and sociable. These inferences may derive directly from experiences in a world in which we encounter people whom we view as warm. We find that many related characteristics tend to accompany that warmth. In addition, our implicit assumptions about the characteristics of others who are warm probably derive partly from how the behavior of those who are "warm" affects us (Harvey & Smith, 1977).

Aside from the research on nonverbal communication cited above (particularly that of Smith-Hanen, 1977; Spiegel & Machotka, 1974; and Haase & Tepper, 1972), virtually no operational definitions of this construct have been developed to understand its operation in the medical setting. In fact, the research on this component has encouraged a tautology. Warmth is believed to bring about positive effects for patients—their feelings of being cared for, supported, respected, and befriended. Yet, the presence of warmth is most often determined by patients' perceptions of feeling cared for, supported, respected, and befriended. As we review the literature on the effects of this interpersonal factor on patient outcome variables (particularly cooperation with medical recommendations), it is very important to keep in mind that the research has been based primarily on the patients' perceptions, and that this issue is still in need of a good deal of theoretical and empirical work.

A number of studies have examined patients' perceptions of warmth, caring, acceptance, positive regard, and friendliness of their practitioners. For example, patients' perceptions of their practitioners' conduct have been found to be the most important predictors of patient satisfaction with medical treatment (Doyle & Ware, 1977; Aday & Anderson, 1975). In another study, mothers revealed that what they liked best about nurses was not the information and advice they provided, but rather their friendliness, interest, and understanding (Conant, 1969).

Patients' perceptions of the warmth, friendliness, and politeness of their practitioners have also been found to correlate with patient compliance. Alpert (1964) for example, found that patients were more likely to fail to keep their appointment in an outpatient clinic if they felt there was no physician there who cared about them with whom they could talk openly and personally. Nelson, Gold, Hutchinson, and Benezra (1975) found a positive relationship between schizophrenic patients' compliance with treatment and their perceptions that their physicians were interested in them. Similarly, Hurtado, Greenlick, and Columbo (1973) found in research on patients in a prepaid multispecialty group practice that appointment keeping was related to their positive appraisal of the interpersonal aspects of treatment. Studies of "doctor shopping" have found that patients are likely to change physicians if they feel their physicians do not care about them as people and show them no warmth and positive feeling (Kasteler, Kane, Olsen, & Thetford, 1976; Gray & Cartwright, 1953). Patient commitment to the therapeutic relationship with his or her physician in a family-practice center has been found to be highly related to the patient's perception that he or she was cared about by the physician. Many other studies have reported positive correlations of patients' satisfaction with the friendliness, warmth, and caring of their practitioners with patient compliance to treatment (Becker, Drachman, & Kirscht, 1972; Kincey, Bradshaw, & Levy, 1975; Caplan & Sussman, 1966). Finally, in one study of outcome, patients' perceptions of their physicians' warmth were positively related to improvement in drug treatment (Rickels et al., 1971).

The precise behavioral definitions of practitioner warmth, friendliness, and positive regard require further examination, although a few studies have attempted to operationalize them and to assess the outcome variables that result. The existing research using this approach has been carried out primarily by Barbara Korsch and colleagues (Korsch, Gozzi, & Francis, 1968;

Francis, Korsch, & Morris, 1969; Freemon, Negrete, Davis, & Korsch, 1971). These researchers investigated various aspects of physician-patient verbal communication in a pediatric clinic and emergency-room setting. Conversations between mothers and pediatricians (800 in all) were tape-recorded and coded according to the specific behaviors exhibited. Patients' case records were reviewed, and the mothers in the study were interviewed immediately after the visit with the doctor as well as a week or two later at their homes. Composite ratings of mothers' compliance and satisfaction were derived from the case records and the interviews. Physician behavior was then compared to compliance and satisfaction of the mothers. Mothers were significantly more satisfied with the visit when the pediatrician was judged by independent raters of the tape recordings to be friendly and concerned. Patient satisfaction with the interpersonal treatment they received was a moderately good predictor of compliance. Perhaps most importantly, mothers' perceptions of the physicians' friendly behavior correlated positively and significantly with their compliance with the treatment, as did the *objective* measures (ratings) of physicians' behavior. The greater the friendliness and solidarity expressed by the physician to the mother during the interaction, the more likely was the mother to be highly compliant in following the recommendations for the child's care. Similar research has been reported by Davis (1971) in which he found patients' noncompliance to be significantly correlated with physicians' high degree of disagreement with the patient during the medical visit, as well as their formal behavior, which conveyed rejection of the patient. Relatedly, physicians' expressions of angry or hostile feelings toward patients were predictive of patients' avoidance of follow-up interviews and their refusal to enter long-term treatment (Salzman, Shader, Scott, & Binstock, 1970; Milmoe et al., 1967). Likewise, in the field of psychotherapy a few studies have shown that the practitioner's warmth (or lack of it) may affect patients' compliance. Therapists who expressed derogatory feelings about clients and who were uninterested in clients' problems were more likely to have their clients drop out of treatment (Baekeland & Lundwall, 1975).

Factor 4: Reassurance and Positive Expectations

Pictures, sketches, and descriptions often appear of the old-time family physician who attends patients in their homes. He is portrayed as supportive and fatherly, worthy of enormous trust. He reassures patients and their families. He quells their anxiety. In Eric Cassell's book, *The Healer's Art* (1976), the supportive role of the physician is illustrated. Cassell begins his discussion of the physician-patient relationship with a description of an incident he experienced as a resident in training at Bellevue Hospital in New York City:

> I had a midnight call from the psychiatric ward: an old woman was having difficulty breathing. I found the patient gasping for air, her skin blue from lack of oxygen; she had full-blown pulmonary edema (water in the lungs) resulting from a blood clot in her lung. I sent the nurse for the urgently needed oxygen and drugs, but in those days, because of staff shortages and inexorably slow or inoperative elevators, a critically ill patient on a psychiatric ward in Bellevue at midnight might just as well have been in the East River: the wait for the necessary equipment would be interminable. I stood at the bedside feeling impotent, but the old woman's face and her distress pleaded for help. So I began to talk calmly but incessantly, telling her why she had the tightness in her chest and explaining how the water would slowly recede from her lungs, after which her breathing would begin to ease bit by bit and she would gradually feel much better. To my utter amazement that is precisely what happened. Not only did her fear subside (which would not have surprised me) but the noises in her chest disappeared under my stethoscope, giving objective evidence that the pulmonary edema was, in fact, subsiding. By the time the equipment came, things were already under control and the patient and I felt as though together we had licked the devil.
>
> I was, of course, immensely relieved and pleased, but I didn't know what to make of it. Now, twenty years later, I understand much better what had taken place in the middle of that night. I had felt helpless because none of the things I identified with a doctor's job of curing the sick were available; I had none of the technology which, to me, was essential to being a good doctor. What I didn't know then was that desperation and fear had led me unknowingly to function as a healer, a role traditionally played by physicians as far back as Hippocrates. [Cassel, 1976, pp. 13–14]

Recently, researchers have begun to document empirically the profound effect of psychological factors on physical states (Pelletier, 1977, 1979). Anxiety, fear, and distress can affect health and well-being, and can significantly influence patients' responses to illness and pain. Psychological factors can mediate the outcomes of medical treatment such as surgery (Janis, 1958; Langer, Janis, & Wolfer, 1975). In recent years, too, there has been an important recognition that social factors in the practitioner-patient relationship and aspects of the therapeutic interaction can affect patients' psychological, and hence their physical, states (DiMatteo & Friedman, 1982; Friedman & DiMatteo, 1979). Consider, for example, the study by Jarvinen (1955) in which he found a significant increase in the sudden deaths of coronary patients during or shortly after ward rounds conducted by the medical staff. Ward rounds are typically rather formal procedures during which physicians "display" their patients, describing and discussing them in medical terms and generally ignoring them as people. Patients often report feeling anxious, depersonalized, and even dehumanized. This study demonstrated that such distressing interpersonal treatment may actually jeopardize the patient's health. Jarvinen found that ward rounds increased patients' fear and anxiety to dangerously high levels, thus significantly increasing the risk (and the incidence, as documented by the researchers) of another heart attack. This phenomenon was examined further by Lynch and colleagues (1974), who found that human contact in frightening, upsetting, or negative emotional situations has major effects on the cardiac rhythms and electrical impulses of the hearts of cardiac patients. This research suggests that upsetting circumstances in the physician-patient relationship, as well as distress and anxiety brought about by impersonal treatment may have a potentially detrimental effect on the patient. This research emphasizes the importance of reassurance and "bedside manner" in the care of patients, for the sake of their physical condition.

Reassurance "consists of a general optimistic and hopeful attitude and specific statements based on data and/or experience designed to allay exaggerated or unfounded fears of the patient. For reassurance to be effective, the physician should know the sources of the patient's fears. They often are based on an incorrect understanding of the disease or proposed procedure" (Leigh & Reiser, 1980, p. 294).

Although not studied directly, the hypothesis that reassurance can influence patient compliance is supported by indirect evidence and is therefore tenable. The physician can positively affect the outcome of such technical procedures as surgery by providing reassurance to the patient (Egbert et al., 1963, 1964). This reassurance, particularly if it leads the patient to greater treatment success, may also reduce the patient's fears regarding the treatment, and hence enhance not only the outcome but also the patient's trust in the physician. We noted earlier that trust is likely to enhance patient compliance. Trust can also serve to insure that patients' reports of information are reliable (Ben-Sira, 1976, 1980), thus optimizing the practitioner's choice and presentation of recommended treatment options.

Perhaps the best-known phenomenon relating physiological and psychological variables in medicine is called the "placebo effect." Beecher (1955) has defined the placebo as an inert substance that may have both physiological and psychological effects on the patient. Of course, these effects can be positive or negative. That is, the practitioner's expectation for both the good and bad sequelae of a treatment can be effectively transmitted to the patient, and can influence his or her reactions. (On the average, an outcome is 35% more positive [or negative] in a placebo control group than in a no-treatment control group, as reported in reviews by Beecher [1959] and Shapiro [1960].) The placebo effect results partly from the character of the practitioner-patient relationship. The practitioner who imparts confidence and who is supportive and reassuring to the patient is likely to bring about the positive therapeutic effect of the substance administered, thus enhancing the patient's belief in its efficacy. It is particularly important to note that practitioners have the interpersonal power to reduce or completely eliminate such problems as patients' negative side effects, which may reduce their compliance directly or indirectly by supporting their belief that following the regimen is too costly. We will see in later chapters that expectations may have important effects on patient compliance. The practitioner's faith in a regimen is likely to translate into positive outcomes for the patient, and hence his or her belief in the efficacy and benefit of treatment.

In Hippocrates' time, placebo effects had already been recognized. This positive therapeutic treatment was advocated in the Hippocratic writings (*Corpus Hippocraticum*). In the early days of medicine, substances and procedures (for example, bleeding, cupping, or purging) used for treatment were ineffective and often dangerous. Yet, patients often regained their health. Shapiro (1960) noted that the placebo effect was the primary reason that medicine survived as a profession. When the technological aspects of modern medical care began to grow, however, physicians, nurses, and other health professionals relied less and less upon interpersonal behavior as a therapeutic medium. Health professionals even today underestimate their own potential impact on the patient's condition. Goodwin, Goodwin, and Vogel (1979) found that practitioners used the placebo effect inappropriately. They reported that they usually gave placebo medications to patients they disliked, or to those whose pain was believed to be psychogenic in origin. When the placebo effect did occur, it was misunderstood by the practitioners. Instead of viewing the placebo as a positive adjunct to therapy and as indication of a potentially successful form of treatment, the practitioners took the placebo effect as evidence that their patients' pain had no physiological basis. Unfortunately, practitioners often fail to recognize that the administration of "something" may help to reduce their patient's anxiety, and in doing so reduce pain and discomfort.

The incorporation of the positive therapeutic effect of the practitioner's reassurance and interpersonal behavior along with the techniques of modern medicine is likely to enhance greatly the efficacy of treatment and patients' cooperation with it. Technical medical care might even be ineffective unless reassurance and trust in the therapeutic relationship are strong (Cousins, 1979; DiMatteo & Friedman, 1982).

Factor 5: Practitioner Self-Disclosure

The practitioner's self-disclosure is likely to be an important factor in the estalishment of trust in the therapeutic relationship. Self-disclosure is likely, for example, to break down some of the interactional barriers between practitioner and patient that may arise from the differences that often exist between them (e.g., education, social and occupational status) and from the pressures toward professional dominance—pressures that encourage detached aloofness and an authoritarian stance. Appropriate self-disclosure, of course, does *not* involve the practitioner's portrayal of weakness or unresolved distress. (On the contrary, emotional difficulties and lack of strength or self-control should be dealt with by the practitioner outside of his or her relationships with patients, perhaps with psychotherapeutic intervention.) Rather, self-disclosure from practitioner to patient should portray the practitioner as strong and able to deal persistently with uncertainty. The disclosure should show the practitioner as a model for the patient's behavior.

If it is appropriate in timing, dosage, and content (Weiner, 1980), self-disclosure can enhance the therapeutic relationship and hence patient cooperation. First, the practitioner should disclose to the patient any errors in treatment that might be detected (Greeson, 1972). In a similar fashion the practitioner should disclose to the patient his or her obvious impairment (for example, significant fatigue or illness). Such disclosure helps to acknowledge the patient's observations, and it communicates concern and respect to the patient. Trying to hide what is obvious sets up barriers between practitioner and patient, communicating a lack of respect for the patient and destroying trust. Second, self-disclosure can help the patient to understand the normality of some of his or her own behavior (e.g., having difficulty remembering to take pills) and to recognize that there is indeed a chance of eventually gaining control over a given problem. For example, the practitioner might mention: "Oh, I really have trouble resisting desserts, too. It's tough, isn't it? But I figure it's worth it to resist them and to work toward maintaining a normal weight." Third, disclosing similar experiences can help to establish a basis of similarity between practitioner and patient that might help considerably to enhance the practitioner's interpersonal influence and capacity to persuade the patient.

In counseling and psychotherapy research, a limited amount of practitioner self-disclosure has been found to promote clients' perceptions that the therapist is genuine (Carkhuff, 1969) and to increase clients' self-disclosure (Jourard, 1971; Truax & Carkhuff, 1965). Self-disclosures that emphasize similarity between practitioner and patient (therapist and client) strengthen interpersonal attraction and social influence (Murphy & Strong, 1972; Strong & Dixon, 1971). The moderate use of similarity self-disclosures in therapeutic situations (first visit) also increases the chances of clients returning for a second session (Giannandrea & Murphy, 1973). Other research has shown that a moderate level of self-disclosure that involves the sharing of feelings and experiences similar to those expressed by the client have enhanced the client's evaluations of the quality of counseling received (Cash & Salzbach, 1978). Of course, the effects of self-disclosure depend heavily upon content and timing (Dies, 1973). Very personal information, or that which conveys weakness on the part of the practitioner, and disclosure that detracts attention from the patient or client, is not appropriate. Certain specifiable conditions prevail in determining the benefits of self-disclosure in the therapeutic relationship.

THE ART AND THE SCIENCE OF MEDICINE

> Medical science is intrinsically and essentially a *social* science, and as long as this is not recognized in practice we shall not be able to enjoy its benefits and shall have to be satisfied with an empty shell and a sham.
>
> [Saloman Neumann, 1847, pp. 64-65, cited in Rosen, 1972]

Traditional medicine has been dominated by a dualism that separates body and mind (Engel, 1977b; Friedman & DiMatteo, 1979). Diseases of the body have been thought to reside in the purely physical realm, treated exclusively with the scientific principles that pertain to physical matter. Problems of the mind, including psychopathologies, addictive behaviors, and noncompliance with medical treatments have been thought instead to reflect distorted or uncooperative personalities. That physical and psychological factors might influence one another, or that both might be influenced by yet another realm—social factors—is an idea that has typically met with resistance.

A related dichotomy that is similarly espoused is that between the science and the art of medicine. Art is typically viewed as dependent upon personal qualities of the caregiver rather than upon principles that can be taught and examined. Such a viewpoint relegates the art of medicine to an attitude (such as "samaritanism" [McDermott, 1977]) or even to a semimystical realm while pointing to such disciplines as biology, chemistry, or pathology as science. The art and the science of medicine (which are sometimes referred to as the "interpersonal or expressive" and the "technical or instrumental" aspects of care, respectively; Bloom, 1963) are often presented as phenomena of entirely different character.

Empirical research on these two aspects of medicine presents quite a different picture, however. DiMatteo and DiNicola (1981) found that physicians' technical and interpersonal skills were always judged to be highly related to one another, regardless of the source of evaluation. In past research (reviewed by Ware, Davies-Avery, & Stewart, 1978) consistently high correlations were found between *patients'* evaluations of physicians on the technical and interpersonal aspects of the care they delivered. The argument could be made, however, that patients were unable to judge the technical quality of their care and so judged both dimensions equally. DiMatteo and DiNicola (1981) replicated the high correlations among patients' ratings, and found similar ones among the ratings made by supervising and peer physicians. It is highly unlikely, of course, that these latter correlations reflected merely the *inability* of the raters to make distinctions among the two aspects of care, since supervising and peer physicians are certainly likely to be able to distinguish between the art and the science of medicine (if such a distinction actually existed). Interestingly, research has shown that patients *can*, in fact, make the distinction between these dimensions *if* the medical-care encounters they evaluate actually represent such a distinction. The fact that in their evaluations of medical care, physicians and patients make very slight distinction—if any at all—between technical and interpersonal skill suggests the existence of a substantial correlation between technical skill and interpersonal skill in the actual practice of medicine (Barro, 1973; Ware, Kane, Davies, & Brook, 1980; Barnlund, 1976).

Many skills are required for the successful formulation of an accurate diagnosis and effective treatment regimen in caring for a patient. Not the least of these involves the interpersonal factors of respect, genuineness, and empathy, which establish the trustworthiness and expertness of the practitioner and enhance his or her capacity to influence patient compliance with the treatment regimen. (This influence may be applied through the various channels examined in detail in the following chapters.) Thus, practitioner competency is likely to involve scientific technical knowledge translated into practice through interpersonal skills and the art of medicine (DiMatteo & DiNicola, 1982).

Skill in the Art of Medicine

Patients' thoughts and feelings are inextricably intertwined with their physical condition. It is estimated that about 35 percent of visits to primary-care physicians in this country are primarily for psychosocial care. At least as many more are for illnesses to which psychosocial factors are relevant (Baker & Cassata, 1978). Thus, clinical medicine depends upon the ability of the practitioner to understand and to help thinking, feeling, human beings: "A pair of kidneys will never come to the physician for diagnosis and treatment. They will be contained within an anxious, fearful, wondering person, asking puzzled questions about an obscure future, weighed down by the responsibilities of a loved family, a job to be held, and bills to be paid. . . . The clinician must learn the facts about it all, comprehend it all, and develop a plan of management for all of it. Otherwise, his approach is superficial" (Tumulty, 1970, p 21).

How do practitioners develop the interpersonal aspects of care of the patient? The answer is suggested in Tumulty's statement, quoted above, and in the following from communication specialist Barnlund (1976): "Commitment to humane values is rarely enough, any more than the simple desire to relieve suffering automatically confers diagnostic or surgical talent. Skill must be acquired to translate respect for patients as persons and the capacity to engage them communicatively as equals. Communication skills must be cultivated that respect patients' intelligence, acknowledge their needs, accept their feelings, value their opinions and promote collaboration in decision-making" (Barnlund, 1976, p. 723).

The notion that the interpersonal aspects of patient care comprise a skill that can be developed and trained has received some empirical support. First of all, studies of the relationship between practitioner personality and components of the art of medicine have characteristically produced very weak and equivocal results. Likewise, in the same studies, attempts to link intellectual variables (such as scores on the Medical College Admissions test, as well as premedical and medical grades) to the art of medicine have produced near zero correlations, or findings that are inconsistent across studies (Flom, 1971; Gough, Hall, & Harris, 1963, 1964; Richards, Taylor, & Price, 1962). On the other hand, the research reviewed in this chapter suggests strongly that the art of medicine consists of a set of definable skills that *can* be learned by practitioners and incorporated into their care of patients:

> Attention to a scientific approach to feelings has special pertinence for clinical medicine, the practice of which so much depends on the ability of the physician to understand and to help thinking, feeling human beings (Engel, 1977a, p. 222). . . . "The ultimate goal of a scientific approach to patient care is to render rational and accessible to conscious awareness and reporting the basis for the decisions and the means of their implementation. . . . They must be predicated on reliable data correctly interpreted and on principles amenable to scientific study and validation. Such standards must apply as much to minute-to-minute microdecisions as to more major decisions, whether to linger a moment longer at the bedside as well as when and how to propose open heart surgery. [Engel, 1977a, p. 223]

THE PRACTITIONER-PATIENT RELATIONSHIP: SOME FINAL ISSUES

The art of medicine (in general, and as it applies to the enhancement of patient compliance) requires a new orientation for medical care. As Engel (1977a) stated, "The problem facing medical education is thus one of overcoming conventional attitudes and acknowledging the fact—for it is a fact—that human behavior, feelings, transactions and relationships—and hence patient care—are indeed amenable to scientific inquiry; that it is possible to make precise observations and to provide accurate verbal descriptions thereof, to characterize and classify data, to establish reliability, to draw inferences and to develop hypotheses that can be put to test" (p. 223). Toward this end, Engel (1977b) proposed that patients' medical problems need always to be understood in the light of their social environment and psychological make-up—an approach he called the "biopsychosocial model" (Engel, 1977b). In this model, the mind-body dichotomy does not exist, for biological, psychological, and social factors in patients' lives are all expected to influence each other. Gradually, such an approach is likely to be accepted throughout medicine, as the dichotomies prove ineffective for dealing with patients as people.

Many of the important and relevant findings of psychosocial research are new, and many of them are scattered unsystematically throughout the literature. Our goal in this book is to integrate a number of large bodies of research on the application of social-psychological principles to the problem of patient noncompliance. Issues of interpersonal rapport between practitioner and patient are of course only part of the entire picture of relevant variables—a single, though critically important, part of the biopsychosocial model. It might be argued (and must be validated by future research) that without practitioner-patient rapport and trust, the remaining issues in this book can never be effectively dealt with in the therapeutic relationship.

In this chapter, we have attempted to examine the many aspects of the art of medicine that are likely to be relevant to the practitioner's capacity to influence patients' compliance. We have recognized throughout, however, that a number of weaknesses presently exist in the empirical literature. As Caterinicchio (1979, p. 81) explained: "Surprisingly little is known about the situational and interpersonal process-related variables which contribute to the development and maintenance of a successful treatment relationship between patient and practitioner. Consequently, the study of the therapeutic process lacks even a strong theoretical orientation; and there is a serious lack of empirical testing of even the most commonly used theoretical concepts and constructs. In short, there exists a substantial data void concerning the situational and interpersonal variables responsible for the evolution of the treatment process." Despite repeated calls for such research (see Hulka, 1979; Becker & Maiman, 1980), a full understanding of the process of interaction between practitioner and patient as it affects patient compliance remains a critically important research goal.

4

Perceptions of Illness, Prevention, and Treatment: The Patient's Perspective

> A person's health-seeking behavior is, to a great extent, based on his or her *perception* of a bodily state, rather than on the body's true, physical condition. [Janis & Rodin, 1979, p. 488]

> The study of the patient's perspective is an indispensable aspect of the analysis of health and disease. [Mechanic, 1968, p. 115]

A phenomenon often approached with fascination by practitioners, lay persons, and social scientists alike is the tremendous variation among people in their responses to what appear to be similar medical conditions. While one individual may hardly acknowledge a symptom, another (with perhaps an even milder form of the same condition) will withdraw from his or her particular daily responsibilities, refrain from going to work, exhibit emotional distress, and display significant social and psychological disability (Mechanic, 1968).

Many explanations have been proposed to account for these differences in individual responses to illness conditions. These explanations include such diverse factors as consistent variation in individual levels of pain tolerance (Beecher, 1959), differences in economic status (Waitzkin & Waterman, 1974; Koos, 1954), differences in personality (Cohen, 1979), differences in cultural patterns of expressiveness (Zola, 1966, 1972), and differences in ability to cope with stress (Cohen & Lazarus, 1979), to name just a few. Of course, more than one of these factors may influence a given individual's particular development and expression of illness behavior. While we will consider other factors such as culture in Chapter 5, here we focus as closely as possible on the individual's own perspective—particularly on beliefs and attitudes regarding illness and medical care.

The term "illness" has no simple definition (Rosenstock & Kirscht, 1979). On the one hand, it refers to a purely physical concept that involves a specific pathogen or tissue damage. Most researchers refer to illness in this particular sense as "disease" (Engel, 1977). On the other hand, illness has both social and psychological definitions, other than disease. Sociologically, illness refers to an individual's inability to perform the roles for which he or she has been socialized (Parsons, 1951). Psychologically, illness refers to the actual behavior of the particular ill person—for example, descriptions of pain and discomfort, private or expressed feelings of depression, and the like (Mechanic, 1968). How, then, do we decide if a person is "really" ill? Must there exist demonstrable disease? Need the individual be incapacitated socially? Kosa and Robertson (1975) have argued rather persuasively that a person is ill when he or she defines himself or herself as such and seeks some form of medical treatment. Illness, then, involves the patient's personal and subjective perceptions (which are in turn influenced heavily by the patient's important reference persons and social norms).

Clearly, however, to define oneself as ill is hardly sufficient to maintain the sick role (see Chapter 2). In order to enjoy the social benefits of being legitimately sick (such as exemption from social responsibilities), one must first convince a physician of one's impairment. However, because impairment is sometimes ambiguous, and because the definition of illness is so dependent upon the individual's behavior and subjective perceptions, legitimation may be granted for a long time before doubts about its validity begin to surface. That a person can both act and be defined as sick without objective supporting evidence of disease suggests that illness is, in essence, a psychological and social phenomenon. Central to its meaning are the perceptions of the individual. Therefore, we contend that a full understanding of medical noncompliance, patient satisfaction with medical care, and even the outcome of medical technical ministrations, requires a clear understanding of the patient's perceptions of illness, prevention, and treatment.

PERCEPTIONS OF ILLNESS

Whether or not an individual seeks medical care usually has little to do with his or her objective physical condition. Sociologists David Mechanic (1968) and Irving Zola (1973) have noted that most individuals, at most times in their lives, experience clinically significant physical symptoms of one kind or another. Within this framework it has been suggested that health, for most people, consists of little more than "compensated illness" (Wilson, 1970).

Many people seek medical advice for nonspecific stomach, body, and head aches and sometimes simply for "not feeling good" (Garfield, 1970). These are conditions that other people, and even these particular seekers of care at other times in their lives, experience and choose to ignore. Many extensive surveys (reviewed by Mechanic, 1968, and by Zola, 1973) have shown that apparently healthy people from all walks of life possess some treatable and medically significant symptoms. Yet, according to White, Williams, and Greenberg (1961), less than one-third of the persons who report experiencing clinically significant illness episodes consult physicians. Thus, it remains a clinical truism that there is minimal relationship between the existence of symptoms and the actual seeking of medical care. This fact sometimes annoys and perplexes physicians, especially when it manifests itself in the patients' choice to ignore important warning signs of such conditions as myocardial infarction, cancer, and diabetic gangrene (Cohen, 1979). As we noted earlier, however, when we considered the general problem of medical noncompliance, people are subject to their perceptions and it is by way of these perceptions that more or less rational decisions (in this case, to ignore a symptom or to seek care) are made.

The path from recognition of a symptom to the practitioner's doorstep is long and complex, influenced strongly by psychological (perceptual) and social factors. These factors affect whether a symptom will be ignored, tolerated, self-medicated, or brought to the attention of a medical practitioner. Zola (1973) has suggested that a symptom is finally acknowledged as illness and medical care sought when the patient can no longer tolerate or accommodate it. Zola has identified five nonphysiological "triggers" for the decision to seek medical care: (1) the occurrence of an interpersonal crisis; (2) *perceived* interference with social or personal relations; (3) social sanctioning (by other people who legitimate the condition); (4) the *perceived* interference with vocational or physical activity; and (5) the similarity of symptoms to one's previous experiences. Four of these triggers (all but the third) depend upon the patient's perception of his or her own physical or emotional state or on a decision about the cost versus the benefit of relieving the symptom. (The third so-called trigger focuses on perceptions of the social environment, which will be examined in Chapter 5).

In order to illustrate these concepts, Zola (1973) presented the case of Mrs. O'Rourke, a 49-year-old licensed practical nurse. After being hit on the side of the head with a baseball, she experienced loss of vision in one eye. Despite this loss of vision, which interfered significantly with reading, Mrs. O'Rourke did not seek medical care for four months. The trigger, in her case, was the comment from another person that her "eyelid was drooping." The drooping, she believed, detracted from her appearance, and so she sought medical advice. Her condition was subsequently diagnosed as permanent partial blindness. Neither the interviewer nor the examining physician noted any "drooping" of her eyelid. For Mrs. O'Rourke, the five triggers may have operated in the following manner to bring her to the practitioner for treatment: (1) another person challenged her concept of her appearance, thus provoking a minor interpersonal crisis; (2) the "dropping of her eyelid," in Mrs. O'Rourke's own perception, interfered with her ability to relate to other people; (3) she presumably received some encouragement from others to have her eye problem checked; (4) she perceived that the drooping eyelid (but *not* the loss of vision) interfered in her vocational activity (nursing) which required a high degree of contact with people; (5) presumably (although we cannot be sure), Mrs. O'Rourke had experienced temporary loss of vision before, or knew others who had, and perceived this condition as not serious. Drooping of the eyelid, on the other hand, may have been something she perceived as quite important.

Patients' perceptions of their symptoms differ tremendously. A patient's inability to tolerate a symptom usually results from a particular situation that may or may not be related to the symptom (e.g., "I can't read") or from a perceived implication of the symptom (e.g., marred appearance) rather than from a worsening of the symptom. Social and/or psychological factors usually trigger the seeking of medical care. In regard to this, King (1972) suggested that the practitioner must pay as much attention as possible to the "crisis" and to the "triggers" that brought the patient in for treatment. To the patient, these triggers are usually as important as the physiological condition, or even more important. By understanding the character and degree of importance attached to each trigger, the practitioner can gain tremendous insight into the patient's beliefs, attitudes, values, and social-environmental influences. Also, as Zola (1973) observed, patients may terminate treatment with a practitioner who does not adequately attend to the specific problems they brought in, even if those problems have no relationship to what is medically wrong with them (e.g., Mrs. O'Rourke's concern about her drooping eyelid).

Lastly, regarding this issue, the patient's description of his or her symptoms may actually signal the real problem, which may be primarily psychosocial. Marsland, Wood, and Mayo (1976) and others have noted that a large proportion (50 to 80 percent) of visits to primary-care practitioners are concerned with primarily psychosocial problems (e.g., depression stemming from marital conflict, or anxiety and occupational stress) or with problems that have very strong psychosocial components (components that serve as triggers for the seeking of care, or as sequelae to physiological distress). The psychosocial problem may thus serve as the "hidden agenda" in the presentation of any medical problem.

ILLNESS AS A PSYCHOLOGICAL COPING RESPONSE

The day-to-day difficulties of life can significantly influence illness behavior. In fact, Mechanic (1968) has noted that all illness is in one sense "psychosomatic," because "distress" is very often a more influential factor in seeking medical help than the actual character of the treatable, medical symptoms. Balint (1957) was among the first to argue that the presentation of somatic complaints often masks underlying emotional problems. For example, a complaint of illness (particularly something relatively trivial) may be one way of seeking reassurance and support in a socially acceptable manner. As noted above, this "hidden agenda" (the emotional issue underlying the physical complaint) is a phenomenon well known to medical practitioners.

Patients are often compelled to couch their psychosocial distress in physical terms because of generally negative societal reactions toward people who cannot cope emotionally with their lives. Sociological surveys of reactions in the general population (Phillips, 1963) demonstrate significantly less positive evaluations of (and greater preferred social distance from) people who seek mental-health services than of those who seek counseling from a family physician. The social stigma attached to the receipt of mental-health services tends to inhibit patients from using them. Instead, patients quite often turn to their primary-care physicians for help with their "problems in living." Because the primary-care practitioner is likely to expect a presenting problem of a physical nature, the patient with a psychosocial dysfunction will typically present a somewhat vague, ambiguous set of symptoms (e.g., fatigue, stomach ache). As mentioned above, studies of primary medical-care settings suggest that a large percentage (50 to 80 percent) of patients' presenting problems are in part or completely psychosocial (Marsland, Wood, & Mayo, 1976).

Mechanic (1968) has suggested that patients may be *unaware* of their problem in its psychological, undisguised form, or may simply lack the appropriate vocabulary to express it meaningfully. Mechanic and Volkart (1961) examined this complex relationship in more detail and suggested that perceived stress (operationalized in their study as loneliness and nervousness) manifests itself in illness behavior (the seeking of medical care) primarily among those who are already inclined to seek medical services (that is, by frequent users of medical care). The use of medical-care services by these individuals is related to their expectation that they will receive emotional relief, comfort, and support from the medical encounter.

An interesting discovery was made by Follette and Cummings (1967; also Cummings & Follette, 1976) who found that the provision of preventive psychotherapy to patients in a health-maintenance organization can result in decreased use of medical services. Cummings and Follette (1976) found that only one psychotherapy session (with no follow-up psychological care) could result in as much as a 65 percent reduction in medical utilization. With two to eight psychotherapy sessions, utilization was reduced by as much as 75 percent over five years. Psychological intervention seems to have allowed practitioners to view patients' *real* concerns, and to offer understanding, support, and suggestions for change. Thus, the important role of psychological (perceptual) factors in the presentation of bodily symptoms is demonstrated in this dramatic intervention in which a clear distinction between psychological concerns and bodily complaints was encouraged.

As we noted earlier, there are profound individual differences in sensitivity to and interpretation of bodily symptoms. Interpretations depend quite heavily on perceptions and attributions. (Attributions are defined as inferences about the manner in which environmental events appear in causal relationship to one another.) Consider the medical student who experiences various symptom complexes and attributes them to some pathological process (Mechanic, 1972). This behavior (also known as hypochondriasis, or specifically in this case "medical students' disease") occurs in approximately 70 percent of all medical students at some point during their training (Woods et al., 1966; Hunter et al., 1964). Social stress and anxiety combine with bodily symptoms (which are often the result of fatigue) and detailed (but often incomplete) information about a disease with similar symptoms to produce a self-diagnosis. This self-diagnosis is typically accompanied by increased fear and anxiety. The researchers concluded that the syndrome's occurrence depends upon the coincidental juxtaposition of the medical student's emotional arousal, the presence of particular (usually vague) bodily feelings, and new information that seems relevant to the existing symptoms. Mechanic (1972) has argued that hypochondriasis is likely to occur in any individual for whom these conditions exist, particularly if he or she is highly identified with someone who is experiencing or has experienced the medical problem. Identification can result from physical or psychological intimacy or proximity, or from similarities in age, sex, life style, and other factors. Hypochondriasis is likely to be intensified by the anxiety that develops from and is exacerbated by feelings of low self-esteem and fears that one cannot cope with adversity (Lazarus, 1966).

Psychological factors (viewed from the perspective of the patient), then, can have an important effect on perceptions of illness. Illness can, in fact, be used as a psychological coping response in an attempt to deal with or make sense of a problematic life situation. Hypochondriasis is an extreme example of how perceptual factors influence decisions about illness and guide the person's attempt to cope with problems. This analysis leads us to the primary purpose of this chapter—to explore the role of patients' perceptions, indeed of psychological factors in general, in determining patients' responses to recommendations for treatment, and to methods for health maintenance and illness prevention. As we will see, the research data strongly suggest that thoughts, beliefs, opinions, and ideas influence in large part patients' responses to medical recommendations and their willingness to invest in their future health.

PSYCHOLOGICAL FACTORS AND PATIENT COMPLIANCE

Psychological factors play a particularly important role in determining patients' responses to bodily symptoms. Patients' perceptions, their interpretations of the situation, their beliefs, and their present needs and desires influence the extent to which they attend to their symptoms and their decision to seek a medical definition for them. Perceptions also affect a patient's willingness to accept medical help once it is offered and to comply with regimens for medical treatment or for disease prevention.

Haynes (1979) conducted an extensive literature review in which he examined the relationship between characteristics of particular diseases and patient cooperation with treatment. In general, he found that objectively defined "disease factors are . . . relatively unimportant as determinants of compliance" (Haynes, 1979, p. 51). Further, many studies have found virtually no correlation between *objectively measured* disease severity and patient cooperation with the prescribed treatment (Haynes, 1979). It is of interest to note that in studies reviewed by Haynes, it was found that minimal or no association existed between compliance and the severity and duration of symptoms, previous bouts with the disease, recency of the last attack, and previous hospitalization and its length. Thus, objectively assessed physical features and manifestations of disease have little bearing on compliance with treatment, just as they have little bearing on definitions of illness and the desire for medical care.

Patient Personality and Treatment Compliance

The personality of an individual is defined by many as a psychological factor that consists of deep-lying, early-learned, and largely unconscious traits (and associated behavior patterns). While this is not the only possible definition of personality (Pervin, 1980), popularly accepted definitions typically emphasize its stability and unchangeability. The personality of the patient, as defined in these stable terms, is the factor most likely to be blamed by physicians in their attempts to understand patient noncompliance with treatment. Davis (1966) surveyed 50 fourth-year medical students and 81 senior (faculty) physicians, asking them to state which factors they believed were general causes of patient noncompliance with medical regimens. Sixty-one percent of the junior physicians and 67 percent of the senior physicians believed the patient's "uncooperative personality" to be the primary cause of patient noncompliance. Of all the factors noted, patient personality was the most likely explanation offered. Patients' legitimate difficulties in following the advice were chosen much less often. These difficulties included the patient's inability to understand the doctor's advice, problematic life situations, and the financial inability to afford to follow the advice. Thus, because of physicians' obvious predispositions to focus on the psychological factor of basic personality, it is important to understand the role that this factor actually plays in patient compliance.

Empirical research on the relationship between patient personality and compliance with preventive and rehabilitative treatment regimens is relatively sparse. There is a myriad of personality characteristics that might potentially be studied in relation to patient compliance, but only a few of these have been empirically examined. In addition, few empirical studies exist for each individual personality characteristic that *has* been examined. Thus, it is difficult to assert the stability of any particular finding. In general, though, the evidence is *not strongly* in favor of patient personality as an important factor in compliance. Neither, however, is personality (in the sense of basic traits) totally uncorrelated with compliance behavior.

In their excellent compilation of compliance research, Haynes, Taylor, and Sackett (1979) examined all the empirical research to date on personality factors and patients' cooperation with treatment. From their tabular summaries, we have identified the various personality factors so far studied that relate positively to compliance behavior, those that relate negatively, and those for which the correlations are close to zero. Some of the findings are equivocal, with some studies showing positive and others showing negative correlations. Personality characteristics that show an equivocal relationship or a nonexistent relationship to compliance are: dependency, depression, anxiety (trait), extroversion, self-concept and self-esteem, feelings of alienation, and somatization. Positively related to compliance are: (1) patient articulateness, intelligence, responsiveness, cooperativeness, and gratefulness (among patients at a general medical clinic; Davis, 1968); (2) futuristic orientation (among rehabilitation patients [Diamond et al., 1968], and in a study of preventive health measures [Suchman, 1967]; (3) "stable" personality (in a general internal-medicine practice [Barnum, 1974], and among compliant patients and those discharged against medical advice in a general hospital [Jankowski & Drum, 1977], and among patients in a study of smoking status [West et al., 1977]).

Patients who were noncompliant were characterized as: (1) impulsive, distressed and demanding (in a study of smokers in treatment [Jacobs, 1972]); (2) authoritarian, overbearing (among general medical clinic patients [Davis, 1968]); (3) neurotic (in a treatment to enhance self-control [Barnum, 1974] and among patients of private practitioners [Hammel & Williams, 1964]); (4)

impulsive, immature, avoidant of responsibility (in a study that correlated psychological tests with oral contraceptive use [Bakker & Dightman, 1973]); (5) unreliable (in a study of admission characteristics correlated with dropout from alcohol treatment [Baekeland et al., 1973] and in a study of drug effectiveness for depression [Glick, 1965]); and finally (6) having a lower frustration tolerance (among chronically ill patients having hemodialysis [Czaczkes & Kaplan, 1972; and Kaplan & Czaczkes, 1972]).

A major conceptual problem exists in many of the studies of personality and compliance. Many have employed as their measures of "personality" *not* objective, standardized personality tests, but rather evaluations made by practitioners and interviewers. These evaluations were, of course, likely to reflect the evaluators' stereotypes of patients who are noncompliant (e.g., patients who do not comply are characterized as irresponsible). It becomes difficult, then, to determine whether the ratings of personality were predictors of noncompliance or reflections of the evaluators' expectations. The role of patient personality in compliance with treatment, therefore, still remains unclear. This question demands research that employs objective definitions of personality variables and uses prospective designs.

To date, then, little substantial evidence exists to implicate personality factors (in the sense of traits as unchangeable psychological characteristics) as causal agents in patient compliance. A nagging question remains, however, regarding *why* physicians might posit a significant role for stable psychological factors in patient compliance. Certainly clinical observation suggests that patients differ among themselves in their characteristic approaches to self-control, and in their attempts to enact prescribed behaviors and to avoid proscribed ones. Observation over long periods may suggest to clinicians that each individual's behavior is relatively consistent. If patients tend to persist in their noncompliant behavior—be it avoidance of exercise or continuance of compulsive smoking—the practitioner might easily come to attribute patient behavior to stable characteristics and traits *within* the patients themselves.

The limited strength of personality variables in predicting and explaining patient compliance may stem from the very definition of personality as basic, unchangeable, deep-rooted, and primarily unconscious. A broader emphasis on personality, namely on the notion of "social personality," may be needed. According to Jessor, Graves, Hanson, and Jessor (1968), such an emphasis on socially learned cognitive systems (including beliefs, attitudes, values, and expectations) may further the understanding of personality as it relates to individual action. These cognitive systems are as much the result of learning in later life as they are of earlier learning. Thus, they can be changed. They may be somewhat available to conscious awareness, as well, and may manifest themselves in speech and action more readily than do unconscious, deep-seated traits. They can also be understood quite well within the context of the individual's past and present sociocultural environment.

As we will see in the following section, various models of health behavior have been developed that emphasize such psychological characteristics as Jessor et al. (1968) proposed. These models focus particularly on patients' beliefs, perceptions, and motivations. An examination of those models and a careful look at one in particular—the Health Belief Model—will help to delineate the role played by psychological factors in patient compliance. As we consider these models, it is important to keep in mind that we are again dealing with patients' perceptions. The patient's perspective is all-important to the understanding of health behavior and compliance with medical regimens. As we saw earlier, whether or not a person seeks medical help has little to do with his or her objective symptoms. Rather, action is more dependent upon the person's perceptions of those symptoms and of related factors such as the interpersonal environment or the cost of care. In general, compliance and health behavior are also dependent upon the patient's beliefs and perceptions of illness and medical care.

In this chapter, we examine patients' beliefs and attitudes about health, disease, and medical care in terms of their effect on patient compliance and preventive health behavior. These are certainly not the *only* cognitive factors that influence health behavior (for example, one's world view regarding the probability of total nuclear devastation might affect one's willingness to engage in preventive health action), but they are the most extensively studied. They also appear to be factors that are most directly modifiable by health professionals in their care of patients.

A few definitions and distinctions are in order before we consider the various social psychological factors that affect patient behavior in the health-care arena. The first distinction is that made by Kasl and Cobb (1966). They refer to *preventive health behavior* as those actions taken to prevent the occurrence of disease. These include activities such as exercising, eating nutritious meals, refraining from smoking, and wearing seat belts in an automobile. *Illness behavior* involves those actions that are undertaken after the onset of symptoms. They include ignoring the symptoms, asking friends about them, seeking medical care, withdrawing socially, and the like. Illness behaviors are those that involve defining symptoms as illness. Finally, Kasl and Cobb define *sick-role behavior* as that which the person exhibits after the diagnosis has been made. Included in this category are compliance behaviors traditionally studied in research on compliance, such as taking medication, following a special diet and exercise regimen, and refraining from an activity that might exacerbate the medical condition.

In research on these three presumably separate aspects of health-related actions, the distinction has proven unnecessary. It happens that the variables that correlate most prominently with one type of behavior tend also to correlate with another. In other words, little difference has been found among factors identified as predicting preventive health behaviors, illness behaviors, and sick-role (compliance) behaviors (Cummings, Becker, & Maile, 1980), although considerably less research has been done on illness behavior than on the other two. Some researchers make the distinction among them, but we feel that as yet there is little systematic evidence that the processes by which these various behaviors come about have noticeable variance among themselves. In our analyses of the factors that influence these health-related behaviors, we will note the specific individual behavior to which we are referring (for example, taking medication or engaging in an exercise program). We will also note whether we are referring to compliance or to preventive health behavior when the distinction seems appropriate. Often, however, we will note in general discussion the factors that are prominent in predicting "health-related behavior." This should be taken to refer to all three categories.

Proposing the existence of a construct called "preventive health behavior" and attempting to evaluate the contribution of particular psychological factors to it have one difficulty: research suggests that "preventive health behavior" may not be a single construct. Baumann (1961) has pointed out that a major problem in attempting to evaluate health attitudes and behaviors in general stems from the fact that individuals differentially perceive various behaviors as related to their concept of health. People often engage in certain behaviors (for example, exercise) because they enjoy themselves, and not specifically because such behaviors will promote health. Furthermore, the behaviors typically classified as health behaviors tend to vary from the maintenance of proper diet, to brushing one's teeth, to voting in an election for fluoridated water (Steele & McBroom, 1972). If it could be empirically demonstrated that these widely varying behaviors are intercorrelated, a construct called "preventive health behavior" could be validly proposed. This may not be the case, although further research is needed.

With regard to the intercorrelation of preventive health behaviors, Langlie (1977) noted a basic deficiency in the research. She called attention to the fact that very few studies to date have examined a wide variety of health maintenance and safety practices (most of which do not involve any contact at all with the health-care system). In her own study, Langlie (1977, 1979) found only moderate positive correlations among the various health-protective behaviors that she labeled "direct risk prevention" (driving behavior, pedestrian behavior, personal hygiene, and smoking behavior). She also found only moderate positive correlations among those behaviors defined as minimizing "indirect risk" (seat-belt use, medical check-ups, dental care, immunization, exercise, and nutrition). Further, these moderate correlations existed only *within* the two groups of behaviors, not between them. Indirect and direct risk prevention bore little relationship to one another. In addition, these correlations were obtained only in the data from respondents who had engaged in those health behaviors over a significant period of time. Other studies have shown very low or near-zero correlations among preventive health behaviors (Mechanic, 1979). As we will see, however, despite the lack of correlation among them and the low cohesiveness of the health behavior construct, many health-related behaviors (whether preventive or compliance oriented) tend to be associated with similar general psychological factors—namely beliefs and attitudes.

BELIEFS, ATTITUDES, AND HEALTH-RELATED BEHAVIORS

Two constructs—beliefs and attitudes—are central to the understanding and prediction of health-related behaviors. (A related concept is that of values, whose role is discussed in Chapter 5.) Stang and Wrightsman (1981) have defined beliefs and attitudes in the following manner. A *belief* is a hypothetical construct that involves the assertion of a relationship between some attitude object (a person, a situation, or a behavior, such as smoking) and some attribute of that object (e.g., causes cancer). An *attitude*, according to Stang and Wrightsman (1981), is a hypothetical construct used to explain consistencies within people in their affective reactions to (feelings toward) an attitude object. The term "attitude" has been defined in a number of different ways. According to Ajzen and Fishbein (1977), most investigators agree that an attitude represents the person's evaluation of the entity in question. Attitudes, according to Ajzen and Fishbein (1977; 1980), are evaluations made on the affective (or feeling, or emotional) dimension. Thus, an attitude reflects an affective evaluation of the attitude object. Most theories of attitudes agree that attitudes are learned (and therefore changeable), and that unless systematically changed, they are relatively enduring and consistent over time. Attitudes are also thought to motivate behavior. People *act* in part because of and in synchrony with their attitudes (Stang & Wrightsman, 1981). The most predominant theories propose that attitudes consist of three component parts—a cognitive component (made up of beliefs), an affective component (the individual's evaluation of the attitude object, usually positive or negative), and a behavioral orientation to the object. The components of cognition (belief), affect (feeling), and behavioral orientation are usually present in all theories that attempt to link psychological constructs with overt behaviors. In this chapter, we have chosen a particular way to conceptualize these variables based primarily on the theory of Ajzen and Fishbein (1980). This conceptualization posits that the belief component is antecedent to the affective-attitudinal component, and that the behavioral orientation is an outgrowth of attitudes and social norms. The behavioral orientation, as we will see, is referred to as an intention. Thus, these three traditional components of attitudes actually appear in the Ajzen and Fishbein (1980) formulation, albeit in a slightly different configuration than is proposed in the classical theory of attitudes.

A classic finding in social psychology is the often noted discrepancy between people's attitudes and behaviors. Rather low or nonsignificant correlations between attitudinal predictors and behavioral criteria have been accumulating for over 50 years (Ajzen & Fishbein, 1977). These findings conflicted with the theories of early social psychologists (e.g., Allport, 1935) who defined an attitude as a state of readiness to exhibit a behavioral response. Attitudes were thus believed to provoke behavioral responses. While early research demonstrated that people who behaved quite differently from one another were also found to have different attitudes, research that attempted to show that attitudes are actually behavioral predispositions has been unsuccessful. An individual's negative attitude toward smoking, for example, only slightly increases the likelihood that he will change his behavior and stop smoking. Serious doubts have thus been raised for many years regarding the ability of attitudes to correlate highly with behavior (La Piere, 1934; Corey, 1937; Fishbein & Ajzen, 1975; Ajzen & Fishbein, 1980).

Most attitude researchers have been unwilling to relinquish completely the assumption of an existing link between an individual's attitude toward an object and his or her behavior with respect to that object. They have attempted to reconcile the relatively low correlation between the two by conceptualizing the attitude-behavior relationship in a somewhat more complex way. New approaches have begun to make a more adequate distinction between beliefs, attitudes (defined affectively), intentions to perform behaviors, and the behaviors themselves. In the past, these distinct concepts were not separated from one another, particularly in the measurements employed. Theoretical and empirical work that has examined these constructs as distinct from one another has been able to identify how these psychological factors interrelate and how they may influence behavior. Rosenberg (1956), for example, showed that a person's affective response (his attitude) is influenced by his belief that the object, person, or concept that he is evaluating will or will not lead him closer to his valued goals. From this kind of multidimensional approach, Ajzen and Fishbein (1980; Fishbein & Ajzen, 1975) developed their "Theory of Reasoned Action."

The Theory of Reasoned Action is currently one of the most promising models offering a general explanation and prediction of behavior. This model has been successfully applied to health behavior as well. Throughout this and the next two chapters, our discussion of patients' perceptions and the relationship of these to health behavior will make use of the Theory of Reasoned Action. In this chapter, we consider beliefs and attitudes, while in Chapter 5 we examine social normative factors that are part of the model. Chapter 6 deals with intentions. We find Ajzen and Fishbein's model (1980) to be an excellent framework within which to organize the literature that relates psychological and social factors to patient compliance and preventive health behavior.

In these discussions, we examine social and psychological factors in patients' decisions to cooperate with medical or preventive care. We have tried to maintain a relatively simple conceptual orientation, keeping in mind the central notion that people's basic perceptions of health and health care manifest themselves in beliefs and attitudes, and then ultimately in some form of behavior. Our adherence to a relatively simple conceptual orientation is supported by the findings of Cummings, Becker, and Maile (1980). Their research has shown that complex definitions and minute distinctions made among the many health-related variables considered in the literature may be unnecessary. The actual number of truly distinct constructs relevant to health actions is small. (In the Cummings, et al. [1980] study, judges, who were themselves model-builders, partitioned a set of 109 variables into groups according to their similarity. The six factors that emerged were: (1) accessibility to health care; (2) evaluation of health care; (3) perception of symptoms and threat of disease; (4) social-network characteristics; (5) knowledge about disease; and (6) demographic characteristics. This study provided a first step toward developing a unified framework for explaining health actions.)

What people believe about their health and health behavior does indeed influence what they do about it. This idea is well supported in the literature. Beliefs are multifaceted. They include the individual's beliefs about health care (such as the benefits of treatment, and the quality of medical care provided), and beliefs about the threat of disease (symptoms, susceptibility, consequences). Beliefs about the expectations of other people, formalized in terms of subjective social norms, are also important and are examined in Chapter 5.

THE THEORY OF REASONED ACTION

The Theory of Reasoned Action, formulated by social psychologists Martin Fishbein and Icek Ajzen (1975), asserts that human social behavior (including cooperation with medical regimens and preventive measures) is not controlled by unconscious motives; it is not thoughtless. Rather, the theory holds that people *decide* to engage or not to engage in a given action by carefully considering its implications. Behavior is under volitional control and is a function of the person's intention to perform or not to perform the particular behavior. Ajzen and Fishbein make a firm distinction in their theory between attitudes (which are affective in nature) and beliefs (which are cognitions based on information about the relevant topics). Beliefs regarding the value of the goal and one's expectation of attaining it combine to

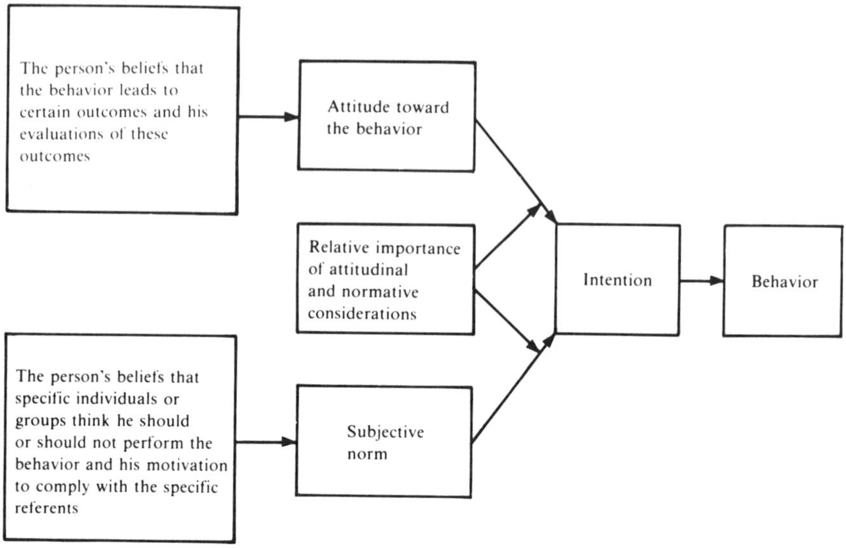

Note: Arrows indicate the direction of influence.

Fig. 4.1. Factors determining a person's behavior.

Source: **Icek Ajzen and Martin Fishbein, *Understanding Attitudes and Predicting Social Behavior*, © 1980, p. 8. Reprinted by permission of Prentice-Hall, Inc., Englewood Cliffs, N.J.**

produce an attitude toward the behavior. (The "value × expectancy theory" [Rotter, 1954] is extremely relevant here, for as we will see, the factors that best predict health behavior—the components of the Health Belief Model, and the construct Locus of Control—fit well in this framework.) Attitudes and beliefs regarding social expectations also accommodate this framework quite well. Together, beliefs (and attitudes) and social norms bring about behavioral intentions, which, under the right conditions, operate to predict behavior (see Figure 4.1). We note in Chapter 7 that the connection between intentions and health behaviors is not at all simple. There, we examine how the correlation between intentions and behaviors can easily be attenuated by difficulties in following the treatment regimen, in gaining access to medical services, or in engaging in self-control.

According to Ajzen and Fishbein's (1980) theory, "beliefs influence attitudes and subjective norms; these two components influence intentions; and intentions influence behavior" (Ajzen & Fishbein, 1980, p. 80). "According to the theory of reasoned action, behavioral change is ultimately the result of changes in belief" (p. 81). Thus, belief changes are needed to bring about changes in attitudes or in perceptions of norms. Then a resultant change in intentions must occur if subsequent behavior is to be altered. In the Ajzen and Fishbein model, it is necessary to determine the degree to which an intention is under attitudinal versus social-normative control. Changes can then be brought about.

In Ajzen and Fishbein's theory, beliefs are thus considered central to predictions of health behavior. It is within their framework that we examine the overwhelming empirical evidence in support of health beliefs as contributors of compliance and preventive health behavior, and in later chapters consider beliefs as the most appropriate focus for behavior change efforts.

Models of Health Behavior

In their study of individuals' responses to health advice, nearly all researchers have focused some attention on attitudes and subjective perceptions. Some researchers have sought to formalize the operation of beliefs, attitudes, and related subjective responses (among other factors). Many different frameworks have been developed by sociologists and social psychologists.

In Table 4.1, we present the models that are most notable in terms of the frequency with which they are cited in the literature, and in terms of the evidence available to support their predictive validity. Work by Becker and colleagues (Cummings, Becker, & Maile, 1980; Becker et al., 1979) has been very useful in compiling this list of models and their component parts. The models in Table 4.1 appear to contain a number of common elements, among them: (1) perceptions of threat from disease, and (2) beliefs in the cost versus benefit (a general evaluation) of health care. (Most also contain a factor involving social norms, considered in detail in the next chapter.) The model developed several decades ago called the Health Belief Model is included in the table (under the reference, Rosenstock, 1966). The Health Belief Model (HBM) contains all the relevant elements regarding perceptions that exist in the other models, and it has the most research support of all the models involving beliefs. We therefore examine the Health Belief Model in detail in our delineation of the role of beliefs in the determination of health behavior.

THE HEALTH BELIEF MODEL

The Health Belief Model (Rosenstock, 1966; Becker, 1974) hypothesizes that people seek and comply with health-care regimens (preventive regimens, such as health screening, or rehabilitative regimens such as treatment for a diagnosed disease) only under certain specific conditions. They must possess some minimal level of health knowledge and motivation toward health. They must also believe that they are vulnerable to a threatening illness condition. They must be convinced that the treatment can be efficacious (that is, that it

Table 4.1. Theoretical Models of Compliance and Health Behavior.*

		PREDICTORS		
Model: Author and Reference	Health Variable Predicted	Patients' Perceptions and Beliefs	Social-Normative Factors	Other Factors
Andersen (1968)	Use of medical-care services	• health beliefs (about medical care, physicians, and disease) • perceptions of own health status • responses to illness	• family composition • social structure (employment, education level, occupation)	• family resources • availability of medical services
Anderson and Bartkus (1973)	Choice of health-delivery service	• appraisal of the adequacy of care • perceptions of own symptoms • sensitivity to own symptoms	• perception of friends' appraisal of care • sociodemographic factors	• availability of health service • having a regular family physician
Antonovsky and Kats (1970)	Use of preventive dental care	• value and saliency of health (amount of money spent on health, time spent discussing health) • "effective motivation" • knowledge of disease • anxiety about health action		• financial difficulties

Fabrega (1973)	Decision to seek medical care (illness behavior)	• recognition and labeling of symptoms as illness • negative valuation of illness • treatment plans and costs (perceived benefits versus costs)	
Green (1975)	Adopting health behaviors	• perceived advantages of health action • health behavior is compatible with existing values and needs • complexity of the health action	• social pressure and social participation
Hochbaum (1958)	Preventive health behavior (screening)	• belief in possibility of contracting disease • belief in benefits of health action • perceptions of care (cost, location, opinion of quality of care) • appearance of symptoms	• "social forces"
Kar (1978)	Health behavior (use of contraceptives)	• awareness of service and perceptions of service • personal aspirations • values • prior experience with health services	• sociocultural factors (including social norms) • social status and demographics

Table 4.1. cont. on p. 130

Table 4.1. (*continued*)

		PREDICTORS		
Model: Author and Reference	Health Variable Predicted	Patients' Perceptions and Beliefs	Social-Normative Factors	Other Factors
Kasl and Cobb (1966a)	Health behavior	• importance of health • perceived susceptibility • perceived severity of condition • past utilization of health services • cost of action vs. cost of no action • perceived efficacy of health action	• "social characteristics"	• information
Kasl and Cobb (1966b)	Sick role and illness behavior	• importance of health • perceived susceptibility and severity • value of action versus cost of no action • pain and distress • tolerance for pain and disability	• social characteristics	

Suchman (1966)	Use of medical care for illness episode	• scientific knowledge about disease • skepticism about illness • dependency on illness (for various gains)	• social-structure index (includes friendship solidarity and attention to family tradition)	
Kosa and Robertson (1969)	Health and illness behavior	• assessment of symptoms • anxiety (specific and free-floating anxiety) • knowledge		
Mechanic (1968)	Illness behavior	• symptom salience, frequency and persistence • own tolerance for symptoms • perceived severity • need for avoidance • competing needs • interference with social activities • information and knowledge about symptoms • monetary and psychological cost associated with treatment	• social and cultural assumptions about symptoms	• available treatment resources
Rosenstock (1966) (Health Belief Model)	Health-, Illness-, and sick-role behavior	• perceived susceptibility to illness • perceived severity • belief in benefits of health action		

Table 4.1. cont. on p. 132

Table 4.1. (*continued*)

		PREDICTORS		
Model: Author and Reference	Health Variable Predicted	Patients' Perceptions and Beliefs	Social-Normative Factors	Other Factors
		• belief in costs of health action [and added by Becker & Maiman, 1975: • general health motivation • locus of control • cues to action]		
Langlie (1977)	Preventive health behaviors	• Health Belief Model variables above • health locus of control • attitude toward providers of care	• neighborhood and family socioeconomic status • interaction with nonkin and kin • marriage • residential mobility	• situational constraints

* Note that many of these frameworks are not really "models" in the technical sense, but tend to be lists of relevant variables.

is indeed possible to obtain control over the disease), and that the cost of such control (in the form of recommended preventive or treatment actions) is not too high in view of the benefits. These conditions are the following: belief in *susceptibility* to and *severity* of the disease, belief in the *efficacy* of treatment (that something can be done about the medical problem), and self-efficacy (one's own ability to deal with the problem), and finally perceptions of the *cost* of treatment (in terms of time, money, energy, interest, fear, embarrassment, and the like). These factors originally constituted the Health Belief Model as formulated by Rosenstock (1966) and as described in detail by Becker (1974).

In its original form, the Health Belief Model was developed from the phenomenological theory of the "life space" first formulated by the psychologist Kurt Lewin (1951) (see review in Becker, 1974). The developers of the Health Belief Model (Hochbaum, Kegeles, Leventhal, & Rosenstock; see Rosenstock, 1974) were social psychologists who worked within the public health service. Their basic concern was to determine why people avoided preventive measures (such as immunizations) and health screenings even when these were provided at little or no cost. Because the researchers were committed to building social-psychological theory as well as to solving practical problems, they carefully developed their studies of health beliefs within a theoretical framework.

The phenomenological orientation on which the Health Belief Model is based asserts that current dynamics within the individual (rather than historical issues) affect health behavior. It is the person's present beliefs and expectations that influence what he or she will do. In the framework of Lewin's life-space theory, it was assumed that the individual gravitates toward regions that are positively valued and away from regions that are negatively valued. In their framework, these researchers viewed disease as a negatively valued aspect of the life space, and assumed that people avoid that region as long as their avoidance does not cause them to move into an even *more* negative region in the life space. It was hypothesized that an individual will seek to comply with preventive and rehabilitative health regimens as long as the relief from or prevention of disease is seen as more positive than the difficulties encountered and the effort required to attain prevention or cure. Of course, the individual also must feel threatened by the disease (having high susceptibility and severity) and must feel that he or she has some power to overcome it. Thus, in the light of their expectations (for engaging in preventive care or following compliance measures), people make decisions. Becker (1979) has noted that the core dimensions of the Health Belief Model may be found in similar models of decision making under uncertainty, such as those by Tolman (1955), Rotter (1954—the value × expectancy theory), Atkinson and Feather (1966), and Edwards (1961).

Becker (1974) and colleagues (Becker & Maiman, 1975, 1977) have added some additional factors to the Health Belief Model that seek to explain preventive health actions and behaviors related to compliance with treatment. They have focused attention on health motivations, which include *concern* about health matters (the salience of health in general) and the individual's willingness to seek medical care (or conversely, to avoid it). In addition, Becker and colleagues added some important factors that they call "modifying and enabling factors." These include demographic variables (which are sometimes relevant, as we will show in Chapter 7). The modifying factors include primarily the patient's attitudes toward care (including evaluation of the physician, the treatment facility, and the interaction with health professionals). They also include such factors as the structure of care (cost, accessibility, and prior experience with the regimen). In addition, "cues to action" include internal reminders such as the symptoms themselves, and external reminders such as media presentations or reminders from loved ones. These factors were added (by Becker and colleagues) to the basic structure of the Health Belief Model in order to improve the model's predictability (Becker & Maiman, 1975, 1977). Of course, in its revised form, the model does not involve *only* health beliefs.

In terms of the predictability of health behavior, the addition of these new variables enhanced the model's validity, albeit giving the model a certain unwieldiness. The need for these additional variables points to the fact that beliefs and subjective perceptions are simply not sufficient to predict health and compliance behaviors accurately. The additional factors of the health professional–patient relationship, the structure of care, and the barriers and supports to health behavior were added to the model in a somewhat haphazard fashion in order to make it more complete. The additional variables, in many cases, have been assessed with single measures, although they are complex issues. The revision of the Health Belief Model thus contains some poorly conceptualized variables, unclear in their theoretical formulation and weak in their empirical measurement.

In the following discussion, we present a review of the components of the original Health Belief Model, focusing on the specific role played by the patient's perceptions (beliefs) as contributors to health-related behaviors. We include the one component of the revised Health Belief Model (health motivation) that has received strong empirical support. (The original HBM components are perceptions of susceptibility, severity, cost, and benefit.) The other components of the revised model (e.g., cues to action, patients' evaluations of practitioners and medical care, the practitioner-patient relationship) are examined in detail in other chapters within our broad theoretical framework. Despite its limitations, we hold that the Health Belief Model (particularly in its original formulation) functions as a very important component of the broader picture of the determinants of health-related behavior.

The strength of the Health Belief Model lies in its excellent delineation of the important role of the patient's subjective perceptions.

Health Motivation

In the expanded Health Belief Model (Becker & Maiman, 1975), the factor of health motivation represents the patient's degree of interest in and concern about health matters. It focuses on the *value of health concerns* to the individual. A few representative studies demonstrate the usefulness of this concept of health motivation. In a study of mothers' health beliefs and the relationship of these to children's clinic visits, Becker, Nathanson, Drachman, and Kirscht (1977) found that mothers who had an active orientation to preventive care brought their children to more well-child clinic visits than did those who did not have this orientation. Mothers who had a fatalistic attitude, or an antiprevention orientation, more frequently appeared for treatments of illness or accident. In a study of mothers' compliance with a medication regimen for their asthmatic children, Radius et al. (1978) found that mothers' general health motivations correlated significantly and positively with the medical regimen for their children's asthma. These health motivations were comprised of their general concern about their children's health (e.g., worries about the child's health, giving the child vitamins, owning a fever thermometer), as well as their preventive orientation (belief that illness and illness episodes are preventable). Likewise, weight loss of obese children was positively and significantly correlated with their mothers' health motivations (concern about the child's health, engagement in special health practices). Finally, in a field experiment testing the effects of threatening communications and mothers' beliefs on weight change in obese children, Kirscht, Becker, Haefner, and Maiman (1978) found that mothers' general concern with the child's health correlated significantly positively with the child's weight loss at first and last follow-up visit. Thus, some strong evidence suggests that interest, concern, and motivation for health (or the value of health) are strongly related to both preventive measures and compliance with medical treatment regimens. (It is important to note, however, that at least some of the operationalizations of this variable involved a belief in the efficacy of health care which is actually a separate component of the Health Belief Model [benefits]. Health motivation is probably best thought of purely in terms of the value placed on health.)

Perceived Susceptibility

Much empirical research (since the time of the original development of the Health Belief Model) has demonstrated the existence of positive correlations between feelings of personal susceptibility to illness and the enactment of preventive behaviors and compliance. Belief in susceptibility to a specific disease has been found to correlate with a person's participation in screening for that disease (for breast cancer: Fink, Shapiro, & Roester, 1972; for cervical cancer: Kegeles, 1969; Flach, 1960; for other cancer: Haefner & Kirscht, 1970; for tuberculosis: Haefner & Kirscht, 1970; Hochbaum, 1956; for heart disease: Haefner & Kirscht, 1970; and for Tay Sachs disease: Becker et al., 1975). Belief in susceptibility also correlates with obtaining immunization against various diseases (Glasser, 1958; Leventhal, Hochbaum & Rosenstock, 1960; Ogionwo, 1973; Rosenstock, Derryberry, & Carriger, 1959), as well as engaging in various other preventive measures such as bringing a child to a clinic for preventive care (Becker et al., 1977). In addition, once a person has contracted a particular disease, his or her feelings of resusceptibility tend to correlate positively with engaging in methods for preventing another attack (Heinzelmann, 1962; Elling, Whittemore, & Green, 1960; Becker, Drachman & Kirscht, 1972). In other compliance studies, beliefs in susceptibility have been found to correlate with following a medication regimen for hypertension (Kirscht & Rosenstock, 1977), adhering to a diet (among obese children: Maiman et al., 1977; Becker et al., 1977; Kirscht et al., 1978), and following a medication regimen to prevent or control asthma attacks (Becker et al., 1978). (Two studies have brought this finding into question, however [Gordis, Markowitz, & Lilienfeld, 1969; Tash, O'Shea, & Cohen, 1969]. In these studies, individuals who complied with treatment and health services were found to rate their susceptibility to disease *lower*—instead of higher, as would be expected—than did their counterparts who did not comply. In these retrospective studies, it is likely that the noncompliers judged their vulnerability to disease on the basis of their having ignored the medical recommendations. In general, *prospective* studies have found that patients' beliefs in their susceptibility to disease correlate positively with their later compliance. Prospective studies have been carried out only in the past few years, however, and they still constitute a considerably smaller proportion of the studies than would be ideal.)

Perceived Severity

Medical estimates of the actual severity of disease are typically not predictive of patient cooperation with treatment regimens (Haynes, 1979). Individuals with medically serious conditions are not more likely to comply with physicians' recommendations than those with benign, innocuous conditions. What matters in influencing the patient's behavior is his or her *belief* in the severity of the medical problem that he or she presently has or might contract as a result of abandoning the recommended treatment. The patient's belief in the severity of disease is significantly correlated with obtaining dental care (Kegeles, 1963; Tash, O'Shea & Cohen, 1969), taking measures to prevent accidents (Suchman, 1967), seeking medical care in response to a variety of symptoms (Battistella, 1971), and bringing a child to the doctor for well-child, prevention-oriented visits (Becker et al., 1977).

Becker (1979) noted that some studies have examined perceptions of severity in relationship to the use of screening programs and found no linear relationship. He suggested that this may have resulted because very low or very high levels of belief in severity (and associated low or high fear and anxiety) may interfere with the recollection of the regimen instructions, as well as with efforts to follow those instructions (Ley & Spelman, 1967). (We will consider the effects of fear-arousal on patient compliance further in Chapter 6, when we examine fear-arousing persuasive messages.)

Perceptions of Costs and Benefits

Not surprisingly, compliance is influenced by patients' perceptions of the "costs" associated with prevention and with following treatment. This tends to be true of a wide variety of compliance criteria, including the receipt of immunizations. Rosenstock, Derryberry, and Carriger (1959), for example, found that regardless of other beliefs and other factors (such as considerations of susceptibility), people would not obtain polio vaccinations if they doubted the safety of those vaccinations. Belief in the "cost" of medical care and preventive regimens thus involves more than the belief that the regimen will be financially costly. "Cost" also involves pain, discomfort, and risk. These latter concerns are classic reasons for the avoidance of dental care (Antonovsky & Kats, 1970; Kegeles, 1963; Tash, O'Shea, & Cohen, 1969).

Haynes' (1979) review examined various forms of cost and their relation to compliance. Financial cost (Alpert, 1964; Antonovsky & Kats, 1970; Donabedian & Rosenfeld, 1964) and negative side effects (sometimes, though not typically: see Chapter 7) (Caldwell, 1970; Kirscht & Rosenstock, 1977; Weintraub, Wu, & Lasagna, 1973) tended to be cited by patients as factors that interfere with compliance. Similarly, in a recent study of attitudes toward prevention, it was found that the majority of patients randomly surveyed in a family-practice center were willing to obtain preventive health services, but only about half of them were willing to spend any money for those services (David & Boldt, 1980). As Haynes (1979) has pointed out, compliance decreases as the overall complexity and cost of the regimen increase. Of course, costs are typically evaluated subjectively and are assessed by the patient in relationship to his or her existing resources for dealing with the requirements of the treatment regimen.

Related to this issue is the fact that patients' beliefs in the benefits of care (including the efficacy of the treatment) are important predictors of compliance and preventive health behavior. For example, the patient's belief that a screening procedure can actually identify a disease in its early, treatable stages is positively correlated with the patient's participation in screening. This has been found to be true for cervical cancer (Kegeles, 1969), tuberculosis (Hochbaum, 1956), and other forms of cancer (Haefner & Kirscht, 1970). Those who believe in the preventive capacity of immunizations are also more likely to obtain them (Becker & Maiman, 1975; Ogionwo, 1973).

A patient's compliance with medical regimens or with various preventive measures tends to be influenced by his or her belief in their efficacy (Donabedian & Rosenfeld, 1964; Feinstein, 1976). This is true, for example, of beliefs in the ability of penicillin to prevent the occurrence of rheumatic fever (Elling, Whittemore, & Green, 1960; Heinzelmann, 1962; Becker, Drachman, & Kirscht, 1972). In general, patients who expressed strong positive beliefs about the value of adherence to their own doctors' instructions (that is, believed that those instructions would help to reduce health risks) were more compliant than those who did not. This was also true of individuals who believed in the benefits of medical intervention in general (Kirscht & Rosenstock, 1977; Becker et al., 1977; Becker et al., 1978; Hartman & Becker, 1978).

THE PRACTITIONER'S ROLE IN HEALTH BELIEFS

It is important to note an important issue that was emphasized during the development of and early research on the Health Belief Model (Becker, 1974). The physician or other health professional, in understanding the role of beliefs in medical care, compliance, and preventive health behavior, is in an excellent position to change those beliefs (and the attitudes that result from them) by tailoring interventions to suit the particular needs of each patient. While the Health Belief Model does not by itself provide a sufficiently complete basis for understanding health behavior and for planning intervention strategies, it does identify several crucially important determinants of health behavior (Berkanovic, 1976).

The findings of research on the Health Belief Model are not independent of but rather are quite closely connected with the issues discussed in earlier chapters on the communication of information and on rapport in the practitioner-patient relationship. For example, in attempting to influence patients' beliefs regarding their susceptibility to and the severity of a disease, the health professional might provide some facts and statistics on the prevalence of disease and help the patient to achieve a realistic appraisal of them. Some realistic appraisals of the costs and benefits of care might also be provided, toward the goal of altering these health beliefs that affect behavior. Patients' motivations to comply, their beliefs in the efficacy of medicine, and their trust in their own individual practitioner are likely to be influenced by the quality of the practitioner-patient relationship. This relationship was considered in detail in Chapter 3 but its relevance may become fully clear only after we examine both the role of patient attitudes and beliefs in their health behavior and the role of the practitioner-patient relationship in changing those attitudes and beliefs. This issue will be considered further in Chapter 6.

Cues to Action

The revised version of the Health Belief Model, as outlined by Becker and Maiman (1975), includes a component called "cues to action." These cues include such diverse entities as mass-media campaigns, advice from others, one's own symptoms, reminder postcards and calls from the practitioner, the illness of family members, and newspaper articles, to name but a few. A cue to action is anything that prompts the individual to engage in a health behavior. It can be one of two types: an internal cue (such as a bodily state or symptom) or an external cue (such as a reminder). Cues to action are dependent upon *perceptions* because they serve to "remind" the person of the need to engage in a particular health behavior, and help to prompt that behavior. Cues to action are, however, not really perceptions or beliefs such as we are considering in this chapter. Cues to action do not "filter" data, as do patients' beliefs and perceptions; cues to action *are* the data. As such, various cues to action are considered elsewhere, notably in Chapter 7, where specific supports for behavior change are examined.

THE LOCUS OF CONTROL

An important component of the Health Belief Model involves the individual's belief in the efficacy of health-oriented actions. The success of a program of preventive health behavior, and the achievement of compliance with a treatment regimen depend, to a significant degree, on the target individual's belief that his or her state of health is within the realm of control (be it the individual's control, or that of the practitioner). The belief in a certain degree of correlation between one's behavior and its outcomes is the basis of the notion of locus of control, derived from the social-learning theory of psychologist Julian Rotter (1954). Rotter's theory states that a person's potential for enacting a behavior (for example, his intention to take medication) is jointly affected by his expectancy that the behavior will lead to a particular outcome (e.g., that it will control hypertension and prevent stroke) and the value of that outcome. The value of an outcome such as controlling hypertension and preventing stroke is likely (as Becker and others have shown in the Health Belief Model) to be at least partially dependent upon the person's belief in the severity of the disease and his own susceptibility to it. The value is also dependent upon the person's motivation toward and concern for health as well as on his belief in the degree to which benefits of the health behavior (e.g., peace of mind) outweigh the costs (e.g., remembering to take the medication). As Becker (1979) noted, however, one aspect of perceived benefits does involve a belief in the efficacy of treatment. Thus, the Health Belief Model involves components of a "value × expectancy" theory of health behavior, although these are not completely developed or explicitly spelled out.

Locus of control is a complex psychological construct that has been well studied both generally and as it relates to health specifically. The concept is important because in order to understand fully the importance of beliefs in the efficacy of care, we must first examine the notion of *generalized expectancy*. This involves the expectation that reinforcement is under one's own individual control (termed "internal locus of control"), or, in contrast, the expectation that reinforcement is under the control of outside forces such as fate, chance, or powerful others (termed "external locus of control"). If an individual's locus of control is considered along with his or her health values and is combined with social-normative factors, it is likely to result in an accurate prediction of behavioral intentions.

The locus-of-control construct is proving to be quite important in empirical research on health behavior. Wallston and Wallston (1978) reviewed a great deal of research on the relationship of Rotter's (1966) measure of locus of control (a scale measuring generalized expectancies) and various forms of health behaviors. Because social-normative factors were not included, and because various barriers may have prevented the actual enactment of the health behaviors measured, each correlation between locus of control and health behavior was typically low to moderate in size. These findings were suggestive, however, of the importance of locus of control in a comprehensive model of compliance and health behavior.

Many studies have shown that individuals with an internal locus of control (who generally believe that reinforcement is contingent upon an individual's own behavior) are more likely to be nonsmokers than smokers (James et al., 1965; Straits & Sechrest, 1963) and to quit smoking or modify their smoking behavior (Steffy et al., 1970). It is interesting to note that the locus of control construct allowed differentiation among people according to their smoking behavior without a need to consider other factors such as values. Wallston and Wallston (1978) suggest tailoring treatments for smoking to individuals on the basis of their locus of control, since their beliefs in the determinants of their health—their own control versus that of fate or powerful others—may vary so much.

Research on the use of contraception also suggests that locus of control is a good predictor of health behavior. Users of contraceptives have been found to be more internal in their locus of control than nonusers (Mac-

Donald, 1970; Lundy, 1972; Phares, 1976), although this is not an unequivocal finding. Locus of control is also a factor in weight and weight loss. Overweight individuals are more likely to be external in their locus of control (O'Bryan, 1972; Manno & Marston, 1972).

In a self-control weight-loss program, Balch and Ross (1975) found that individuals with an internal locus of control were more likely to complete the weight-reduction program and lost more weight than those with an external locus-of-control orientation. Other researchers failed to find differences, however (Wallston et al., 1976), which suggests that more research in this area is needed. It is particularly important to evaluate a suggestion by Phares (1969) that weight-loss programs might best be developed for individuals partly on the basis of their locus of control. It might be particularly useful to gear programs for "internals" to self-control, and to gear programs for "externals" to social-normative factors and support from others. A study by Saltzer (1978; reviewed below) suggests the potential usefulness of this approach.

Internal locus of control has also been found to be related to greater (self-reported) seat-belt use (Williams, 1972a), and preventive dental care (Williams, 1972b). Among already ill patients, locus of control has been a good predictor of sick-role behavior. Seeman and Evans (1962) found that tuberculosis patients with an internal locus of control knew more about their condition, were more inquisitive with health professionals, and were less satisfied with the amount of information they received about their condition.

Wallston and Wallston (1978) report that the relationship between locus of control and compliance behavior is somewhat weak and sometimes equivocal. As we noted earlier, this is probably because locus of control must be combined with the value of health (general or specific) and with social-normative factors in order for it to have a substantial degree of predictive power. The Health Belief Model contains both value and expectancy variables, but the measures of efficacy (generalized or specifically related to health) are typically weak. The combination of generalized and specific locus-of-control (expectancy) measures and health-value measures is likely to achieve a better prediction of preventive and sick-role behavior than health-belief and locus-of-control measures alone. The study of value × expectancy theory and its relationship to prevention and compliance is, therefore, very important in the pursuit of psychological factors that influence health behavior.

Measures of Locus of Control

The Health Locus of Control Scale (HLC) was developed in a similar way to Rotter's IE scale to measure locus-of-control expectancy as it specifically relates to health (Wallston et al., 1976). The Health Locus of Control Scale was designed to focus on beliefs regarding an individual's ability to exert control over his or her health, versus the dependence of health on uncontrollable factors such as fate, chance, or powerful others. Conceptually, Health Locus of Control has been valuable, but empirically it has been somewhat disappointing for a number of reasons. The original scale reliability of .72 dropped to between .40 and .54 in subsequent research. Later, too, it was found that the scale contained a number of distinct dimensions. Also, the HLC contained scales that included beliefs about personal as well as general control over health. The personal control ideology involved the individual's belief that he himself could control his health. General control involved the belief that health is, in general, controllable. A revision of the HLC to a multidimensional Health Locus of Control Scale (MHLC) (Wallston, Wallston, & DeVellis, 1978) has proven to be a more promising approach methodologically as well as conceptually. The MHLC reflects three dimensions of beliefs: *internal* health locus of control (belief that one can control many aspects of health with one's own behavior; for example—"I am directly responsible for my health"); *powerful others* health locus of control (belief that health professionals keep one healthy, or that they control health, and that regular contact with them, following their orders, etc., is the best way to stay healthy). The final dimension is *chance* health locus of control which indicates the individual's belief that his health or illness is a chance happening. This scale, with three aspects of expectancy, has considerably higher reliability than the HLC. Research on the validity of these three aspects of the construct of locus of control, however, is still somewhat limited. Wallston, Wallston, and DeVellis (1978) suggest that the eventual use of this scale in examining delay in presentation of suspicious signs of cancer, reactions to side effects of drugs, and trust in the physician might prove quite valuable. As these researchers note, belief in an internal health locus of control may require interventions for health-behavior change that involve self-direction, while an emphasis on decision making by health professionals might be best for those with a powerful-other locus of control. Of course, those who believe that health is mostly a matter of chance may fail to comply with any approach.

The Differential Treatment of Internals and Externals

Measures of health locus of control are beginning to prove beneficial for determining the most effective methods for changing health behaviors. A few studies have examined the potential effectiveness of such an approach. Cromwell et al. (1977), for example, studied participation of myocardial infarction patients in self-treatment. It was found that those in "congruent conditions" (that is, internals given high participation, and externals given low participation) fared better physically than patients in incongruent conditions. Saltzer

(1978) studied the role of personal attitudes and social pressures as they interacted with internal-external locus of control to influence weight loss. Subjects were asked to indicate their "weight locus of control" as well as their pattern of personal attitudes and social norms with regard to health and physical appearance. The finding was that "there was a consistent pattern of personal attitude as the stronger component of behavioral intentions for the internals, and subjective norms as the stronger component of behavioral intentions for the externals" (Saltzer, 1978, p. 124).

In concluding this discussion of the concept and measurement of efficacy expectations, we suggest the need for much further research on the relation of generalized (as well as specifically health-related) locus of control, particularly in concert with measures of values toward the goal of understanding the formation of behavioral intentions. These issues require understanding in order that appropriate interventions might be planned to change health behavior. This is an important area for attention from psychologists who are oriented to health research, as well as those particularly interested in the impact of attitudes, beliefs, and expectations on behavior.

ATTITUDES AND HEALTH BEHAVIORS

Earlier in this chapter, we outlined the Theory of Reasoned Action proposed by Ajzen and Fishbein (1980). According to this theory, beliefs combine with expectations to form attitudes. An attitude is an affective response to a person, object, or concept. Specifically, an attitude toward a health behavior is a judgment based on beliefs and expectations regarding the goal to which the behavior will lead. An attitude is determined by evaluation of the behavior as positive or negative combined with the expectation for its attainment. Attitudes may correlate with behaviors but they do not bring them about singlehandedly. Rather, attitudes combine with social-normative influences (each weighted by its relative importance) to produce intentions to perform the behavior.

How do attitudes in this framework fare in predictions of health behavior intentions? Although the research has not been very extensive in this area, positive evaluations of health behavior tend, *when combined with social-normative influences*, to be good predictors of intentions to engage in a variety of health behaviors (for example, family planning [Fishbein, et al., 1980; Smetana & Adler, 1980] and weight loss [Saltzer, 1981]). In fact, the joint consideration of beliefs (and related attitudes) and social norms in determining intentions to perform health behaviors has resulted in much better predictions than in the cases in which beliefs or expectations alone were used to predict behaviors. We will consider this point again a number of times throughout the remaining chapters of this book. The present chapter has been devoted to an examination of empirical evidence for the influence of psychological variables such as health beliefs and locus of control on health behaviors. As we have seen, however, a more complex framework is needed to consider the many factors that might influence the patient's intention and subsequent ability to carry out a particular health behavior.

AN EMPHASIS ON BELIEFS AND ATTITUDES: IMPLICATIONS FOR RESEARCH AND PRACTICE

By using the Health Belief Model and other psychological constructs examined in this chapter, we have sought to explain preventive health and compliance behaviors partly in terms of the beliefs and attitudes held by patients. We have emphasized the need to combine such cognitive factors with other variables such as social norms. We have seriously questioned the validity of approaches to patient health behavior that posit a single diagnosis, cause, and treatment of noncompliance. Health-related behavior and compliance with medical regimens have multidimensional causes.

The Health Belief Model and the Theory of Reasoned Action fulfill the important function of helping to organize and present for research examination many hypothesized connections between patients' behaviors and their thoughts and feelings. The phenomenological orientation at the core of such an analysis of thoughts and feelings forces researchers and practitioners to stop for a moment and consider the distinct possibility that compliance or noncompliance represents a rational choice made by the patient. Many writers have referred to noncompliance as "irrational behavior," particularly in the light of the difficulties that the patient may have gone through to obtain a medical recommendation (Stone, 1979). Yet, within a phenomenological orientation, it makes perfectly good sense for a patient to be noncompliant if he is unconvinced that a particular illness is serious (within his own value system), or believes that he himself is unlikely to contract the disease (probably for reasons unknown to the practitioner). It is also not surprising that the patient, who believes that the costs of treatment in time, money, or embarrassment are not worth the trouble to him in contrast to his evaluation of the benefits, will fail to comply. An approach to patient compliance that emphasizes rationality and patient choice also suggests the probable value of interventions (for health-behavior change) that focus on beliefs and attitudes. While in the field of public health (and other areas of study concerned with health behavior) few of these interventions have been undertaken (Becker, 1979), in other fields, notably social psychology, research evidence abounds to support the fact that attitudes and beliefs in general can indeed be altered. Methods for change have been studied extensively. (These methods are examined in Chapter 6, and their application to health practice is carefully considered.) Becker (1979) has noted, however, that little research has been devoted to changing health beliefs and attitudes specifically, and to determining the precise quantity and quality of effort needed to achieve a successful intervention. This is an important issue that deserves serious research consideration.

Methodological Issues in Research

As we have noted, the role of beliefs and attitudes appears to be promising and important, particularly when combined with other factors such as social norms and social roles in patients' lives, and various behavioral barriers and supports. Yet, some methodological considerations continue to limit the faith that can be placed in these phenomenological variables.

Future research on health beliefs, for example, should consider more varied health settings, different populations, and different illnesses (particularly chronic). The generality of the Health Belief Model in fact remains to be demonstrated (Becker, 1979). The Health Belief Model has been, by far, the most heavily researched of those that involve a phenomenological approach but its empirical investigations have been primarily retrospective. That is, patients have been asked about their beliefs (in severity, susceptibility, cost, benefits) *after* they have engaged (or not engaged) in the prescribed health behaviors. In his review of research on the Health Belief Model, Becker (1979) noted that there exist only a few major prospective studies. These prospective studies have provided preliminary evidence to support the Health Belief Model. At present, however, there is too little data available to answer some important questions regarding its validity (Taylor, 1979). Specifically, it can be argued that retrospective data demonstrate only that beliefs and behavior co-vary. Behavior might just as easily cause beliefs as vice versa. Indeed, at least two psychological theories would predict an effect of behaviors on attitudes and beliefs. Festinger's (1957) theory of cognitive dissonance notes that individuals adjust their beliefs to be consistent with their behaviors in order to avoid the discomfort of cognitive dissonance. Thus, a person might decide that he is susceptible to a particular disease in order to provide himself with some justification for having complied with the related health regimen. Bem (1967) has argued that this resolution might be explained simply by the fact that people observe their own behavior and infer their attitudes and beliefs from it. They may decide that since they have complied, they surely must believe that compliance behavior has some benefit. Thus, health behavior might change as a result of some factor that is unrelated to beliefs (such as giving up smoking to please a loved one or to save money) and the belief (that smoking is dangerous to one's health) may then be adopted.

Because of the possibility that behavior may bring about changes of attitude and belief, it is important that experiments be conducted in order to demonstrate the validity of the Health Belief Model (Becker, 1979). Experimental studies should attempt to modify one or more of the phenomenological variables prior to the observation of the subsequent health behaviors. Becker (1979) and Taylor (1979) have noted that this research should have high priority considering the theories and empirical evidence that suggest that behaviors cause attitudes. Such a possibility, of course, seriously questions the contention of the Health Belief Model that health beliefs bring about health-related behaviors. This issue must be resolved.

It should not be inferred from our methodological discussion that the Health Belief Model's validity has never been supported empirically. On the contrary, some prospective (Leventhal et al., 1960; Kegeles, 1963) and experimental studies (Haefner & Kirscht, 1970; Kegeles, 1969) have been conducted and were found to be supportive of the predictions made by the Health Belief Model. It is quite clear, however, that more evidence is needed before principles of the Health Belief Model (or of any approaches that emphasize beliefs and attitudes) can be put into practice in health care with confidence.

Conceptual Issues for Future Research

The developers of the Health Belief Model have been the literature's foremost proponents of the need for a multidimensional approach to health behavior. In fact, they have emphasized that beliefs are by no means the sole (or even the major) determinants of health behaviors (Becker, 1979; Becker & Maiman, 1977). Additional elements such as the practitioner-patient relationship, social-normative factors, interpersonal expectations, and the lay-referral network (see Chapter 5) have been identified as important co-determinants of health behaviors.

Proponents of the Health Belief Model do not make clear, however, precisely how patients' beliefs might fit into a multidimensional model of health behavior. Such clarification is crucial to understanding the role played by health beliefs in patients' preventive and compliance behaviors, and to assessing the degree of impact on health behavior that might be expected from changing health beliefs. Within the framework of the Ajzen and Fishbein (1980) model, the interplay among health beliefs, attitudes, and social norms (considered in Chapter 5) in determining a patient's intention to enact a particular behavior can be systematically examined. Of course, whether or not the individual is actually able to translate the intention into behavior will be dependent upon his or her behavior-change skills and upon the supports and barriers encountered in behavior-change attempts. The predictability and modifiability of intentions suggest some important implications for efforts to change behavior.

The Health Belief Model is also limited because it deals only with disease avoidance and does not consider motivation for various aspects of health that are independent of the threat of specific disease. A study of attitudes *toward* various health practices is thus an important goal, for some crucial questions presently remain unanswered. To what extent, for example, do people engage in exercise simply because it "feels good," or avoid obesity for reasons of aesthetics or distaste for an obese appearance? Such attitudinal factors must be understood not only for their theoretical importance and for the enhancement of empirical prediction, but also to promote the design of more effective interventions to improve health behaviors.

Research on attitudes and beliefs in predicting and understanding health behavior has generally been limited to the study of one-time commitments or fairly short-term compliance behaviors. No studies to date have followed chronically ill or even health-conscious people for many years, assessing their changing beliefs and health attitudes, and determining how these co-vary with behavior. Although the primary focus of health behavior research is to promote long-term compliance and lifetime commitment to health, the difficulties of carrying out longitudinal studies have so far precluded a complete understanding of the achievement of long-term change. These answers are now desperately needed.

Based on Lewin's Field Theory (Lewin, 1951), the Health Belief Model contains an important basic assumption—that health is valued positively and illness valued negatively by all individuals. It is hypothesized that people seek to avoid diseases to which they feel themselves susceptible, and that they believe are severe. It may not always be the case, however, that a person who believes himself to be at risk for the development or exacerbation of a medical problem will engage in behaviors designed to reduce the risk. Under some conditions, illness is valued positively (Mechanic, 1968, 1972). Illness may serve to exempt an individual from some (possibly long-term) obligation (such as caring for a disabled parent, or keeping a job, or going to school). Consciously or unconsciously, the individual prefers illness to fulfilling the obligation or asserting his decision not to do so. Illness might also bring with it secondary gains in the form of attention, sympathy, compensation benefits, the satisfaction of self-destructive desires, or a socially acceptable outlet for emotional problems (Mechanic, 1968). Examination of this possibility is likely to provide greater insight into behavioral responses that seem to have minimal or even a negative relationship to health beliefs. Relatedly, the point at which an individual's health beliefs begin to undermine his or her willingness and ability to take health action is not known. A person's belief in his own susceptibility to disease and in its severity may be so strong that his fear and anxiety give rise to massive denial. This is particularly likely when the disease is one as emotionally charged as cancer. The literature on delay in seeking care for symptoms of cancer (Antonovsky & Hartman, 1974) and myocardial infarction (Gentry, 1979) points to the important role played by patient anxiety in avoiding diagnosis and treatment. A complete understanding of the role played by *all* levels of perceived susceptibility and severity (including the very high levels) in seeking versus avoiding health care is needed if such a major problem as patient delay is to be overcome. The manner in which health beliefs and attitudes operate under conditions of threat or actual occurrence of serious illness is therefore an important area for study.

Much of the latter part of this chapter has been concerned with recommendations for research on the topic of health beliefs and their relationship to behavior. A major reason for this emphasis involves the large number of important questions that remain to be answered. The connection between attitudes, beliefs, and behaviors in general has been an important subject of concern to social psychologists since as early as the 1930s, but as yet a limited amount of research on these psychological constructs has been devoted to understanding health behaviors and responses to medical treatment. Only very recently have psychologists begun to examine issues of health, and to apply their knowledge of beliefs and attitudes to solving problems in the health field. Scientific psychological knowledge about beliefs and attitudes may be extensive, but precisely how these constructs operate in the special world of health and medical care is yet to be discovered.

As we will see in the next chapter, the constructs of norms, roles, and social values have been examined in the realm of health care. These constructs belong not only to the domain of psychology, but have also been of major concern to sociologists who have examined medical issues since the initial development of the field (Kendall & Reader, 1972). Thus, the relation of social influences, norms, and roles to health, illness, and medical care has been studied fairly extensively. Therefore, conclusions about medical care and health can presently be drawn somewhat more comfortably with regard to social factors than with regard to attitudes and beliefs. While research on these latter psychological constructs is likely to support in the medical realm the predictions based on general psychological research on these constructs, only further empirical study will determine this for certain.

5

Norms and Compliance: The Effect of the Patient's Culture

THREE PATIENTS

In his classic book, *The Doctor and His Patient*, sociologist Samuel Bloom (1963) described Mrs. Tomasetti, a patient whose compliance behavior was enmeshed with her culture. Mrs. Tomasetti, age 55, was a diabetic whose difficulty in following her low-carbohydrate, low-fat diet was a major source of distress to her physicians. She faithfully followed a complex regimen of medication, but her diet posed a significant danger to her health. A medical student assigned to her care found that Mrs. Tomasetti's ethnic background was of great significance. A woman of Southern Italian background, Mrs. Tomasetti valued food highly. Eating played a central role in her life; it brought solace and comfort. Heaviness was associated with health. Mrs. Tomasetti also lived in an atmosphere that encouraged eating. She provided all of the meals for her large family of children and grandchildren. Family members and friends often dropped by to visit her in her kitchen. Her restricted diet was therefore a threat to full and spontaneous involvement in her social network.

In Chapter 4 we introduced Mrs. O'Rourke, who was described by Zola (1973). Mrs. O'Rourke's head injury remained untreated when it first occurred, even though it caused her pain and some blurred vision. Her decision to seek care resulted neither from her experience of pain from her head injury nor from her fear of damage to her sight. Instead, Mrs. O'Rourke sought medical care because of a concern for her appearance; someone told her that her eyelid was drooping.

Finally, Oscar Smithgard, age 48, smokes heavily. His doctor has warned him that his weight and genetic history combine with his heavy cigarette smoking to predispose him to a heart attack. Smoking also increases his risk of lung cancer. Despite his sporadic efforts to quit, however, Oscar continues to smoke more than two packs of cigarettes a day. His wife and teen-age children also smoke. In fact, in the Smithgard family, cigarette smoking is an acceptable way to "calm your nerves." The family members are in need of a coping mechanism, for they are almost constantly in conspicuous conflict about issues ranging from financial problems to discipline of the youngest child. The longstanding marital conflict now affects them all. Since smoking is accepted (in fact encouraged) in the family, and since it fulfills an important need in Oscar's most intimate social group, it is likely that Oscar will find it very difficult to quit smoking.

The health behavior of these three patients—Mrs. Tomasetti, Mrs. O'Rourke, and Mr. Smithgard—is not completely under the control of their own thoughts, attitudes, and beliefs. Their behavior is also guided by the beliefs and expectations of other people. Mrs. Tomasetti, for example, believes her doctors when they tell her that uncontrolled diabetes is dangerous. She feels susceptible to the complications that her disease might bring about, and she believes that the health consequences are severe. She believes in the efficacy of the proposed treatment. She takes her medication faithfully but the diet is much more difficult to follow. Primarily because of her Southern Italian background, Mrs. Tomasetti derives much of her identity within her family from her reputation as a good cook. Her kitchen is warm and comfortable, and there she engages in social exchange with her family and friends. Although influence by her ethnic group on her behavior is by no means immutable, altering her behavior to go against cultural values and expectations is likely to be very difficult.

Mr. Smithgard's beliefs are equally strong, and are contrary to his behaviors. The death of a friend from lung cancer convinced him of the validity of the warnings he had heard about smoking. His own chronic cough also warns of the seriousness of potential health problems and his susceptibility to them. Mr. Smithgard's beliefs and attitudes toward smoking are negative, and so he should be able to quit. His family, however, is a very powerful force holding him back.

Mrs. O'Rourke's situation illustrates a somewhat different issue, although it too demonstrates the influence, albeit indirect, of culture and social norms on health behavior. Mrs. O'Rourke looked to other people for an evaluation of her physical condition—a judgment about whether or not it required medical attention. Her decision to seek care was prompted not by how she felt or by what she believed, but rather by other people's evaluations of her appearance. Mrs. O'Rourke's self-definition of illness was prompted by social-normative factors.

In Chapter 4, we examined the influence of patients' beliefs and attitudes on their decisions to seek medical care and to follow their treatment regimens. In this chapter, we consider another aspect of the perceptions and beliefs of patients—the expectations of other people. We examine social expectations and patients' attempts to accommodate social demands. This social-normative perspective helps to explain, among other phenomena, the influence of social expectations on the individual's claim to be ill, the factors prompting the individual's exemption from usual social obligations, and the role played by other people in influencing patient cooperation with prescribed treatment regimens. Throughout this chapter, we will demonstrate that health behavior is not determined solely by the individual's psychological characteristics, beliefs, and attitudes. Rather, we will see that health behavior also derives from the person's experience of his social world—what he believes other people want him to do, and how central those people are to his self-definition and self-evaluation.

Before we consider health behavior specifically, let us examine some general background issues concerning the influence of other people on an individual's behavior. With this background, we will be better able to understand the influence of family, friends, social class, and ethnic group on cooperation with medical regimens.

THE SOCIAL GROUP

Socialization

Socialization is a process by which persons (as children or adults) acquire the knowledge, skills, and dispositions that identify them as members of a particular social group or society. A social group is a collection of other persons to whom the individual is related or compared in some way (for example, age, sex, social class, neighborhood, club, or family). The concept of socialization is basic to our discussion of the individual's relationship to others because it refers to the process by which an individual adopts the values and behaviors of other people (Brim & Wheeler, 1966; Hogan, 1973). Through the process of childhood socialization, a child's behavior is influenced and controlled so that it will be acceptable to others. Socializing agents have a high frequency of contact with the child, and by means of rewards and punishments they orient the child toward particular values and patterns of behavior.

Socialization does not end after childhood. Through complex interpersonal relationships, each person develops as a member of a group (or groups) and the individual's behavior becomes acceptable to group members. According to psychology's social learning theorists (Bandura & Walters, 1963;

Merton & Rossi, 1957; Brim & Wheeler, 1966), any group can have tremendous control over an individual's motivations and behavior because of the rewards and punishments associated with the process of socialization. Throughout childhood, the individual has been reinforced for conformity to others' expectations. Then, years later, he is motivated to live up to the standards of the group, and his sense of well-being and satisfaction depends upon conformity. The individual's self-appraisal depends upon the evaluation of others, primarily because of their former control over rewards and punishments. The grown individual remains subject to the desires of the group (for example, the culture, social class, or family) because his self-esteem depends heavily upon fulfilling its desires.

Norms

The group's control manifests itself in the form of a group *norm*. Any value shared by members of a culture that acquires the status of a group "standard" is called a "norm" (Rokeach, 1973). A norm is a commonly occurring group pattern of behavior and/or belief. It comes to be accepted and expected among members. Objects of attitude, desire, and need are compared by members to the group norm to determine whether or not they are acceptable. Conformity with the group by means of adherence to the norm is (usually subtly) rewarded. Nonconformity is punished. For example, marriage to someone outside one's ethnic group may bring subtle criticism (though perhaps not overt ostracism). Likewise, dieting to become slender when one's culture values overeating and heaviness might incur a similar response.

The Pressures toward Uniformity

Groups have enormous power to control the thoughts and behaviors of their members. Social psychologist Leon Festinger (1950, 1954) argued that people grant such power to groups by relying on them for social information, particularly when "objective" checks on reality are not available or would be too costly to obtain. The individual thus is not required to engage in the behavior in order to find out what others' reactions will be. Instead, by consensus, members of the group define that reaction.

Festinger (1954) posited people's intrinsic need to validate their view of issues that defy direct objective appraisal. Thus, they turn to the views held by others. Because there are no objective standards for such, people actively seek social evaluation of their behavior, beliefs, and values. They compare these to the norms of their culture—their social class, sex, age group, family, and so on. This form of evaluation is termed "social comparison." By means of social comparison, the individual reaches a state of agreement with the group.

Festinger (1950) also noted that groups are motivated to achieve uniformity because cohesiveness is necessary if the group is to reach a goal. Group members attempt to persuade one another in order to achieve the conformity necessary for the continued existence of the group. Thus, the group pressures dissenters toward agreement and cohesiveness.

The individual's use of group norms for the purpose of identifying an external reality is called "informational influence." On the other hand, conformity to group pressures that arises out of fear of disagreeing with others and bringing on their disapproval is called "normative influence." Research on conformity (e.g., Asch, 1952, 1958; Deutsch & Gerard, 1955) has found that both types of influence are in operation (Harvey & Smith, 1977). Individuals rely on both the approval of others in their group and the information provided by the judgments of others.

Symbolic Interaction

The perspective of a *symbolic-interaction* approach to human behavior emphasizes the importance of group norms, but at the same time regards the individual as a creative, thinking entity rather than as one who reacts mechanically to the influence of social forces (Cockerham, 1981). The symbolic-interactionist perspective views society from the standpoint of the person's interaction with other people (Mead, 1934; Blumer, 1969; Charon, 1979). This approach assumes that human behavior is directed by the person on the basis of shared, communicated symbolic meanings (Denzin, 1970). Interactional behavior between persons results from a creative process, and the person is *not* at the mercy of the social environment but rather acts upon and changes it.

The philosopher/social psychologist George Herbert Mead conceptualized the self as an entity that is formed and developed as a result of interaction with other people in society (Blumer, 1969). It is only in relation to others that an individual can define himself or herself. Related to this, Charles H. Cooley (1964) formulated the symbolic-interaction notion of the "looking glass self." He maintained that a person's self-concept is the result of social interaction in which he sees himself reflected in other people's attitudes toward him. In other words, we see ourselves as others see us, and we imagine their judgments of us. We also experience some feelings about ourselves as a result of how we are reflected by others. Thus, symbolic interactionists view the group as an entity with which the individual interacts actively and from which he derives a sense of identity and self-worth. Other people serve an important function in defining the individual.

In the symbolic-interaction framework, reality is not something possessed by the group for which the individual searches. Instead, whether or not a particular behavior is "good" or "right" or "appropriate" depends upon an ongoing process of definition, interpretation, and response. Reality is socially constructed by the perceptions and actions of all the individuals involved. Thus, in this framework, the individual continually interacts with members of the group in order that they may create a shared reality. This symbolic-interaction framework suggests, too, that social norms can be altered by means of active involvement by the individual in his or her social group.

We see, then, that the group is considered by social psychologists and sociologists to be of central importance although the precise reasons proposed for the group's importance vary. All tend to agree, however, that the group provides the individual with a self-definition, a basis for social comparison, and/or the information needed to make a decision. In addition, once it has served as the socializing agent, the individual's social group may continue to exert considerable power over him or her throughout life.

A Broader Perspective on Norms

The relationship between what people feel they *ought* to do and what they do is by no means simple. In everyday routine, according to many theorists (e.g., Hewitt, 1979), people rarely focus on social norms alone as determinants of their behavior. Rather, people are also concerned with achieving certain valued goals. Their behavior is determined partly by norms but also by their own beliefs and attitudes. In Chapter 4 we found that beliefs and attitudes are particularly important to health behavior. Therefore, we must consider the role of normative factors in relationship to attitudes and beliefs in determining health behaviors.

Another important related issue that must be kept in mind throughout this chapter is the fundamental distinction between one's *membership* group and one's *reference* group. While the membership group is that to which the individual actually belongs, the wishes of its members (embodied in the membership-group norms) may matter very little (or not at all) to the person. Instead, the norm of his or her reference group—the group used by the person as a basis of comparison for self-appraisal—may be the most compelling. Thus, the individual's behavior may be largely predictable only from the norms of his or her reference group (Hyman & Singer, 1971; Kando, 1977; Merton & Rossi, 1957).

A COMBINED MODEL OF BELIEFS AND SOCIAL NORMS

Despite their importance, normative factors rarely operate simply or alone. In the extreme view, Hewitt (1979) stated that norms enter consciousness only when they are violated. Otherwise, they are not consciously acknowledged. Less extreme positions are proposed by Ajzen and Fishbein (1980;

also Fishbein & Ajzen, 1975) and by Triandis (1977) in their predictive models of human social behavior. These models propose that beliefs (and their related attitudes) must be combined with the individual's perceptions of his social norms in order to predict and understand social behavior.

According to the "Theory of Reasoned Action" (Ajzen & Fishbein, 1980), a behavioral intention is defined as an individual's subjective probability that he will engage in or perform a particular behavior. An intention results from the combined operation of attitudes toward a behavior (influenced by beliefs and expectations) and subjective norms concerning that behavior. This latter component involves, as we have seen above, the individual's belief that members of his reference or membership group (whichever is more salient) feel that he should engage in a particular behavior. A subjective norm, according to Ajzen and Fishbein (1980), involves the generalized important "others," while a normative belief involves a belief about a specific individual or a specific group. Normative beliefs are similar to subjective norms except that the former refer to specific individuals or groups in the environment of the person, while the latter are more global and refer to general expectations.

Not every membership group or reference group will be relevant for every issue. Only "salient" groups will influence the subjective norm. Thus, in order to assess the role of norms in the person's intention to act, one must first elicit from the individual some estimate of the salience of the groups that possess those norms. The individual's family may or may not be more salient in a particular situation than his or her colleagues at work. Thus, the normative belief (that is, the degree to which the salient norm group is positive or negative toward the action) must be combined with the individual's motivation to comply with the norm (the salience of the norm group) in order to assess the strength of this component in determining the intention to act.

In Chapter 6, we examine in detail the assessment (and alteration) of subjective norms. Ajzen and Fishbein (1980) noted the importance of accurate measurement of attitudes and subjective norms in the prediction of intentions to act. They state (p. 76) that the predictions may be in error if beliefs, attitudes, and subjective norms lack correspondence in their measurement. They also note that behavioral intentions are not necessarily strongly related to behaviors—an issue that must be understood in studies of predictions of behavior. We consider this in Chapter 7.

The formal theoretical model proposed by Triandis (1977) focuses somewhat more broadly on social factors than does the model of Ajzen and Fishbein (1980) in determining behavioral intentions. Social factors, according to Triandis, involve not only the norms to which people are subjected but also the roles they play. Roles are sets of behaviors that are considered appropriate for persons holding particular positions in a group. Of course, a person may belong to any number of different groups and thus have many different social roles (e.g., Greek-American, businessman, father). Sometimes (and for some individuals at all times) these roles are in conflict with one another. Other social factors in Triandis' (1977) model include both specific behavioral contract arrangements (e.g., acceptance by the group for giving up smoking), and the individual's self-esteem (which is determined by his or her feeling that the behavior is consistent with self-definition). Regarding this latter point, the individual may use a definition of self that is derived from the reference group in order to decide upon the appropriateness of a particular behavior. In this theory, then, there are many ways in which the physical or psychological presence of other persons will influence behavioral intentions.

In the following sections, we examine the manner in which health behaviors (via intentions) are affected and influenced by social-normative factors, just as we considered the importance of attitudes in Chapter 4. We will examine the role of family, social class, ethnicity, sex, and age on health behavior and compliance. In doing so, we will avoid simple delineation of the specific expectations of various groups. Rather, we will conceptualize the general issues that are of importance. In our conceptualization, we will examine variations in the responses of different groups to illness, their acceptance of responsibility for health care, and their willingness to accept certain preventive or rehabilitative treatments. Our goal is not to provide a catalogue for clinicians, but rather to note some important general issues that should be understood by health researchers and practitioners alike. Because of the central importance to human functioning of reference groups and conformity with their norms, these concepts must be understood. No practitioner can realistically expect compliance with a regimen that goes against the patient's social norms. Thus, practitioners and researchers must be sensitized to some important issues regarding social norms in the formulation of behavioral intentions.

Our examination of social-normative factors in compliance and health behavior presented on the following pages focuses on research findings and their interpretations within a theoretical structure. Unfortunately, the research in this area has been somewhat sporadic and has some noticeable limitations. Without belaboring them, we do point out these limitations and examine some of the issues that must be addressed in research. We also point out some clinical applications of the empirical research, and suggest ways in which health professionals might assess the role of various social norms in their patients' lives. Finally, we argue for the importance of the health practitioner's respect for the patient's subjective norms (whether they be from his ethnic group, family, social class, or the like). Only with the respect that derives from knowledge and understanding can the practitioner hope to become a reference person for the patient—someone whose wishes and recommendations carry as much normative pressure for the patient as the patient's membership and reference groups. In this chapter, we construct a theoretical basis for the discussion in Chapter 6 of the health practitioner as a reference person for the patient, and of the power to effect change that is inherent in the health professional's role.

SOCIAL FACTORS IN HEALTH, ILLNESS, AND MEDICAL TREATMENT

In the process of treating disease and enhancing health, practitioner and patient must deal with a constellation of symptoms. Usually, the job of the practitioner is to search for a diagnosis that fits the symptoms and to develop an appropriate course of treatment. Traditionally, the practitioner has focused on the primarily physiological and biological processes related to the symptoms, and may also have inquired about some stress-related psychological factors. It is a rare clinician, however, who will focus attention on aspects of the patient's life beyond the one-to-one encounter (Hunt, 1978). The reluctance of practitioners to deal with these issues may stem from their lack of knowledge about the operation of social factors in health and illness. It is critically important, however, for practitioners to recognize that considerable research has demonstrated that from the definition of illness through the final stages of rehabilitation, the patient is immersed in and affected by his social context.

Effective health promotion and disease care demand an understanding of the norms and shared values of the patient's culture. We refer to "culture" in the general sense (see Mechanic, 1978). Culture consists of the designs for adapting to the social and physical environment that characterize life for a particular population. The concept of culture is a "sensitizing word" (Mechanic, 1978, p. 34) that gives us a way to view the patient's social world and to understand health and illness behavior. Culture refers to shared behavioral patterns within any ethnic group, social class, gender, or age cohort. The concept allows us to see differences in behavioral trends between one group and another. Cultural ideas and activities are, to a large extent, communicated from one generation to another. Individuals are socialized to adhere openly to norms or shared values of the culture. Therefore, the practitioner's understanding of the norms of the patient's culture and the extent of the patient's immersion in that culture can be critical to understanding the patient's response to medical advice (Becker & Maiman, 1980; Cummings, Becker & Maile, 1980). (Note that nearly all the models of compliance and preventive health behavior presented in Table 4.1 contain a social-normative or cultural component. Cummings, Becker, and Maile's (1980) condensation of these factors identified a category of social factors composed of the individual's perception of the attitudes of friends, relatives, and other salient persons concerning a particular health action, as well as knowledge of others' past health behaviors.)

ILLNESS BEHAVIOR AND THE SICK-ROLE

> An individual's interpretations of symptoms and complaints are strongly affected by personal and social circumstances, including consideration of others' expectations of the interpretations. [Coe, 1978, p. 108]

In Chapter 4 we noted that individual differences in the ways in which people respond to symptoms can be quite marked. In this chapter we further examine this issue of differences in illness behavior. "Illness behavior . . . refers to the varying perceptions, thoughts, feelings, and acts affecting the personal and social meaning of symptoms, illness, disabilities, and their consequences" (Mechanic, 1977, p. 79). When faced with certain signs of disease (including its confirmation by medical experts), some individuals will accept the role of a sick person while others will reject that role entirely. Some will accept medical care while others will be ashamed and fearful and will reject nurses, physicians, and hospitals. While different biological sensitivities may account in part for these variances in illness behavior, they cannot do so completely. These variances are also attributable to differences in early experience with illness and symptoms, to the varying capacities of people to cope effectively with their environment, and to the varying social definitions that they apply to symptoms. All of these factors are particularly influenced by the expectations of other people—expectations that are formalized in terms of cultural- and reference-group norms. Patterns of illness behavior are complex and varied, and they mirror the many complex social factors in patients' responses to medical treatment.

Studies of illness behavior point consistently to the role of illness in serving adaptive needs. Symptoms of various disease states are very prevalent in the population at large, but only a small number of these symptoms are actually presented to practitioners for treatment (White, Williams & Greenberg, 1961; Mechanic, 1977; Zola, 1973). In addition, a person's decision to seek care at one particular time and not another is usually due to factors that have little relation to the symptoms (see Chapter 4). Rather, the decision is likely to result from social validation or social pressure to seek care, or from various interpersonal difficulties. The process of defining himself or herself as ill may release the individual from obligations, pressures, and responsibilities. Illness may also enhance supportive measures from others. It may provide a legitimate excuse for failing to meet social obligations; it may provide a needed self-definition. Further, whether or not illness behavior is used by the patient to serve these larger social needs will depend to a great extent upon whether he or she has learned to do so, and on the extent to which others find this behavior acceptable, as explained by Mechanic (1980):

> If individuals use doctors as a means of dealing with distress in their lives, then it is reasonable to ask why they do not simply report what is truly bothering them, rather than present various physical symptoms. Here social and cultural values become important. It is apparent that some patients have a highly developed psychological vocabulary and can discuss what concerns them in psychodynamic terms. Others lack such a vocabulary and, indeed, may not even consciously recognize the sources of their discomfort. Such patients may have been raised to feel that open expression of feelings of distress is disapproved and seen as an expression of weakness. A number of studies has found that these patterns of expression vary by culture, ethnicity, social class, and urban/rural origins. [p. 15]

Illness behavior can be influenced strongly by cultural norms. The social context and the expectations of one's group are likely to help relieve confusion and ambiguity regarding how to respond to symptoms. Whether he or she chooses to ignore them, or to seek medical care, or to follow the advice of physicians, or to become overly incapacitated and a burden to his or her family will depend significantly upon the influence of the individual's culture (involving family, social class, and ethnicity). The current expectations of his or her reference group will operate in an important way. In addition, the extent to which the individual will follow prescriptions to engage in preventive measures, or instead follow a self-indulgent life style, will depend significantly upon the norms imposed by the social environment (Guttmacher, 1980).

Related to this issue is the *sick role* and the cultural factors that influence it. Sociologist Talcott Parsons' (1958) original conception of the sick role specified the behaviors expected from its occupant. The sick person is regarded as not responsible for his or her incapacity. He or she is exempt from normal social-role obligations, and is expected to seek competent help and comply with the medical recommendations. In practice, however, social and cultural norms often take priority over these theoretical sick-role expectations (Segall, 1976; Mechanic, 1966). The attitudes of family, friends, and associates can have a substantial impact on the course of sickness and disability. For example, a family member's sickness might as easily affect family relations positively as it might strain or harm them. Improved family relations as a result of illness is an example of *secondary gain* from illness, a positive outcome that may encourage the individual to retain his or her illness (Mechanic, 1966, 1978). Measures to treat and overcome the disease in such a case are likely to be ignored. Others too may benefit from and encourage illness behavior. For example, a husband whose occupation has taken him away from his family may, as a result of illness, become increasingly functional in family roles and more considerate of other family members. As his work involvement lessens and his family involvement increases, the family may benefit significantly and hence exert subtle pressures to maintain the father's illness as a means to promote family harmony.

Finally, it is important to recognize that adherence to the sick role's requirement of compliance with recommendations is strongly influenced by social values. The value of good health is normally judged in relation to other values. While good health is normally high on the list of important life values among middle-class persons, it ranks low among lower-class persons whose priorities involve more basic necessities such as a decent place to live, food, and transportation. As Koos (1954) noted, in lower-class cultures good health competes with many other unfulfilled needs, primarily those involving economic survival. Cultural norms also influence expectations that one will be able to control one's environment, and because of this, cultural norms may strongly influence an individual's attempts to take personal responsibility for his or her health. Finally, norms of social class, ethnicity, family, age, and sex can affect the individual's orientation to a life of activity, mastery, and long-range planning versus one characterized by passivity, fatalism, and a focus on the immediate present. These factors are extremely important in the area of preventive health behavior in general (Antonovsky, 1972; Antonovsky & Kats, 1970; & Rosenstock, 1969) and in attempting to understand delays in seeking help for signs of serious medical problems (such as cancer: Antonovsky & Hartman, 1974) in particular.

So far, we have considered the general issues necessary to help us understand how social and cultural norms may come to affect both preventive and rehabilitative health behavior. The remainder of this chapter will focus on issues that are specifically related to the origins of these important norms—the ethnic group, the social class, the family, and the individual's sex and age cohort. While we cannot consider all aspects of social and cultural norms, we will examine some relatively well established normative factors that influence health-related behavior.

THE FAMILY AND HEALTH BEHAVIOR

From the standpoint of the social-psychological study of medical-care compliance and preventive health behavior, the family is of central importance. The family constitutes the most important social context within which illness occurs, and is dealt with (Litman, 1974). The family serves as the primary unit in hygiene and health care (Pratt, 1976). Of course, the concept of family is not exclusively applied to the traditional nuclear family consisting of both biological parents and their children. Such a constellation presently constitutes a rather small proportion of the population in the United States (Goldenberg & Goldenberg, 1980). Family constellations are now more likely to take on the form of single-parent families or blended families (remarried parents, each with their own children). In considering the family here, we refer to the intimate social network of the individual—the persons with whom the individual has strong psychological bonds, with whom he or she lives, and from whom the individual derives some identity and self-definition. We define the family as the center of biological reproduction, emotional development, socialization, and/or the organization of status and roles in relationship to other individuals in the community. Thus, the family can take on many forms. Despite their diversity, however, the various family constellations do not differ greatly among themselves in many important areas of health care (Wingert et al., 1968). Thus, with respect to health care we may consider the various family constellations in one general category.

Precisely how family functioning influences health has been a matter of theoretical concern among sociologists for more than three decades (Richardson, 1945). Only rather recently, however, have methodologies for family research become available (Haggerty, 1965; Kosa, Alpert & Haggerty, 1967). In addition, while family sociologists have learned quite a lot about family issues in general (e.g., kinship structure, power relationships, socialization patterns), "such major issues as familial response, adjustment and behavior in health and illness have generally escaped the empirical involvement and theoretical interest of the family sociologist" (Litman, 1974, p. 495).

Based upon theories of general family functioning, Haggerty (1965) developed a model that encompassed three major theoretical categories: (1) the family's influence on health through past medical experiences and attitudes toward health; (2) family influence through internal functions related to interactions, internal role relations, dominance structure, and child-rearing practices; and (3) external functions related to others in the community, social mobility, social isolation, and recreational activities. Litman (1974) has reviewed the existing literature on family health and illness behavior and has categorized the findings according to the form of influence from the family (for example, through norms or direct requirements, or through constraints such as economic limitations). Here we present a scheme similar to those outlined by Haggerty and Litman.

Family Influence on Health Norms

In the field of social epidemiology, considerable research has implicated the family as hereditary link, causal agent, and source of communication of disease (Dingle, 1959; Kellner, 1963). Not surprisingly, members of family units are likely to fall prey to one anothers' illnesses (Pratt, 1973). Of course, norms of family behavior also significantly affect the definition and reporting of illness episodes. While the direct spread of infectious agents may occur more easily in the family group (Haggerty & Alpert, 1963), the direct spread of *illness definition* may occur among family members as well (Mechanic, 1966).

This latter point, of course, emphasizes the importance of shared reality in the family, particularly as far as the issue of illness is concerned. Whether certain symptoms are defined as illness and brought to the attention of a physician or other health professional will be determined by the consensus of family members and close friends (Richardson, 1970; Knapp, Knapp & Engle, 1966). Individuals consistently report their physical symptoms first to their family members and intimates. This relied-upon network of nonprofessionals has been referred to as the *lay referral system* or the *lay referral network* (Freidson, 1960, 1961; McKinlay, 1973). The family also imposes norms for the appropriate use of various remedies such as medication (Osterweis et al., 1979). Finally, the family (particularly the wife and mother) is normally the source of illness definition for the children and other members (Aho, 1977; Robinson, 1971; Mechanic, 1964). Thus, the family provides norms for decisions regarding the onset of illness and the need for medical care.

Family resources influence health behavior and compliance with medical regimens. These resources include the family's capacity to tolerate stress and disruption, as well as the capacity to afford financial cost. (We will consider this last factor in Chapter 7, where we examine direct barriers to compliance). What is relevant here is that the family's resources also operate indirectly by establishing norms for the definition of illness and for adoption of and compliance with the sick role. In seeking to protect the interests of the family as a whole, the members will adopt more or less stringent definitions of their own personal health and illness (Muller, 1965; Tucker, 1970).

Finally, family norms influence individual beliefs about the severity of various illnesses, susceptibility to these illnesses, and benefits versus costs of treatment. These considerations will, of course, include the benefits and costs of continued adoption versus relinquishing of the sick role (Morris, Hatch & Chipman, 1966; Parsons & Fox, 1952; Becker & Green, 1975; Baric, 1970).

Illness and Family Functioning

Another important way in which illness behavior, health behavior, and compliance are influenced by the family involves the role of illness as both cause and consequence of family dysfunction. Regarding the former case, the literature is replete with evidence that illness disrupts the family. Family members may all experience significant strains when any one member becomes acutely or chronically ill. Expectations for each person's behavior undergo some change as a result of illness (Hill, 1958; Klein, Dean, & Bogdonoff, 1968), and family members may find it necessary to develop new patterns of interacting with the individual who is ill (Klein, Dean, & Bogdonoff, 1968; Salk, Hilgartner, & Granich, 1972; Gordon & Kutner, 1965). Of course, the extent of the disruption is likely to depend upon the seriousness of the illness and on other factors that remain, as yet, unexplored. Litman (1974) noted that while we know that in some cases family solidarity may be enhanced by illness while in others it is likely to be broken down, we know as yet very little about the circumstances under which one or the other is likely to occur, or about the consequences of either. We might predict that certain effects of illness on family functioning may threaten the patient's chances for compliance and successful rehabilitation. An example is a patient's inability to assume his former role (or a new, related role) in the family, which may reduce the incentive value of getting well, and thus reduce the patient's tendency to comply with the treatment regimen. The family's adjustment may therefore have a significant impact on the patient's motivation for recovery, and hence on the patient's cooperation with the treatment.

The family structure and patterns of functioning (or dysfunction) may have a significant effect on the health and sick-role behavior of its members in yet another way. Theoretical approaches that emphasize family dynamics in the understanding of self-destructive behaviors such as alcoholism and drug abuse suggest that the family environment is an important cause of these behaviors. Alcoholism and drug abuse may help the individual cope with significant family dysfunction, to gain power over others in the family (when affiliative behaviors do not work), or to reduce anxiety from strained family interactions. (We saw an example of this in the case of Mr. Smithgard.) Recurrent crises in various illnesses (for example, childhood asthma) may reflect the patient's attempt to improve family members' cooperation with one another and thus reduce or deflect interpersonal tension in the family (Minuchin, Rosman, & Baker, 1978). Studies also show that negative or upsetting interactions among family members may have astoundingly negative effects on health and the outcome of medical care (Mathis, 1964; Lynch et al., 1974; Lynch et al., 1977).

The ill member of a family might also serve as the family scapegoat, absorbing the blame for the family's interactional and emotional difficulties that cannot be faced as such (Vogel & Bell, 1968). The scapegoat allows the family to channel tensions that would otherwise destroy the family's cohesiveness. For example, parents may resist the cure of a child with enuresis by unconsciously subtly reinforcing and supporting the behavior. Their unstated goal might be to guarantee their continued projection of their own marital frustrations and anger onto the child. They may use the enuresis problem to avoid facing their own emotional or interactional difficulties. Bursten and

D'Esopo (1965) showed that this situation also occurs among adults whose illness may promote a stable equilibrium in their troubled family.

In summary, then, we see that in many ways the family is central to compliance and health behavior. The intimate social context of each patient is of critical importance to researchers in their attempts to understand general issues in compliance and health behavior, and to practitioners who attempt to treat their patients effectively.

SEX AND AGE NORMS FOR HEALTH BEHAVIOR

An analysis of research that is directly concerned with compliance behavior (reviewed by Haynes, Taylor, & Sackett, 1979) suggests that there is no clear-cut direct relationship between the two demographic factors, age and sex, and responses to medical care. In studies of age and compliance reviewed by Haynes, Taylor, and Sackett, (1979), 29 citations reported a positive correlation of age with compliance, 14 reported a negative relationship, and 77 reported no relationship at all. Likewise, 65 studies showed no relationship between compliance and sex, while the 28 that did show a relationship were more or less equally divided between showing males and females as the better compliers. These findings have led researchers to conclude that there are no stable relationships between age or sex and compliance with medical care (Haynes, Taylor, & Sackett, 1979).

Nevertheless, the presence of some significant related findings suggests the possibility that age and sex *do* sometimes influence health behavior. It is important, then, to examine some health issues as they relate to these variables. One of the most consistent findings of health-survey research is that women report symptoms of physical (and mental) illness, and use physicians and health services significantly more than men (Nathanson, 1975). At the same time, however, in Western Europe and North America, women's life expectation at birth exceeds that of men by five to seven years. Women are considered *constitutionally* more resistant to infections and to degenerative diseases (Madigan, 1957; Childs, 1965), but they have higher rates of illness conditions, restricted activity, bed disability, and physician visits. (These statistics, of course, exclude episodes related to pregnancy or delivery.)

The lack of an adequate biological basis for the difference in rates of health-care utilization and illness adoption suggests that alternative explanations may be found among sociocultural variables that affect illness and sick-role behavior (Nathanson, 1975). Specifically, the following explanations have been suggested: (1) women report more illness than men because it is culturally more acceptable for women than for men to express discomfort; (2) the sick role may be more compatible with women's other role obligations. These explanations, as Nathanson suggested, posit a difference in response to symptoms and hence emphasize a social-psychological explanation of the sex difference in pattern or use of health services. Thus, while in terms of medication taking or following specific medical treatment regimens the sexes do not appear to differ in their rates of compliance, they do differ considerably in their definitions of illness and in their patterns of utilizing health services and medical care.

Finally, increasing age usually brings increasing limitations owing to chronic illness and disability (Mechanic, 1978). Hospital admission rates and length of stay are positively related to age. Yet, despite a higher degree of illness and greater utilization of health services among older persons as well as their differing expectations for physician conduct and the delivery of medical care (DiMatteo, Prince, & Taranta, 1979; DiMatteo & Hays, 1980), compliance behavior patterns seem to be unaffected by age norms. Of course, it is possible that a higher degree of utilization of service by older persons may result from norms that render the seeking of health services by older persons acceptable. On the whole, however, age does not seem to be an important normative factor in compliance and health behavior.

SOCIAL CLASS NORMS

> To a considerable extent, the best known conceptions of the sick role reflect a middle class value pattern on which physician and client agree; this pattern emphasizes the merits of individual responsibility, deliberate striving and grooming of the self toward health, mastery and activism in the carrying out of normal social roles. . . . Health is to be sought and illness expeditiously cured. The fate of misfortune is not to be passively bemoaned or stoically accepted. [Bloom & Wilson, 1972, p. 332]

The active orientation toward illness, as Bloom and Wilson noted, is a social-class norm. It is an expectation held by a relatively advantaged sector of our society—those who are comfortably housed, well fed, educated, and employed. There is considerable evidence that individuals of lower socioeconomic class face greater risks of illness than do individuals of higher social class (Mechanic, 1978). Evidence has shown consistently that the lower classes have higher mortality, morbidity, and disability rates (Syme & Berkman, 1976). Persons of lower-class backgrounds are less likely to seek medical care for (and thus are more likely to tolerate) such basic indicators of disease as pain, swelling, and bleeding (Koos, 1954; Saunders, 1954). Persons of lower social class are less likely than those of higher social class to engage in preventive health behavior (Green, 1970; Rosenstock & Kirscht, 1979), and in some studies (16 out of 40 reviewed by Haynes, Taylor, & Sackett,

1979) are less likely to comply with therapeutic regimens, particularly those which involve keeping clinic appointments. (Hertz & Stamps [1977] noted, however, that this finding may have had much to do with the "block scheduling" of appointments typically used in low-income clinics—a system that requires all patients to arrive at the clinic at a given time and wait their turn throughout a four- to five-hour time period. These researchers found that compliance with appointments was markedly improved by giving each patient his or her own particular appointment time.) Part of their tolerance for symptoms probably stems from a lack of resources (time, money, transportation), as we will see in Chapter 7. These limitations do not *fully* account for the responses of the poor to illness and medical care, however. Much of their health-related behavior stems from expectations and norms within their social group. Motivational and life-style features of the lower class, as well as a tendency to reject a future orientation (Horton, 1967), often render their patient-practitioner interactions uneasy. Lower-class patients may even reject and fear the medical establishment (Samora, Saunders, & Larson, 1961; Shuval, 1970; Norman, 1969; Cartwright, 1967).

Another explanation has been proposed by Suchman (1964, 1967) and examined empirically by Langlie (1977). The explanation considers the lower-social-class individual as immersed in a parochial group structure that exhibits traditional family values, ethnic exclusivity, and friendship solidarity. Popular or folk-health orientations are likely to exist, and adherence to the group's norms is likely to supersede adherence to the norms of the medical profession. Relatedly, Green (1970) suggested that higher social status is related to greater health-oriented behavior because of (1) the greater interaction with nonkin (unrelated persons) who exhibit health behavior, and (2) the greater reliance among the middle and upper class on "scientific data." Rundall and Wheeler (1979) evaluated the results of almost 800 interviews with adults regarding their use of preventive health services and involvement in preventive care. The data revealed a surprisingly negligible *direct* effect of income (socioeconomic status) on preventive care, but a positive *indirect* effect of income via attitudes. That is, income level affected the individuals' perceived susceptibility, which in turn affected health behavior, but an explanation based on financial constraints was not supported. Rundall and Wheeler thus argued that health behavior is affected by a "culture-of-poverty." Low-income persons believe themselves to be less susceptible to illness than they really are, and they have no usual source of care that might convince them otherwise or provide them with needed preventive health services.

It is important to keep in mind that people in the lower social classes have a greater general vulnerability to illness than people in higher social classes. According to Syme and Berkman (1976), the lower-class environment is highly stressful, though not enough is yet known about what specifically constitutes the stress. Risks seem to be associated with the greater geographic, cultural, and social mobility of the poor, and the pressures of the poverty environment. The specific coping responses available to and typically chosen by lower-class patients (such as cigarette smoking and obesity—USDHEW, 1973; Khasla & Lowe, 1972) often further enhance risks to their health.

The extent to which health behavior is influenced by economic limitations or limitations from the "culture of poverty" (beliefs, values, norms of the lower class) is not an easily resolved issue. Clearly, values do differ among the classes. For example, Larson and Sutker (1966) found that lower-social-class persons were more likely to attach importance to being clean, owning a home, having insurance, and living in a good neighborhood while middle- and upper-social-class persons valued being in good health, having a good education, being respected by people, having children, and having friends. Health is more important to middle- and upper-class persons than to lower-class persons, although this may be because the lower classes have a large number of competing survival needs. Upper- and middle-class values are more "growth oriented" (in an economic and psychological sense) because basic needs are already satisfied. The health professional's understanding and recognition of these differences in values may be critically important (although difficult to achieve) in providing health care for patients who come from lower social classes and have different values than they do themselves (Twaddle, 1969).

ETHNIC IDENTIFICATION AND HEALTH BEHAVIOR

An individual's adherence to his or her ethnic group norms may affect health behavior and compliance in a number of ways. Patterns of illness and death in particular ethnic groups are often influenced by values related to the organization of the family, of work, of relaxation and recreation (Mechanic, 1978). Behaviors such as smoking, alcohol use, the use of drugs, diet, exercise, and driving motor vehicles influence the major health risk factors prominent in the United States today (Torrens, 1978). The leading causes of morbidity and mortality—heart disease, cancer, accidents, and cirrhosis of the liver—have strong behavioral components in their causes, and these behavioral components are highly related to ethnic habits and norms.

A particularly important component of ethnic group identity is food. Diet has social and sometimes even religious connotations, as well as nutritional ones. Some groups will dictate how foods must be prepared so as not to violate taboos. Changes in patterns of preparing and eating food are therefore not easy to make. As we saw earlier with Mrs. Tomasetti, these changes may significantly disrupt family and group associations (Mechanic, 1978).

In all ethnic groups, eating is an accepted adaptive response to hunger, but the meaning of food and overeating may differ among various ethnic groups. Among the Swedish and the British for example, overeating is not considered an acceptable means of coping with stress, and is not looked upon as a way to gain comfort. Obesity is devalued, and obese persons frowned upon. Among the Pennsylvania Dutch, Southern Italians, and Jews, however, a large appetite is a source of pride, and food is used for comfort and stress reduction. Obesity is equated with health, and thinness is considered suggestive of illness (Bruhn, 1976). There is little doubt, of course, that knowledge of such a connection between food and coping in a particular ethnic group can aid the health-care practitioner to understand the meaning of obesity to a patient. The patient might then be aided more effectively to overcome the difficulties he or she is having in adhering to a dietary regimen.

Ethnic differences in behaviors—particularly health behavior—have their roots in early experience. Ethnic identifications affect child-rearing practices and teach modes of coping with the usual tasks of life. The child acquires from his ethnic and cultural group a sense of self, a sense of community, expressive skills, and psychological defenses (Mechanic, 1978). From an early age, children learn appropriate interpretations of and responses to various aspects of life from their culture. It is now commonly accepted that reactions to pain and distress are socially learned behaviors that are particularly influenced by the individual's ethnic group (Zborowski, 1952; Davitz, Sameshima, & Davitz, 1976; Davitz, Davitz, & Higuchi, 1977).

Ethnic-group beliefs and behavior patterns influence reactions to illness and health care. In some ethnic groups, for example, the orientation of individuals is to the present. Protection against possible future disease, particularly if that protection involves pain, discomfort, or delay of pleasure, may be typically dispensed with. Indeed, the meaning of pain and reactions to it vary systematically as a function of ethnic group. Zborowski's (1952) classic study of ethnic differences in expressions of pain showed that Irish and individuals of old American background were stoical about their pain, were reluctant to describe it in a detailed manner, and were withdrawn and nonverbally unexpressive. The Italian and Jewish patients, on the other hand, communicated their suffering, describing it in an animated fashion. The Jews differed from the Italians, however, in that they were concerned about the implications of their pain while the Italians simply demanded immediate relief. This research has been followed up and supported by later studies, and it suggests the enormous importance of culture in understanding illness behavior.

Ethnic groups may also vary in their acceptance of medical care in the format in which it is usually offered. Mexican-American patients, for example, require the maintenance of dignity and respect in order to tolerate a dependent role such as the one required in the medical setting. They expect to have the opportunity to share decisions with their families, and to be shown respect for their ideas about the causes and cures of illness (Quesada, 1976). If these conditions are not met, patients of Mexican cultural origin are likely to reject modern medicine and turn instead to their folk healers, the *curanderos*, or receive no care at all.

Table 5.1 presents a description of the most prominent health-care expectations and norms of a number of different ethnic groups. These norms and expectations vary widely among themselves. Their similarity lies in the importance attached to the concordance between the behavior of the medical practitioner and the expectations of the patient. When this concordance does not exist, patients are more often satisfied with the care given by their folk practitioners whose ethnic background and values are similar to their own. Folk practitioners typically understand what patients need, what they want to know, and how they wish to be treated (Kleinman, Eisenberg, & Good, 1978). Unlike modern medical practitioners, folk healers within an ethnic group tend to treat the personal, interpersonal, and cultural reactions to disease and discomfort. The patient is recognized as being embedded in a complex family and social system, with certain expectations for behavior (Fabrega, 1972; Litman, 1974).

The importance of ethnic group factors to patient compliance and health behavior suggests that effective care of the patient demands the practitioner's understanding of the patient's ethnic identity and related conception of illness. The practitioner must show respect for the patient's cultural orientation toward illness, and provide complete explanations of the meaning and importance of the modern medical treatments imposed. An excellent example of this approach is provided by Kleinman, Eisenberg, and Good (1978), who viewed medicine as clinical social science and argued for the relevance of cultural anthropology to the provision of modern medical care. They related the case story of a 26-year-old Guatemalan woman who had resided in the United States for ten years. This woman's cultural beliefs had strongly influenced her perceptions of clinical reality and had provoked behavior in her that was confusing and distressing to her physicians and nurses. She was being treated for severe enteritis, and was therefore not allowed oral intake of food. Instead, she was fed intravenously. During her treatment, she became emotionally withdrawn, angry, and uncooperative. Her behavior followed directly from the belief that her medical problem was caused by the witchcraft of her fiancé's sister. She reasoned that because she was not receiving any food by mouth, her physicians had abandoned her or "written her off" as unlikely to live. Further, she believed that she was being prevented from regulating her hot/cold balance of nutrients—the basis of the traditional health beliefs of the medical system in which she grew up. She was unable to talk about her beliefs and ideas because she feared ridicule from her physicians and nurses. When encouraged to talk about her conception of

Table 5.1. Specific Ethnic Group Norms Regarding Health and Illness.

Group	Reference	Norms
American Indian	Primeaux (1977)	• Forces of good and evil are interwoven in all aspects of health care; • Indian medicine emphasizes balance of person with nature and environment (concept of holism). Illness is result of imbalance, not germs; • It is difficult to separate medicine and concepts of God and religion; • Medicine man treats the whole family.
Asian American (particularly Chinese)	Aslam et al. (1979) Lin and Lin (1978)	• Traditional healers treat whole person; • Illness (particularly mental) is regarded as punishment for violation of moral ethics or filial piety; • Illness is due to imbalance of yin and yang; • Reliance on intrafamiliar resources and home care; • Trust and security rarely extend beyond the family; Western concept of citizen responsibility makes sense only when translated into family-relevant terms.
Greek American and Italian American	Pilowsky and Spence (1977)	• Greek (as well as Italian) more likely to report common physical symptoms ignored by some other cultures (sometimes referred to as hypochondriacal); • Belief in the "evil eye" (externalization is used as a style of defense); • Anxiety about health exists; • Sick role is not viewed stringently; entry is easy; • Expressiveness about pain (Italians).
Mexican American	Saunders (1954) Clark (1970) Kiev (1968) Rubel (1960)	• Illness relates to individual's life, community, interpersonal relationships, and God; • Pain is necessary to define illness, making preventive measures difficult; • Folk beliefs and practices such as hot-cold dimension in illness; • Folk-healers (*curanderos*) are important members of the community and culture;

		• Efficiency of the doctor not admired; haste is seen as discourteous; • To maintain dignity, patient wants friendly, calm, cautious, courteous physician; • Need for involvement of whole family in health-care decisions.
Jewish American	Mechanic (1963)	• Response to pain is emotional; concern is with meaning and significance of pain; • Cultural norm involves somatic sensitivity and concern with physical symptoms; self-medication common; • Illness is important part of Jewish culture (cultural jokes about chicken soup as a remedy serve to illustrate this); • Traditional role of illness is to draw family and community together; • Health is associated with parental affection and concern; • That one must eat to achieve health is a strong belief, and so there is a high rate of obesity; • Children exhibit hypochondriac tendencies and anxiety about health; • Physical complaints are regarded as a proper way to express tension and dissatisfaction
Filipino American	McKenzie and Chrisman (1977)	• Medical therapies are combined with folk remedies; • Disease is associated with total life situation and with both natural and supernatural causes; • Spices are thought to have special powers to heal; • Folk remedies endure in the United States because they are well known, accessible, and trusted, relatively inexpensive and are perceived to be successful in solving everyday health problems; • Filipino-American will employ folk medicine both before and after consulting M.D.; • Balance of hot and cold important in health; • In health-care delivery, practitioner should maintain eye contact with Filipino patient lest practitioner be thought to be a witch, or the cause of the illness.

her illness, she was relieved that her ideas were treated with respect, even though her doctors indicated that they did not share those beliefs and would continue their modern medical treatment of her. Her hostile attitude and withdrawn, uncooperative behavior ceased when she was reassured that the doctors had not given up on her.

Health professionals need not know the specific beliefs and health practices of every ethnic group. Rather they need only develop an openness to each patient's own "explanatory model" of illness. Practitioners must question and explore with each patient the various aspects of his or her conception of illness because it is likely that this conception will be both different from that of the practitioner and influenced by the patient's ethnic identity. "Patients often hesitate to disclose their models to doctors. Clinicians need to be persistent in order to show patients that their ideas are of genuine interest and importance for clinical management" (Kleinman, Eisenberg, & Good, 1978, p. 256). These authors also suggest some questions which may help to reveal the patient's hidden explanation of his or her medical problem:

> (1) What do you think has caused your problem?
> (2) Why do you think it started when it did?
> (3) What do you think your sickness does to you? How does it work?
> (4) How severe is your sickness? Will it have a short or long course?
> (5) What kind of treatment do you think you should receive? [Kleinman, Eisenberg, & Good, 1978, p. 256]

The following quotation from Eric Cassell provides an excellent summary of the role of ethnic beliefs regarding health and illness. This anecdote suggests that such beliefs are central to the most basic issues in health care—issues such as what constitutes illness, and how illness might best be treated in a given individual:

> In 1955 a Navaho medicine man who was also a tribal leader spoke at a monthly meeting of white physicians gathered at Fort Defiance. "There are some things which we medicine men know the white doctor is better able to cure than we, such as appendicitis and tuberculosis; we have given up on these. Then there are such things as snake bite, which both the medicine man and the doctor can cure, each using his own method. But there is still a third kind of illness which only the Navaho medicine man can cure—for example, a person might have lightning illness, caused by his being nearby when lightning struck. You white doctors wouldn't know that person is sick and so it wouldn't occur to you to treat that person. But, in the Navaho way of thinking, it is just as important to treat him as it is to treat the person in pain with appendicitis."
>
> It is important to realize that this is the statement of a sophisticated man in a culture that has accepted Western medicine where it is useful. [Cassell, 1976, p. 50]

Ethnic Diversity among Practitioners

The enormous ethnic diversity among patients in the United States necessitates the practitioner's interest in and concern with cultural issues and their relationship to health and illness behavior. This concern is likely to enhance the practitioner's provision of effective health care. Of course, it should not be forgotten that health professionals also differ among themselves in their expectations for appropriate health and illness behavior from their patients. These differences, interestingly enough, are partly attributable to the health professionals' own ethnic backgrounds (Davitz, Davitz, & Higuchi, 1977; Davitz, Sameshima, & Davitz, 1976). This is particularly true of the health professionals' acceptance and understanding of their patients' expressions of pain. In research on nurses from six different cultures, marked differences were found among them in their inferences about patients' behavior, physical pain, and psychological distress. These differences varied according to the nurses' ethnic origins. Interestingly, a nurse was influenced by a patient's verbal and nonverbal expressiveness in inferring the degree of physical and emotional pain only when the nurse's ethnic group differed from that of the patient. For example, American nurses assumed that Japanese and Korean patients—who were very stoical in their expressions—actually suffered less than persons who were expressive about their pain. Japanese and Korean nurses, however, attributed much suffering to their patients, even though the patients were quiet and stoical in manner. This suggests the potential difficulty of trying to understand patients' communications about illness if the health professional does not share their ethnic identity. Thus, the health professional must remain fully aware that ethnically influenced factors such as expressive behavior do indeed affect health care and illness, and that the practitioner's own ethnic identity in relation to the patient must always be fully considered.

SOME LIMITATIONS AND IMPLICATIONS FOR TREATMENT

In studying culture and its relationship to health and illness behavior, we are seeking to infer "cultural patterns," and to make sense out of the great variation among people in their health and illness behavior and their responses to medical regimens. It is important to recognize, however, that cultural patterns are only rough approximations. They are not immutable rules. There can be great diversity of thought and action within any cultural group. As Mechanic (1978) noted, there may exist vast differences in ideals, in conceptions of morality, in patterns of work and leisure, in aspirations, in values, and in child-rearing principles. All of these relate in various ways to health and illness.

A related limitation of this chapter's analysis (and indeed of cultural phenomena and illness behavior in general) is methodological in character. According to Mechanic (1978), when various investigators describe cultural patterns, they often generalize from behavioral observations and infer cultural meanings and values. Mechanic (1978) cites Talcott Parsons'(1958) analysis of health values as an example. Parsons concluded that the emphasis on health in American society is linked to American cultural values such as mastery (over the environment) and an emphasis on progress. He concluded that Americans value the maintenance of good health because health enhances this mastery and progress. He also argued that the values of mastery and progress have in turn enhanced the development of the health sciences in America. Such an analysis is at a high level of abstraction and generalization. Although both statements of causality are equally plausible, the individual assertions are difficult (if not impossible) to support directly. On the other hand, a very different level of abstraction is inferred by the following straightforward finding and interpretation: Zborowski (1952) noted that Italian patients are concerned with the present pain they are experiencing while Jewish patients are concerned with the future meaning of the pain. Both groups are emotionally expressive in contrast to Irish and WASP patients who are unemotional about illness and pain. Zborowski's assertions follow precisely from his data, and are made at a low level of abstraction. These assertions are straightforward reports of how patients behaved. Because of these differences in levels of abstraction and generalization, Mechanic (1978) emphasized that we must always remain aware of the source of data upon which we base our generalizations about health behavior. The "value" of health in a culture, for example, could refer to its importance in the attitudes of the cultural group members or to the amount of money or other resources spent on health care by people in the culture. On the other hand, this value could refer to the extent to which people in the culture engage in preventive health care measures. These measures differ from one another quite extensively. (An excellent example is the United States, where large sums of money—at least 10 percent of the gross national product—are allocated to medical care, and members of the U.S. middle class rank health very high on their list of important values. On the other hand, however, very little money is spent on health maintenance programs and few individuals engage consistently in preventive health regimens [Surgeon General, 1979; Haynes, Taylor, & Sackett, 1979].) Thus, a generalization is meaningless if we do not keep in mind the data on which it is based.

A final limitation of the consideration of social norms and health behavior that we have presented in this chapter concerns the inability of social norms and cultural factors alone to predict compliance and health behavior. In her review of the literature on preventive health behavior, Langlie (1977) noted that the methodologically adequate studies of social-group properties and health have generally found that *both beliefs and social-group normative factors* must be considered. Together they can effectively predict health behavior and compliance. In addition, it is unlikely that health beliefs and social normative variables exert completely independent influences on health behavior, since several of their components are related to one another (Langlie, 1977). For example, feelings of powerlessness to control events in one's life tend to be associated with lower social class (Rotter, 1966). Thus, the norms *and* the beliefs or attitudes, as well as their interrelationships, need to be considered in predicting intentions to engage in health behaviors. Earlier in this chapter, as well as in Chapter 4, we alluded to the need to consider beliefs (and hence attitudes) and social norms jointly, and we consider this issue somewhat further in the next chapter.

We have seen in the present chapter that many aspects of social norms are relevant to compliance and health behavior. Social class, ethnicity, and the family seem to be the most salient in their influence, which is either direct (as is usually the case with the family) or indirect (through values, such as those associated with one's social class). In Chapter 4, we similarly examined the many aspects of health beliefs and their importance to compliance and health behavior. In Chapter 6 to follow, our analyses of beliefs and social norms will be brought together. There, we will review the literature on changing beliefs, attitudes, and subjective norms. We will emphasize the more recent theoretical and empirical work (primarily by Ajzen & Fishbein, 1980) which argues for the importance of this multifaceted approach, whether we are concerned with the prediction of intentions or with their actual formulation. As we have seen so far, and as we will continue to see, however, the precise character of the joint operation of beliefs and social norms has yet to be specified empirically. This will be an important area for future research once the groundwork has been carefully built.

6

Changing Beliefs and Attitudes: The Formation of Behavioral Intentions

In Chapters 4 and 5, we examined the relationship of patients' beliefs and social norms to their health behaviors and compliance with medical regimens. As we saw, the Theory of Reasoned Action (Fishbein & Ajzen, 1975; Ajzen & Fishbein, 1980) posits a joint operation of attitudes and social norms in bringing about behavioral intentions. As we noted in Chapter 5, an *intention* is an individual's subjective probability that he or she will engage in or perform a particular behavior (Ajzen & Fishbein, 1980). The formation of behavioral intentions is the subject of this chapter.

Before we examine various aspects of the formation of intentions, let us consider the Theory of Reasoned Action somewhat more closely. The model was first presented in Figure 4.1. There, and in Chapter 5, attitudes (formed primarily by beliefs such as those in the Health Belief Model) and subjective norms were considered in detail. The Theory of Reasoned Action posits that together they predict behavioral intentions. Both these factors must be weighted in some way, of course, in order to predict intentions successfully. According to the Ajzen and Fishbein theory, any given variable will have an effect on behavioral intentions if it influences the attitude - belief component of the model, or if it influences the social - normative component, or if it influences the relative weights of the two components.

The Theory of Reasoned Action has received rather extensive empirical support, albeit primarily in areas other than health behavior. This supportive research is reviewed by Ajzen and Fishbein (1973; Fishbein & Ajzen, 1975). In the applied area of health care, behavioral intentions—such as to use contraceptives or to follow a diet regimen for weight loss—have been found to adhere to this general predictive model (Smetana & Adler, 1980; Sejwacz, Ajzen, & Fishbein, 1980).

In this book we are concerned with understanding factors related not only to predicting but also to changing health behaviors in order ultimately to achieve patient cooperation with medical regimens. The usefulness of Ajzen and Fishbein's predictive model for achieving the goal of behavior change is therefore important. As we will see in this chapter, although their model is primarily a predictive one, it provides a very useful framework for bringing about changes in behavioral intentions. The factors that influence intentions to act—such as to follow a medical treatment regimen—can be altered, and as a result changes in behavioral intentions can be brought about. According to Fishbein and Ajzen (1975), "in order to change behavior, an influence attempt should be directed at the intention to perform that behavior. To change that intention, however, it will be necessary to focus on attitude toward the behavior and on subjective norms" (p.406). Their conclusion is not based solely on implication or extrapolation from the predictive model. Rather, these researchers have reviewed a large number of studies in support of their assertion. These studies have shown that stated intentions are brought about by changing the appropriate attitudes and subjective norms (Fishbein & Ajzen, 1975). The application of these findings to health situations is still somewhat limited, however, and this topic needs further investigation in the health arena. We do feel, however, that there is enough evidence at present to propose with confidence a role for both attitudes (and hence beliefs) and social-normative factors in changing health behaviors. Still, further empirical work on the factors involved in changing health behaviors will be a significant and much needed contribution.

It is probably useful to note here again, as we have elsewhere, that our analysis of factors in compliance does not have as its goal the building of a precise predictive statistical model. Others have pursued this goal quite successfully (Wallston & Wallston, 1981). Rather, we are concerned with merging an empirical and a "clinical" or individual orientation. We wish to examine what might be done in any given circumstance to bring about change in a patient's behavior. We examine this question within an empirical or statistical framework. Thus, it is clear that we are concerned with the empirical evidence for any given intervention, but at the same time we do not wish to lose sight of the ultimate application of such knowledge—the care of the patient.

Compliance researcher Irwin Rosenstock (1975) has proposed a possible resolution of the tension that may occur between these two disparate approaches to compliance:

> Knowing *why* many patients do not comply with medical advice does not imply any particular strategy for changing their behavior. But the practitioner may be able to develop his own strategy for more effective persuasion if he becomes

clearly aware that in order for patients to comply with advice they need to be interested in their health, to believe and understand the diagnosis, to assess correctly its potential impact, to believe in the efficacy of the prescribed treatment, to find ways of giving or using the medication that are not more trouble than the disease itself, and to know exactly how and for how long to take the medication. [p. 403]

Becker and Maiman (1980) have made a similar suggestion:

> Research has demonstrated that attitudes and perceptions can be altered; and by learning which of these beliefs is below a level presumed necessary for compliance, the provider can tailor intervention to suit the unique needs of each patient. Thus, it is recommended that more attention be paid to both monitoring and motivating the patient along these belief dimensions (e.g., does the patient care about health; agree with the diagnosis, perceive the condition as very serious or not at all serious, feel the recommended therapy will work, fear medication side effects; feel the regimen will be too hard to follow?). Such a "compliance-oriented history" should be reviewed as a critical extension of the usual medical history and be made a routine part of the examination process. [p. 120]

Without doubt, then, there exist some prerequisites to patient compliance. These need to be understood by researcher and practitioner alike. The evidence from theory and research suggests, for example, that one would not institute a specific behavior-change program for a patient without first enlisting the patient's stated intention to comply. It is likely, too, that before receiving an intentional statement from the patient, one would need to be sure that the intended regimen did not go against the patient's beliefs and cultural norms. (Were this to be the case, the stated intention might be unstable or even deliberately false.) In addition, one would not go about searching for clues to the patient's attitudes, beliefs, and norms, or try to change them without first establishing a reasonably good therapeutic relationship with the patient. Without a strong therapeutic alliance, the patient may never truthfully disclose necessary information to the practitioner. Thus, it is necessary that both researcher and practitioner understand the factors we have considered so far in order to formulate intelligent, carefully conceived research investigations and to develop techniques for practical clinical application.

CHANGING BELIEFS AND SUBJECTIVE NORMS

The Assessment of Beliefs

Changes in behavioral intentions must begin with an assessment of the individual's *total set* of beliefs, including (1) beliefs concerning the specific behavior in question, and (2) subjective-normative beliefs. Both of these are considered in the following paragraphs.

First, in order to bring about or formulate a patient's intention to act (for example, to follow a low-sodium diet), we must assess *all* of the patient's beliefs *about the regimen*. This assessment must examine how each belief relates to the outcome of the behavior, and how strong or salient each belief is. For example, Ajzen and Fishbein note some possible beliefs that a person might hold regarding the use of birth control pills. They include the following: (1) birth control pills may cause the individual to gain weight (a belief that has a high salience or belief-strength for the respondent, and is quite negative); (2) they are convenient to use (a belief that also has high salience, but that is valued quite positively); and (3) using them may induce guilt feelings (a belief that has an intermediate level of strength, but only a slightly negative evaluation). By combining the outcome evaluation of each belief with the strength of that belief, one can determine the potential impact of the individual's entire set of beliefs on the formation of an intention. These combined factors, when summed over the individual's entire set of beliefs (concerning birth control pills, for example), will determine the attitudinal component of the model predicting behavioral intentions. Ajzen and Fishbein (1980) typically assign numerical values to the outcome evaluations and to the belief strengths, thereby allowing more precise empirical predictions and the building of statistical models. In the following examples, we illustrate this assessment by using a more qualitative assessment of these factors, such as might be undertaken by the medical practitioner.

The second component to consider in the formation of intentions is the individual's set of *subjective norms.* Each subjective norm has two important parts: (1) the evaluation of the behavior (also called the value orientation toward the behavior) by the normative person or group; and (2) the individual's motivation to comply with the normative person or group. For example, a patient's family may be very positive toward his following a diet that prohibits alcohol, his fellow workers may be only slightly negative, his church-group friends may be slightly positive, and his bowling team buddies may be extremely negative. His motivation to comply with the wishes of his family and his bowling team are very high (possibly causing some conflict for the patient, because the value orientations of the two are in conflict) while his motivations to comply with the wishes of his fellow workers and his church group are rather low.

In Table 6.1 we present a detailed, hypothetical analysis of the case of Mrs. Tomasetti (see Chapter 5) using the various beliefs and social-normative factors that we examined in Chapters 4 and 5.

Changing Beliefs and Forming Intentions

As noted earlier, changes in behavioral intentions can be brought about by pursuing one or both of the following avenues for change. The first avenue

Table 6.1. Analysis of Mrs. Tomasetti's Total Set of Health Beliefs and Subjective Norms.

Goal: Mrs. Tomasetti's statement of her intention to follow her special diet.
Means: Formation of intention will be achieved through analysis of health beliefs and subjective norms, and change in these components (by means of persuasion, etc.) where necessary.

A. *Mrs. Tomasetti's Health Beliefs*

Outcome Belief	*Outcome Value*	*Salience*
1. Not following my diet is dangerous to my health because I have diabetes. (susceptibility)	positive	high
2. Uncontrolled diabetes is a serious condition. (severity)	positive	high
3. The result of controlling my diet is my good health. (benefit)	positive	low
4. I would have to lose my central place in the family if I diet. (cost)	very negative	very high
5. I don't think I can control my eating anyway. (self-efficacy)	very negative	very high

B. *Mrs. Tomasetti's Subjective Norms*

Referent Person or Group	*Value Orientation*	*Mrs. Tomasetti's Motivation to Comply*
1. Family*	very positive	very high
2. Close Friends	positive	high
3. Social Class	neutral	low
4. Ethnic Group*	very negative	very high
5. Religious Group	neutral	high
6. Physician	very positive	low

* Note that a conflict exists between the value orientations of Mrs. Tomasetti's family and ethnic group, and her motivation to comply with both is high. The physician might drastically change this system of subjective norms by raising Mrs. Tomasetti's motivation to adhere to his or her desires.

would require the health professional to persuade the patient to change one or more or his or her beliefs regarding the outcome evaluation and/or the normative persons' evaluation of the behavior. For example, the practitioner might try to persuade the patient that birth control pills are unlikely to cause much noticeable weight gain (thereby lessening the negative outcome evaluation). Likewise, the practitioner may try to persuade the patient that his bowling buddies are not as negative as he might think toward the patient's restriction of alcohol. This approach might be difficult (or impossible) if the facts are clear or immutable. The birth control pill may actually cause the patient to gain considerable weight (as she knows from previous experience), or the bowling buddies may really be quite strongly against the patient's abstinence from beer. Should this be the case, the second avenue to intentions can be pursued. This involves persuading the patient to change the salience of the troublesome belief (to conclude that weight gain is not such an important problem after all) or to change his motivation to comply with the troublesome referent (for example, to conclude that the opinions of his bowling buddies are not so important after all). Thus, the practitioner might try, through persuasion, to change the character of the patient's beliefs, or to change their salience, or both. Needless to say, the origin of those beliefs may need to be taken into consideration, as might the needs (such as security or esteem) that are served by maintaining them.

As noted earlier, in order to alter the intentions of the patient, the health professional must first alter the patient's beliefs (and as a result, his or her attitudes toward the behavior and subjective norms concerning the behavior). No doubt, many naturally occurring factors can bring about rapid changes in people's beliefs—factors such as religious conversions, traumatic events, physical illness, and falling in love. The practitioner whose goal is to change a patient's health behavior is likely to have neither the time nor the inclination to wait for one of these natural catalysts to behavior change. The practitioner usually wants to effect the change within a manageable period of time. The process of persuasion can help to accomplish this goal.

Persuasion is defined as a form of social influence in which one person uses a verbal appeal to change the behavior or opinions of another person (Stang & Wrightsman, 1981). Thus, persuasion represents one important practical, time-limited means available to the practitioner to change patients' beliefs. These belief changes can effect alterations in attitudes and subjective norms, and ultimately behavioral intentions can be formed.

As we saw in Chapter 2, there often exists a barrier in practitioner-patient communication. This barrier typically limits the amount and quality of information given to patients about their medical care. Even the specific regimen in which the patient must engage is often not clearly communicated to him or her, and so the patient remains confused and unsure of what he or she is required to do. Although patient education and the clear communication of information are not sufficient to bring about behavior change in patients, information and communication constitute a necessary first step. Simply stated, people must know of the practitioner's desire for them to change their behavior before they can be expected to do so. Yet, as reported by the Surgeon General (1979), only about 25 percent of smokers are told by their physicians to stop smoking. Only two-thirds of physicians and one-third of dentists now routinely ask if their patients smoke. The report of the Surgeon General estimated that the smoking rate might be somewhat reduced if physicians would routinely ask their patients about their smoking habits and simply recommend that they quit. While this approach may successfully change the behavior of only a few patients, it is likely to lay the groundwork for change for many more. The practitioner's communication of specific behavioral expectations to the patient is likely to be a crucial first step to bringing about changes in beliefs, and hence in behavioral intentions.

Despite the special expertise of health-care practitioners (particularly physicians), their mere communication of information normally cannot alter patients' beliefs. In fact, the limitations in the power of that expertise are the subject of this book. Later in this chapter, we examine the various forms of social power available to the health practitioner, how they operate, and how they might best be used to bring about patient's self-directed change in their beliefs (and hence in their intentions and behaviors). We begin here with one very basic aspect of the change process—persuasion of the patient by the health practitioner.

The goal of persuasion may be one or both of the following: to change one or more of the patient's beliefs about the behavior (the outcome evaluation of each belief, or its salience), or to change the patient's subjective norms concerning the behavior (the evaluation of the behavior by others who are important, or the patient's motivation to comply with their wishes). In the following section, we consider how persuasion might be accomplished using the general methods identified and supported empirically in the social-psychological literature. We will apply them to the health-care encounter. Later in the chapter, we will consider persuasion in a broader context and will examine the social power of health professionals to change their patients' beliefs.

PERSUASION

As noted above, persuasion is a form of social influence in which one individual attempts to effect a change in the behavior or opinions of another (Stang & Wrightsman, 1981). A great deal of research on persuasion suggests that people can indeed be influenced by others to change their beliefs and attitudes. Certain techniques and approaches are required, and these have been extensively studied in social-psychological research. Their application to health-care situations, although still in need of considerable empirical validation, is relatively straightforward.

An extensive program of research on persuasion was carried out by Yale University researcher Carl Hovland and his colleagues during and after World War II (Hovland, 1959; Hovland, Janis & Kelley, 1953; Rosenberg & Hovland, 1960). This research was based on the assumption that people process information rationally. The Yale attitude-change approach specified four factors that determine the extent to which a person will be persuaded by a communication. The person must *attend* to the communication (thus, it must be interesting enough to hold his attention). The individual must *comprehend* the message (note discussions in Chapter 2 on the importance of clear communication of information to the patient). The individual must *accept* the message or arguments used to change his opinion or belief. Finally, the individual must *retain* or remember the message. Thus, attitude-change methods should focus on improving the receiver's ability to attend to a persuasive message, to learn it, to remember it, and to incorporate it into his or her own attitudes and beliefs. The Yale researchers examined the characteristics of communicator, message, and audience that make attending, learning, remembering, and incorporating more likely to occur. Although this research was not specifically directed toward health-related belief change, its findings are in many ways generic and can be applied to health-care situations.

Many different social-psychological approaches to persuasion and belief change exist. These include: the *perceptual* approach [which emphasizes the importance of selectivity of perceptions and frame of reference; see Sherif and Hovland's (1961) social judgment theory]; the *functional* approach [which emphasizes the relationship of the position advocated in the persuasive message to the person's underlying personality needs; see Kelman, 1961; Katz and Stotland, 1959], and the *consistency* approach [which emphasizes the individual's need to maintain internal harmony in his or her belief system; see Festinger, 1957; Osgood & Tannenbaum, 1955]. The approach we emphasize in this chapter is primarily derived from the *learning* orientation to persuasion [which focuses attention on the source, content, and mode of the message, and on characteristics of the audience; Hovland, Janis & Kelley, 1953], but we include elements of the other three theories as well. The underlying framework for our discussion of beliefs, attitudes, intentions, and behaviors is, however, considered to be a *cognitive response* approach [Brock, 1981].

Characteristics of the Effective Persuader

The Yale researchers found that the success of the communicator of a persuasive message (his or her ability to persuade) depends upon the four characteristics examined below.

Expertness. In order to be persuasive, an individual must appear to be knowledgeable about the topic of concern. This was a major finding of the Yale attitude-change research (see also Croner & Willis, 1961), and is often corroborated by popular stereotypes of the persuasive salesman or public speaker (Carnegie, 1956). Certainly the health professional's expertise in areas of health and illness carries certain potential advantages. Throughout recent years, however, this is possibly becoming less and less true. The impression of authority of physicians and other professionals as experts on health and illness has begun to erode (Haug, 1976; Haug & Lavin, 1979). The developing consumer orientation among patients (Reeder, 1972), and the recent emphasis on self-help and alternatives to traditional medicine (Pelletier, 1979) suggest that the expertness required for effective persuasion may no longer be automatically attributed to the health professional as it once was (Eisenberg, 1977). The practitioner's role as an expert must now be earned.

The expertise required of today's practitioners is not limited to technical medical matters. It is estimated that in recent years more than 50 percent of all conditions brought for medical attention involve primarily psychosocial problems. A large percentage of the remaining conditions presented have associated psychosocial factors, either in their etiology or in their sequelae (Marsland, Wood, & Mayo, 1976). Expertness, then, demands an understanding and a working knowledge of psychosocial factors in medical care (DiMatteo & Friedman, 1979, 1982).

Related to expertness is an issue that will be considered again in Chapter 7. The health professional's own health behaviors (particularly the obvious ones, such as smoking and weight control) are likely to affect patients' perceptions of his or her degree of expertise about health. A patient is unlikely to be convinced of the expertise of a practitioner who endangers his or her own health through self-destructive behaviors. The precise operation of this latter factor, however, needs further empirical investigation.

Liking the Communicator. A second characteristic of the effective communicator, identified in the work of the Yale researchers, was that he or she is liked by the audience. Personal attractiveness and liking of the communicator—brought about by rapport with the receiver of the message—was found to be critically important in enhancing persuasiveness. A positive evaluation of the communicator is likely to be important because of its generalization to the message. The new belief may be embraced by the patient because of his or her positive response to the practitioner who advocates the new belief (Berkowitz, 1980).

In Chapter 3, we considered various aspects of practitioner-patient rapport that are likely to enhance the positive evaluation of the practitioner-communicator. We noted in Chapter 3 that verbal and nonverbal behaviors of the health professional in interaction with the patient were critically important, as were communications of warmth, genuineness, and empathy.

Confidence and Enthusiasm. The Yale researchers identified a third characteristic of the effective communicator—enthusiasm and interest, particularly in the delivery of the persuasive message. Effective persuaders are dynamic and believe the information they transmit. They exude confidence. According to Zimbardo, Ebbesen, and Maslach (1977), confidence heightens persuasiveness (particularly at the outset of a persuasive communication) because a confident communicator is assumed to believe his or her own message. Other studies of persuasive communications suggest that dynamism, enthusiasm, and confidence are displayed through nonverbal behaviors such as varying one's voice tone, nonverbal facial expressions and gestures (Berkowitz, 1980; London, 1973; Smith et al., 1975; Miller et al., 1976; Johnson, 1980). Maintaining eye contact with the receiver of the message communicates confidence, as does responsiveness (with verbal and nonverbal behaviors) toward what the receiver says in answer to the communication.

Trustworthiness. Finally, the Yale researchers found that in order for a communicator to have credibility, he or she must be perceived as trustworthy—as not deceiving or manipulating in any way, and as obviously motivated to communicate unbiased information. Two components of trustworthiness have been identified in the research. The first relates to the reliability of the communicator—his or her apparent dependability and predictability. The communicator must be consistent in his or her message in order for the receiver to believe that the message is reliably conceived. A health professional's inconsistency can cause the patient to lose confidence in his or her ability, knowledge, and capacity to make valid recommendations. A second component of trustworthiness involves the communicator's motives. The receiver must believe that the communicator's message is *not* delivered in the communicator's own self-interest, but is instead formulated for the good of the receiver. The patient, for example, must believe that his or her belief change brings no personal gain to the practitioner.

Interestingly, the two aspects of trustworthiness identified in the persuasion research are formalized in the social role of the physician that was proposed by sociologist Talcott Parsons (1951). According to Parsons, the practitioner must be *technically competent* (that is, have an abundance of knowledge from which to make consistent, trustworthy recommendations). The practitioner also must have a *collectivity orientation* (that is, altruistic motives that prevent him or her from acting other than for the good of the patient). In addition, the health professional is expected to be *free of value judgments* about the patient, and is expected to enact his or her role with emotional neutrality, never allowing positive or negative feelings for the patient to interfere with effective treatment. This suggests that the expected role of the health professional in American society embodies the characteristics of trustworthiness necessary for effective persuasion. Whether these expectations are actually fulfilled in the practitioner's behavior is, however, a separate issue altogether.

The Development of Persuasive Characteristics. The characteristics of an effective persuader, as described by the research of Hovland and colleagues, can be developed. Confidence, enthusiasm, expertness, and others that we have considered here can be enhanced through interpersonal behavior. Like the components of the art of medicine, characteristics of the effective persuader can be acquired through appropriate practice and continued self-monitoring (Johnson, 1980). Precisely how to develop these qualities (for example, what constitutes appropriate practice) is yet another important topic for future empirical research on the role of health professional in changing health beliefs and behaviors.

Characteristics of the Persuasive Message

The manner in which the health professional organizes and delivers his or her persuasive message to the patient is likely to determine, at least in part, the effectiveness of the message in changing the patient's beliefs (Johnson, 1980). When presenting a persuasive message, health professionals are often tempted (because of a lack of time or energy) to present only one side of an argument. For example, if the health professional's goal is to convince the patient of the merits of exercise, he or she will probably present only the side of the question that relates to the benefits of regular exercise (or, conversely, the problems that may result from a sedentary life style). It is likely, however, that at some point the patient will encounter the other side of the argument—i.e., that exercise has few beneficial effects on health. Research has found that it is best if the counter-argument is first heard by the patient from the persuader—in this case, the health professional (Zimbardo, Ebbesen, & Maslach, 1977; McGuire, 1969; Insko, 1967). If the patient is told by the health professional only about the positive effects of a particular action, and then learns elsewhere of the negative effects, the patient's belief in the expertise of the health professional may be weakened. The impact of the health professional's recommendations may be lessened. Therefore, a single side of any issue should be presented only when the patient is unlikely ever to encounter an opposing argument (Abelson & Karlins, 1970).

While presenting the various sides of an issue, the health professional should attempt to involve the patient actively in the development of arguments counter to the one being presented. Then, the effective health professional can develop arguments *along with the patient* to discredit those counter-arguments. The patient who has been actively involved in supporting the health professional's communication will be better able to withstand any threats to the new beliefs. In other words, when faced with the other side of the story, the actively involved patient will be better able or more likely to maintain his commitment to the belief encouraged by the health professional (Johnson, 1980; Zimbardo, Ebbesen, & Maslach, 1977).

Threat Communications and Scare Tactics. As we have noted in this chapter, many research studies have demonstrated that information per se is seldom capable of significantly changing beliefs or influencing behaviors. Many health professionals recognize this and try instead to motivate their patients through scare tactics. "If you don't stop smoking, you'll probably get lung cancer," says the well-meaning practitioner, whose subsequent description of the progress of the disease frightens the patient profoundly. Sometimes such fear-arousing messages motivate the patient to change his or her beliefs or behaviors. More often, though, health-threat warnings do not work at all. They may actually reduce the chances that the patient will change (Beck & Frankel, 1981).

Under what circumstances are health-threat warnings effective? Research has shown that their effectiveness depends upon the extent to which the warnings diminish or enhance the patient's perceived control over his or her own health. In fact, a patient's perception of personal efficacy, as well as his or her general belief in the efficacy of health action (often called "response efficacy") together will strongly affect health-belief change. While in Chapter 4 we saw that an individual's degree of perceived efficacy often reflects a generalized expectation, perceptions of efficacy can also be influenced by the communication. Research has found that threatening communications will produce belief change only when: (1) the warnings actually convince people that their health is in danger; (2) the recommended responses are perceived as efficacious (i.e., people are convinced that the threat to their health will be reduced if they take the recommended action); and (3) people believe that they themselves are indeed capable of carrying out the recommended responses (Beck & Frankel, 1981). Thus, the health professional's communication of a fear-arousing message in order to obtain a belief change will succeed only if the patient is convinced that the suggested steps for dealing with the threat are available and efficacious, and that he or she is fully capable of carrying them out. Feelings of lack of control in response to threat, on the other hand, may bring about overwhelming anxiety, helplessness, and even depression (Seligman, 1975).

A fear-arousing message may work quite well if it serves to arouse motivation and some facilitating anxiety in an otherwise complacent, unconcerned individual. Because it has the potential of overwhelming the patient with debilitating anxiety, however, the fear-arousing communication must be used cautiously. Its content is extremely important. The warning should always carry explicit behavioral recommendations. Thus, people who are told of the dangers of smoking, for example, should also be told that while it may be difficult to quit smoking, it *is* possible to do so. An illustration of a specific method for quitting smoking might also be presented. Of course, when considering the use of a fear-oriented appeal, the health professional must take into account the patient's personal characteristics, particularly his or her locus of control and past history. A patient who has experienced repeated failures at self-control may be unlikely to believe in his or her own efficacy. Finally, the health professional should also explore the amount of relevant information the patient has about the problem, because the fear-arousing quality of any factual presentation will depend upon what the patient already knows about the medical consequences of the issues at hand. In sum, the use of a fear-arousing persuasive attempt may be useful in some circumstances, but it demands the careful consideration of many important factors.

Distraction. Research in social psychology has found that distraction (such as a loud noise) can, paradoxically, have the effect of increasing agreement with a persuasive message (Keating & Brock, 1977). While intuitively it may seem that people would be better convinced of a particular belief if they are allowed to concentrate on the appeal without distraction, in fact this is not the case. When people are not distracted during attempts to persuade them, they often spend time thinking of counter-arguments to defend their own opinion against that of the persuader (Festinger & Maccoby, 1964). Distraction forces the person to attend more closely to the persuasive message in order to understand it. The person's active participation in trying to understand the message prevents him or her from developing contrary arguments. Of course, if the distraction is too extreme, the receiver of the communication will not be able to process or understand it at all, and its persuasive intent will be lost (Zimbardo et al., 1970; Insko, Turnbull, & Yandell, 1974).

The following example illustrates the use of distraction in the persuasive communication of information from practitioner to patient. It also suggests an important ethical question:

> While Dr. Evans was talking with Mrs. Arthur about the importance of quitting smoking, the intercom buzzer on his phone sounded. He picked up the receiver, listened for a few seconds, and then said, "I can't talk with you now about it. I'm talking with a patient. I'll have to discuss this with you later." Turning to Mrs. Arthur, he said, "Now, let's return to the smoking issue. You know it's bad for your health don't you, and that smoking has been linked with heart disease and lung cancer?" The buzzer sounded again, but Dr. Evans ignored the phone and continued to talk. "You know, the Surgeon General has evaluated all of the research done at top medical centers around the country. The dangerous effects of smoking are very clear." The buzzer sounded again but Dr. Evans continued. "It is really important for you to quit smoking because your own risk is getting to be quite high. After you quit, your lungs will become more like a non-smoker's again and your heart attack risk will be reduced." As Dr. Evans was talking, Mrs. Arthur was forced to listen very carefully because the buzzer was distracting. What Mrs. Arthur did not know was that the intercom call and buzzers were not actual calls. Dr. Evans activated the buzzer by tripping a

switch on the floor with his foot. He did this to maximize his ability to influence and persuade Mrs. Arthur to change her beliefs about smoking, and eventually to make a commitment to quit.

The use of the buzzer technique by Dr. Evans may be ethically controversial. Although it is used ultimately for the patient's own good, it represents some deception and manipulation on the part of the physician. What difference is there, however, between this technique and others that are used to influence the patient (such as the careful formulation of arguments that are likely to change the patient's mind)? Such ethical considerations are always in the forefront when we consider interpersonal influence and attempts by a persuader to bring about attitudinal and ultimately behavioral changes in another. We examine ethical considerations in detail in Chapter 8.

The Audience: Receiver of the Message

Whether or not a patient is persuaded by a message is also dependent upon the extent to which it can capture his or her attention. The message must appeal to the patient's interests and values for these determine in part what is rewarding to him or her. Thus, a persuasive appeal is more likely to succeed if it addresses the patient's values directly. For example, a patient who smokes and also values thrift is more likely to be persuaded by an argument that emphasizes the economy of not smoking. Aesthetic appeals, depicting smoking as unattractive, are likely to influence people who have aesthetic interests or who value how they look to others. Spiritual appeals are likely to work best with people who have spiritual values. Thus, determining a patient's values is critically important to enhancing persuasion (Johnson, 1980).

Interaction between Message and Audience

Complexity of the Message and the Patient's Active Participation. A persuasive message becomes most effective when it is developed to precisely the appropriate complexity for the patient, and when the patient's active participation in the communication is obtained. Attitude-change research has found that the influence of complex, subtle messages tends to last longer than that of simple messages. When messages are complex (although not too complex to be understood), the receiver must do the work of filling in the missing parts. The patient is thus able to generate his or her own reasons for accepting and acting on the message. As we noted earlier, attitude change is more persistent over time if the receiver of the persuasive message must participate in it actively rather than simply passively receiving it (Berkowitz, 1980; Zimbardo, Ebbesen, & Maslach, 1977). Consider this example:

Rather than tell Mr. Moreno to take penicillin four times a day, nurse-practitioner Debby Andrews actively involved her patient in the persuasive communication of a plan for treatment.

N.P.: According to the sensitivity test from your throat culture, Mr. Moreno, the best medication for this strep infection in your throat seems to be penicillin. Since you have taken it before and are not allergic to it, I'd like to prescribe it for you. Is that all right with you?
Mr. M.: Sure that sounds fine; whatever you think is best.
N.P.: Now, I have found that if my patients take this antibiotic four times a day at regular intervals—for example, about an hour before breakfast, lunch, and dinner and then at bedtime—the best results are obtained. Why do you think that is so?
Mr. M.: Because they remember to take it when it's connected up with something?
N.P.: Yes, that's part of it. Why else do you think that method works best? It has something to do with the ability of the antibiotic to fight the infection.
Mr. M.: Well, let's see. Maybe you want a pretty steady level of antibiotic available in the blood to destroy the infection?
N.P.: Yes. That's exactly right. So, do you see why a four-times-a-day penicillin regimen is important?

Mr. Moreno's participation in the establishment of the four-times-a-day regimen is likely to have contributed to persuading him of its importance.

Repeated Exposure to the Message. Research on persuasion has found that the more times a person hears a message, the more likely he is to remember and be persuaded by it (Moreland & Zajonc, 1977; Bogart, 1967; Zajonc, 1968). The more times a health professional mentions to a patient that it is a good idea to quit smoking cigarettes, the more likely it is that the patient will stop—that is, under certain conditions. Evidence in favor of repeating messages is very strong. Repeating the message gives the person a chance to learn it. In addition, the person can develop a positive attitude toward the message simply as a consequence of repeated exposure to and familiarity with it (Zajonc, 1968).

The conditions must be right, however, if a positive effect is to result from exposure to a message. The positive effects of mere exposure to anti-smoking messages, for example, are more likely to occur if the repeated stimulus is not completely predictable. If the patient hears the same message every time he encounters the health professional, the patient will tend to predict it and possibly then to ignore it. Similarly, if the receiver is bored by the persuasive message, the effects will be detrimental to the goal of persuasion (Harrison, 1977). Finally, repeated exposure can have a "boomerang" effect if a patient for whom the message was intended is initially antagonistic to it, finds it distasteful, or is skeptical of it. After repeated exposure, the individual is likely to feel even more negatively toward such a message (Brickman et al.,

1972). Thus, in order to avoid a boomerang effect, the initial message which is repeated should be neutral or positive in relation to the patient's existing values.

The Sleeper Effect. Finally, an important phenomenon discovered in attitude-change research is known as the "sleeper effect." The desired opinion change occurs sometime after exposure to a persuasive message, but does not happen right away. Usually the person eventually remembers the persuasive message and may change his or her own belief as a result of it. The receiver forgets, however, from whom the message first came (Cook & Flay, 1978; McGuire, 1969; Hovland, Janis, & Kelley, 1953). For example, Mr. Pedley has considered quitting smoking but is not quite ready to take the step to a behavioral commitment. There are still some beliefs to which he holds, and these beliefs prevent his statement of an intention to quit. Mr. Pedley's doctor told him that quitting smoking is easier if he first assesses (perhaps by keeping a diary) the time, place, and situation surrounding each light-up of a cigarette. Mr. Pedley can then determine under what circumstances and in response to what stimuli he feels the desire to smoke. He may not be at all convinced by the practitioner's arguments in favor of this assessment approach. In fact, he does not even remember what the doctor told him. A few months later while talking with his friend about quitting smoking, Mr. Pedley mentions that a good way to start is to keep a record of the times, places, and circumstances under which he smokes. He cannot remember who suggested this to him, but he knows he heard it somewhere.

ALTERNATIVE APPROACHES TO BELIEF CHANGE

Role-Play

An effective technique for changing beliefs is role-play, as illustrated in this example:

> Dr. Flynn tried unsuccessfully for many years to convince Jack Murphy that he should stop smoking. No argument seemed to persuade Jack that smoking was dangerous and that he should make a commitment to overcome his dangerous habit. During one of his routine visits to the clinic for a check-up, Jack was greeted by Dr. Flynn, who suggested that together they role-play a particular situation. Jack was to pretend that he was a patient found to have lung cancer, most likely caused by cigarette smoking. Dr. Flynn was to play the role of the physician communicating the tragic news. Enacting this scenario was upsetting to Jack. As they played their respective roles, he and Dr. Flynn discussed the possible treatments available for lung cancer, the poor prognosis, and the uncertain future for himself and his family. They discussed many details of the

upcoming months of serious illness and terminal care. Jack was so shaken by the role-playing situation that he asked Dr. Flynn to recommend some methods he might try to help him stop smoking. Pretending to be a lung cancer patient was distressing enough to convince Jack that his smoking was dangerous. The role-play helped him to alter his beliefs sufficiently to state an intention to quit.

The role-play technique can be quite successful in persuasion (Janis & King, 1954). Research on the role-play technique clearly supports its efficacy under circumstances in which the individuals take their roles seriously. In fact, the original role-play research required smoking subjects to simulate physician and patient in discussions of lung cancer caused by cigarette smoking (Janis & Mann, 1965). Subjects who were smokers enacted the same kind of scenario as Jack Murphy. Those who had experienced the role-play were more likely than individuals in the control group to change their attitudes toward smoking, to stop the behavior, and to maintain their state of abstinence (Mann & Janis, 1968). There was little change in attitudes or behavior among control-group subjects who simply heard a persuasive message regarding the evils of smoking.

Role-play is actually a set of techniques with varying forms. These techniques operate in different ways to bring about changes in beliefs (Aronson, 1969; Bem, 1972; Gerard, Conolley, & Wilhelmy, 1974). Role-play involves a simulation exercise in which the individual assumes the role of another person or espouses an idea contrary to his own. Having the subject take the role of another person is illustrated by the example of Dr. Flynn and Jack Murphy above. Role-play can also involve the individuals' reversal of their usual roles (for example, the patient would play the role of the physician and try to persuade the physician, who would play the role of the patient). The message might involve such things as the communication of the disadvantages of smoking. This technique forces the patient to participate actively in producing arguments for the desired position or belief. The possibilities for role playing are numerous, and it may require some imagination and creativity for the health professional to design a role-play situation that will work best for an individual patient. Role-play can also be used to help the patient to practice expressing a new belief or attitude (such as refusing the offer of a cigarette) until he or she becomes comfortable doing so.

Role-play techniques are effective partly because they are capable of arousing in the individual the emotion he or she would likely experience in the actual situation being role-played (for example, fear and remorse upon learning of one's lung cancer). The patient may then be motivated to learn what he or she can do to prevent the situation in reality. Of course, as we saw earlier, if the patient's fear is aroused, the health professional must make clear to the patient the precise course of action necessary to avoid the situation that has been role-played. This technique is successful also because it helps the individual to see a perspective other than his or her own, and to understand more fully the issues supported by the persuader. By taking the role of the health professional, the patient may come to understand his or her beliefs more fully.

Positive Expectations

Another important influence on belief change is the practitioner's expectation for the patient. If a health professional feels that a patient is hopeless—that is, that he or she is unlikely to change beliefs or behaviors—the health professional's prediction may work to fulfill itself. The relationship between prediction and outcome may be due in part to the health professional's ability to make predictions. This is not the complete explanation, however. The health professional's behavior toward the patient may actually subtly encourage the patient to fulfill the prophecy. Of course, positive expectations can work in the same way, and health professionals' positive expectations for their patients are likely to contribute positively to altering the latter's beliefs.

A great deal of research in the field of social psychology has documented the powerful effects of interpersonal expectations (Rosenthal, 1969). The earliest research studies were done with rats. It was found that college-student experimenters who believed that their rats were "bright" (that is, could learn to run a maze easily) actually obtained better results from their rats than college students who believed that their rats were "dull." In actuality, all the rats came from the same strain and were equal to one another in learning capacity. The only difference between the bright and the dull rats was the expectation that their trainers held for them. When the behavior of the college-student trainers of supposedly bright rats was compared with the behavior of trainers of supposedly dull rats, notable differences emerged. The trainers of the bright rats gave their rats more attention than did the trainers of dull rats. They touched them more and rewarded them sooner after success in running the maze. Because of the experimental nature of these studies, it could be concluded that the differences in the rats' performance were due to the expectations of their trainers. These expectations influenced the rats through their trainers' behavior toward them.

If expectations can influence the performance of rats, can they also influence the behavior of people? Social psychologist Robert Rosenthal (1976) conducted many studies and also reviewed an overwhelming amount of evidence in support of the role of interpersonal expectations in many areas of human social interaction. One important area involved the performance of elementary-school children. In one experiment (later replicated in different settings), a few children in each class of an elementary school were singled out to their teachers as being promising for "intellectual blossoming" during the school year. This prediction was ostensibly made by psychologists on the basis of tests of intellectual potential. Actually, the children who were singled out in each classroom as special had been randomly chosen. These children were neither more nor less capable than others in their class. At the end of the school year, however, the children for whom their teachers had positive expectations actually gained significantly more points on a measure of intellectual ability than children who were not singled out. Studies of the behavior of teachers with positive expectations for certain students have shown that teachers behave more warmly toward students for whom they have positive expectations. They also give these children more feedback about their answers and a longer time to think of an answer before calling on someone else. Expectations that the children would perform well are translated into behavior that helps them to perform well (Rosenthal, 1976).

This research has important implications for the care of patients. Awareness of the possible effects of their interpersonal expectations may, for example, aid health professionals to avoid holding negative expectations for certain patients. Also, focusing on the positive aspects of patients' abilities and strengths may help a health professional to develop and to act upon expectations for the positive outcome of influence attempts. Believing that a patient can and will change and communicating that belief to the patient through actions and words may ultimately contribute a great deal to changing the patient's beliefs and improving the patient's health behavior.

BEHAVIORS, ATTITUDES, AND SELF-PERCEPTIONS

Behaviors and Attitudes: The Feedback Connection

It is probably not surprising to hear that beliefs (and their associated attitudes) are among the causal factors in the initiation of behavior. Knowing that 45-year-old Mrs. Jones values health and vigor, for example, partly explains why she runs three miles every morning. It may be surprising, however, to suggest that Mrs. Jones values health and vigor partly *because* she runs three miles every morning. The enactment of behaviors can influence beliefs and attitudes. There is a reciprocal relationship between the two.

Social-psychological theories and programs of research suggest that under certain conditions, behavior can bring about beliefs and attitudes. The theory of cognitive dissonance, proposed by social psychologist Leon Festinger (1957), addresses this issue. It is concerned with consistencies and inconsistencies between people's attitudes and behaviors. Festinger's theory proposes that if a person's behavior is inconsistent with an attitude he or she holds at that time, the person will experience discomfort or cognitive dissonance. As a result, he or she will be motivated to seek a resolution that brings the beliefs and the behaviors into line with one another (Festinger, 1964). If the behavior has already occurred, it obviously cannot be changed, and so the individual must change his or her attitudes and beliefs. Thus, if a person finds that he or she has enacted a behavior that is discrepant with his or her beliefs, and that no obvious explanations exist for the behavior (for example, high payment, or coercion), the individual will resolve the dilemma by changing the beliefs.

Social psychologist Daryl Bem has proposed a similar theory to explain how behavior might be a causal agent in beliefs—a finding that appears repeatedly in research studies. Bem (1967) suggests that people infer their beliefs and attitudes from their behaviors. According to this theory, a person may not know what his attitude really is until he observes his own behavior. Thus, Bem's theory would suggest that Mrs. Jones' attitudes about health and vigor derive from her observation that she runs every morning. This theory implies that belief change can occur in response to behavior change.

Evidence suggests, then, that there exists an important reciprocal relationship between attitudes and behaviors. Health professionals might use this "feedback loop" to implement healthy beliefs and healthy behaviors (Bandler, Madaras, & Bem, 1968). Within this framework, the health professional might, upon recognizing the patient's performance of a health behavior, seize the opportunity to encourage beliefs and attitudes that are consistent with the healthy behavior. For example, Mrs. Jones may initially run to keep her husband company, not because she particularly values physical activity and exercise. The change in her beliefs and her self-perception (as valuing exercise, health, and vigor) could be promoted by the health professional's stated admiration of the patient's commitment to health values. The practitioner can help to establish for the patient the connection between behavior and belief. In turn, the patient's beliefs may encourage his or her initiation of more health behaviors. Thus, in the total picture of care, the health professional might initially use persuasive techniques (as above) to encourage Mrs. Jones' positive evaluation of exercise. When she begins to exhibit the new health behavior, the feedback loop may be used to enhance her beliefs in the value of exercise (and her perception of herself as someone who values health).

There is little question that the initiation of behavioral change is a complex and difficult process. Knowing that beliefs and behaviors may influence one another reciprocally suggests some potentially valuable approaches to the initiation and support of health behaviors. Patients' self-perceptions may also play an important role in the belief-behavior feedback loop. In the following section we consider self-perceptions and their potential role in the relationship between attitudes and behaviors.

The Role of Self-Perception

An important principle of the theories of self-perception (Bem, 1967) and cognitive dissonance (Festinger, 1957) involves the freedom of choice associated with the performance of the target behavior. Belief or attitude change is unlikely to result from behavior change that is coerced or compensated very highly. Thus, the patient's perception of the conditions surrounding his or her performance of the behavior is an important factor in the resultant formation of beliefs.

The practitioner has the capacity to influence the patient's self-perceptions, beliefs, and ideas regarding freedom of choice. Focusing on the patient's past behavior, for example, and eliciting a self-perception based on it can be an effective method for developing beliefs consistent with the desired behavioral intention. For example, in a discussion with Mrs. Jones, the health professional might attempt to elicit a description of various forms of exercise in which she has engaged in the past. The health professional might then use this information to point out to Mrs. Jones that she is indeed capable of carrying out a program of exercise. The health professional's emphasis on Mrs. Jones' past exercise behavior as a reflection of the value she places on health and vigor may contribute in an important way to her beliefs and attitudes, and in turn may help to bring about the behavioral intentions desired. The elimination of self-perceptions that are inconsistent with the desired belief and behavioral intention might also be accomplished.

Johnson and Matross (1975) have suggested five steps that the health professional might use in order to elicit a patient's unhealthy self-perceptions (those that thwart the target behavior) and to confront the patient with concrete evidence to refute them. By means of this process, which involves questioning the patient and leading him or her to the desired conclusion, the health professional encourages the patient to arrive inductively at a new view of himself or herself. The view is one that is consistent with the goal-behavioral intention. These five steps, with health-related examples, are:

1. The health professional initially attempts to identify the self-perception or attitude that needs to be changed. One example is the patient's belief that he or she cannot resist physical gratifications (such as eating) and therefore lacks self-control. The health professional's goal in changing this self-perception is to examine the patient's various past behaviors that are incompatible with it. For example, the patient's past successful cessation of smoking, and his or her tendency to overeat only at home could be elicited as incompatible with the patient's self-perception that he or she always lacks self control.
2. The health professional then questions the patient about behaviors related to the attitude or self-perception. For example, the practitioner

might ask, "What are some examples of times when you have controlled your eating?" The initial question must be general, and must focus on the positive aspects of the patient's behavior. The question for the patient is not, "When have you *not* controlled yourself?" but rather "When *have* you controlled yourself?"

3. The health professional then asks for more specific examples of recent behaviors, such as those involving self-control. The health professional might ask, "When have you recently controlled habitual behaviors like smoking or drinking or eating?" If the patient gives an example of his or her *lack* of control, the health professional must acknowledge this information briefly (e.g., "So ice cream is a problem") and then repeat the explicit question about the target issue: "When did you last control . . . ?"
4. The health professional then pursues a detailed examination of the outcome of the past successful behaviors. He or she may ask questions such as: "How did you feel when you stopped smoking? Were you able to breathe better? Was your family proud of you? Did you achieve a sense of personal satisfaction?" The health professional then may suggest how the patient could have acted had he or she not been in control: "You know, you could have just continued to smoke and endangered your health, but you controlled yourself very well and reduced your health dangers. It seems that you do have a lot going for you." This is the first time that the health professional is directive in drawing conclusions and stressing the patient's strengths.
5. Finally, after collecting as many examples as possible, the health professional demonstrates how these form a consistent pattern. This is done by reiterating three or four of the best examples of the patient's past behaviors (including a brief, nonspecific acknowledgment of the negative behaviors). For example, the practitioner might say, "You see, when you really put your mind to controlling yourself, you can do it. It seems that you sometimes lose control—particularly when it comes to eating ice cream at home. But, overall the evidence suggests that you can decide to make a change in your life, and carry out that change with self-control."

The manipulation of patients' self-perceptions is one successful method for belief change, particularly with regard to beliefs in self-efficacy. This method is more effective than simply lecturing the patient because the patient must generate his or her own evidence for beliefs. Self-deprecation, doubt, and belief in one's inability to change usually result from a collection of negative beliefs. Beliefs in self-efficacy are needed in order to develop health-behavior intentions. Therefore, the practitioner must help the patient focus attention on his or her positive actions, and thus modify the patient's self-perceptions. Since the past behaviors cannot be altered, the health professional must guide the patient's interpretation of them and work to bring about the patient's appropriate self-perceptions toward the goal of stating a behavioral intention.

Enhancing the Stability of Beliefs

As we have seen, there are many ways in which a patient's beliefs can be changed. The new beliefs will not endure subsequent external pressures to change, however, unless they are stabilized. For example, a person may be persuaded that smoking is a dangerous habit, but his or her *internalization* of that belief (against smoking and toward a healthy life style) is necessary in order for the belief to persist. The health professional can help the patient to stabilize new beliefs. Johnson and Matross (1975) suggest four ways to do this.

First, the health professional must thoroughly discuss the new beliefs with the patient so that they can become integrated into the patient's total system of beliefs. Once the patient has adopted one new belief, he or she may experience a changed view of other issues as well. For example, if the patient begins to value self-control and healthy action, he or she will probably also develop a new (negative) attitude toward self-destructive behavior. The health professional may need to help the patient resolve inconsistent beliefs and even formulate a new system of values.

Second, the health professional must constantly reiterate to the patient the positive consequences that may result from the new beliefs. For example, if a person makes a strong commitment to stop smoking, the health professional must point out the increased attractiveness, health, energy, and other beneficial consequences. It is more important, though, that the health professional explore the patient's own perceptions of the advantages (such as self-satisfaction) of the new belief. Once determined, these advantages can be supported and emphasized.

Third, the health professional must "inoculate" the patient against attempts to change the new belief. For example, the health professional may challenge the patient's new belief with mild counter-arguments, thereby forcing the patient to think of arguments to defend the new beliefs. The patient's arguments can then be used in the future should challenges arise from others. The health professional might also discuss hypothetical situations with the patient, such as: "What are you going to say when your buddies at work challenge your statement that smoking is dangerous, or when they say that people who don't smoke are cowards?" If the patient is able to work out some possible solutions to these challenges ahead of time, he or she will be better able to deal with them successfully when they arise.

Finally, the health professional must continually work to enhance the patient's feeling of personal responsibility for the belief change. The patient is more likely to maintain the change if it is attributed to his or her own decision, rather than to some external forces. Thus, the health professional must always emphasize the patient's free choice of the belief change.

THE SOCIAL INFLUENCE OF THE HEALTH PRACTITIONER

So far, we have considered various general approaches that are available to the practitioner for influencing patients' beliefs (and hence their attitudes and subjective norms). By applying techniques of persuasion, the health professional can attempt to bring about changes in patients' beliefs concerning the medical treatment regimen (its cost and efficacy), the character of the potential disease (severity, susceptibility), and the social norms regarding the behavior. These changes, in turn, contribute to the establishment of the patient's stated intention to cooperate and to follow the regimen. As we will demonstrate in Chapter 7, certain facilitating conditions must obtain if this intention is to be translated into action. Prerequisite to action, however, is the patient's stated intention to comply.

Techniques of persuasion would not be needed if the practitioner-patient relationship conformed perfectly to the Parsonian model (Parsons, 1951). In that model, the practitioner recommends health behaviors to the patient on the basis of his or her technical expertise and nonjudgmental stance. The patient is motivated to cooperate, since cooperation is one of the expectations of the sick role. In this ideal situation, in which the common enemy is the disease, "doctor's orders" are accepted and followed precisely. As we have seen so far, however, patients' beliefs are seldom precisely in line with those of the practitioner, and patients' social norms can interfere with the acceptance of the practitioners' suggestions. In addition, health professionals are rarely able to change the beliefs (and/or behaviors) of their patients simply because of their authority or social position. It is sometimes argued that in earlier days patients complied with regimens and altered their beliefs and intentions simply in order to please their "good old doc" (Rodin & Janis, 1979). This may be true, but the special trust once considered part of the practitioner-patient relationship appears to have eroded in recent years. Today it rarely exists (Eisenberg, 1977). Patients have begun to try to exert some control in situations (such as diagnosis and treatment) in which they have traditionally been given little control at all (Stimson, 1974). Nowadays, the practitioner's insistence upon submission to his or her authority is often met with resistance (Haug, 1976; Appelbaum, 1977).

Persuasion techniques (examined throughout this chapter) may now be more important than ever in the history of the practitioner-patient relationship. Traditional forms of social power and authority that were once available to the health practitioner (particularly to the physician) are no longer, by themselves, consistently effective. Instead, the practitioner requires a variety of forms of social influence in order to bring about change in patients' beliefs and attitudes. In the following pages we examine some of the more important of these aspects of social influence.

The Process of Social Influence

Social influence has been defined by social psychologists (Raven, 1974; French & Raven, 1959) as a process in which any change taking place in one person's beliefs, attitudes, or behavior has its origin in another person or group. The capacity to influence (or the potential to shape another person's beliefs, attitudes, or behaviors) is called *social power*. Thus, social power is translated into social influence when a change actually takes place in the target individual's beliefs, attitudes, or behaviors. Social interaction and social power are, by their nature, interdependent processes. In the context of social interaction, people influence one another. No less is true of the practitioner and the patient. While the practitioner attempts to influence the patient, the patient attempts also to influence the practitioner. Here we focus on the practitioner's influence on the patient. The reciprocal process of patient influencing practitioner is considered briefly in Chapter 7.

Social power

Social psychologist Bertram Raven (1974) has described six modes of social power. They are informational power, reward power, coercive power, expert power, legitimate power, and referent power. Let us illustrate these forms of social power with examples in which health professional, Dr. Davis, attempts to influence a patient, Mr. Banning. Mr. Banning is a 42-year-old, Caucasian, overweight hypertensive. His treatment regimen involves adherence to a low-sodium diet, weight loss, moderate exercise, and antihypertensive medication twice a day. Mr. Banning presents a compliance problem. His diet remains uncontrolled, he rarely exercises, and his medication taking is sporadic.

Informational Power. "Mr. Banning," said Dr. Davis, "the fact that your cholesterol is 235 puts you at risk already for a coronary. With your uncontrolled blood pressure, that risk is increased 500 percent." Informational power is based solely on the content of the communication. It is the information conveyed that ultimately brings about the social influence. For Mr. Banning, a 500 percent increase in coronary risk is convincing. Once Mr. Banning has been influenced to change his beliefs and attitudes, he will relate the change back to the information, not to Dr. Davis. He will be following the recommendation because he is trying to avoid a coronary, for which he carries a very high risk. Informational power is, by definition, socially independent. The five remaining sources of social power are, however, socially dependent—that is, change is dependent on something about the health professional or about his or her relationship with the patient.

Reward Power. Dr. Davis said, encouragingly, "Tell you what, Mr. Banning, if you make a commitment to monitor your food and medication intake, next time you come in there will be no charge for the visit." Reward power is based on the health professional's capacity to mediate rewards. Rewards can be both material (e.g., money) and personal (e.g., time or positive regard). If asked why he changed his mind and decided to make a commitment to the therapeutic regimen, the patient will refer to the reward. While the patient might use other explanations in addition to the reward, central to the influence he has experienced is the attractiveness of obtaining the reward from the practitioner.

Coercive Power. "Mr. Banning, if you won't make a commitment to monitor your food intake and your medication regimen, I'm afraid I won't be able to treat you anymore." Coercive power is based on the health professional's capacity to mediate punishment—sometimes physical, but primarily interpersonal.

Expert Power. "Take my word for it, Mr. Banning. I know a lot about heart attacks, blood pressure, and health. You ought to stick to the schedule you have for medication, and lose some weight or you will be in deep trouble. I really think you should trust my judgment." Expert power is based upon the patient's acceptance of the health professional's superior knowledge and skill.

Legitimate Power. "Mr. Banning, as your doctor, I suggest that you follow my instructions." Legitimate power is based on the patient's acceptance of the health professional's right to make medical demands of him (typically for his own good).

Referent Power. "Mr. Banning," said Dr. Davis, "your friend Mr. Beaumont is the same age as you are and has similar problems with his blood pressure. He sticks to his treatment regimen, and he's glad he does." Referent power is based on the patient's desire to identify with a particular person or group. In this case, Mr. Banning is motivated to be as compliant as his respected friend, Mr. Beaumont. The health professional also might use himself or herself as a referent. ("I have trouble losing weight too, but I follow this diet and I'm able to resist temptations to eat between meals.") This is only possible, of course, if the patient wishes in some way to identify with the health professional—to be like him or her in any number of ways. Referent power is based upon the patient's own decision to model his or her behavior after that of another person or group. The reference person or group has the power to change the individual's beliefs because of the individual's desire to emulate the referent.

It is important to note that the various forms of social power are usually used in combination and rarely appear alone. Any single communication might contain elements of a number of modes of social power.

Responses to Social Influence

Social psychologist Herbert Kelman (1958) has further extended the analysis of social power to describe three possible responses of the target person (the patient, in this case) to attempts at any form of social influence (that is, any exertion of social power). These responses are: compliance, identification, and internalization. *Compliance* refers to a response made in order to obtain rewards or avoid punishments. Thus, we might expect it to result from the use of reward power or coercive power. *Identification* refers to a response made out of a desire to be like another person or to feel included in a particular group. Identification is thus likely to result from the use of referent power, legitimate power, or expert power because the patient attempts to form a social unit with the practitioner, or else to conform to the role of a patient in response to the professional's expert or legitimate authority. *Internalization* occurs when the patient's responses are based solely on the congruence between the belief or attitude expressed by the health professional and the individual's system of values and beliefs. Of course, usually the patient must make changes in his or her existing pattern of beliefs in order to accommodate the beliefs advocated by the health professional.

Kelman has ranked these three responses to influence according to the degree of permanence in the change they usually produce. Compliance (specifically as defined by Kelman, *not* as used in the health literature and thus far in this book) is seen to induce the most temporary change. (Compliance in Kelman's scheme refers to a coercive event. Compliance as used in the health behavior literature is a broad term referring to the patient's following of treatment recommendations, whether as a result of coercion, identification, or [the ideal] internalization. As we noted earlier in Chapter 1, some theorists and researchers argue that the semantic labeling of patients' health behaviors may, in fact, influence or be a product of the processes which bring about those behaviors.) The continuance of the belief is typically controlled by the mediation of rewards and punishments. Of course, the change is likely to become more stable and to continue over time when the rewards and punishments are self-generated by the patient. If they are instead managed by the health professional, long-term change is unlikely because the health professional's continual management of the patient's rewards and punishments is usually impossible. Identification is typically maintained for as long as the association with the referent person or group is felt to be satisfactory. If, for example (as Rodin & Janis, 1977, suggested), the health professional is the reference person, it is necessary to maintain rapport and satisfactory practitioner-patient communication in order to maintain the change in beliefs. In general, the patient's continued use of any person or group as a referent is necessary in order to bring about continued change. As with compliance, the belief change is dependent upon the continued involvement of the influencing agent. Internalization is the most permanent response to social influence (Kelman, 1958). In order for internalization to occur, the individual must accept the information communicated, and incorporate it as a belief into his or her own personal belief system. The newly adopted belief (or behavioral commitment) must be felt to be congruent with and a logical extension of the individual's entire system of beliefs.

In Table 6.2, these three responses to social influence are examined in terms of their characteristics. The forms of social power that are expected to bring about each response are considered, and the medical-care situations in which the responses are most likely beneficial are presented. The analysis suggests that if the goal of care is to maintain self-motivated, long-term commitment from the patient, internalization would be best achieved. While it is not strictly true that *only* informational power (coupled with persuasion) can bring about internalization, a theoretical analysis of the operation of this form of social power suggests that internalization is the likely outcome. In the short term, referent power (enhanced by rapport) as well as expert power (which increases the acceptability of the message) may also help to bring about the initial change in the patient's beliefs. Long-term maintenance of the new beliefs (and hence, the intention to change behavior), however, is dependent upon the individual's incorporation of the new beliefs into his or her total belief system. Thus, the techniques examined throughout this chapter have as their ultimate goal the patient's internalization of new health-related beliefs, and a resulting statement of an intention to engage in behavior change.

Limitations of a Social Influence Approach

The analysis of patient cooperation with medical regimens in terms of social influence is advantageous. The understanding of social power and its resultant effects on the motivation of patients is particularly useful because it helps to clarify the factors that may enhance patients' internalization of health beliefs and hence their commitment to a behavioral intention based on those beliefs. Limitations exist in the analyses of social power, however,

Table 6.2. Responses to Social Influence.

Response	Societal equivalent	Dependence on relationship with influencing agent	Endurance of behavioral or attitude change	Necessity of surveillance by influencing agent	Requirements of influencing agent	Modes of social influence most likely to result in response	Medical Situations in which response is most beneficial
Compliance	Rules	very high	very low	high	Capacity to mediate rewards or punishments	Reward power, coercive power	Emergency care and acute care
Identification	Roles	high	low	none	Attractive, credible, & trustworthy	Legitimate power, expert power, referent power	Acute care
Internalization	Values	none	high	none	Capacity to present information congruent with target person's values	Informational power, referent power,* expert power*	Chronic care, life-style change, preventive care, self-care

* Probable prerequisites for the acceptance of information.

and so there are some important considerations that limit the operation of social-influence processes in effecting belief change in patients.

The first important issue involves the fact that the various forms of social power are each appropriate only under certain conditions (and hence only under certain circumstances of health-care delivery). Their use is highly dependent upon the goals of care. For example, the form (or forms) of social power that enhance the internalization of health recommendations may be necessary only when the regimen is long term (e.g., for chronic illness). A short-term regimen (one that requires, for example, only ten days of taking medication four times a day) might be quite successfully completed simply through the maintenance of reward power (e.g., "If you take this whole course of antibiotics as directed, I'll see you are motivated to take care of yourself and I'll make your appointments here maximally convenient for your work schedule"). Here too, however, the characteristics of the patient and the regimen will determine whether it is possible to administer and maintain those rewards and punishments. Whether coercive and/or reward power are appropriate will depend a great deal upon whether the practitioner is able to assess the patient's behavioral compliance (separate from the physical outcome), and to administer rewards and punishments (himself or herself, or by delegation of power to another). Thus, the use of various forms of social power will be affected by practical considerations, not only by what is appropriate for the patient at the given time.

With practical constraints put aside, the decision about the relative appropriateness of one or more of the forms of social power will usually depend upon what the practitioner determines to be best for the patient. This is no easy choice, however. In an effort to be nondirective and to use referent power, for example, a practitioner might remain totally unaware of the patient's need for expert power (and although the patient really desires advice, the practitioner will not give it). The decision about what sort of stance to take must be made anew with every patient. The practitioner must know the various forms of power available, their various meanings, and the details of their enactment. An analysis such as that in Table 6.2 might be quite helpful to the practitioner. In regard to the use of social power, Raven (1982) has suggested, "It is reasonable to assume that the choice of a more effective basis of power must be a function of the nature of the practitioner, the patient, their relationship, the type of behavior being influenced, and the situational and cultural variables, all of which must be explored further in careful investigations" (p. 16).

A second limitation is that some of the forms of social power that practitioners try to use together may be inconsistent with one another. For example, expert power might be used to enhance the acceptability of information to bring about belief change, and referent power might be used to establish the practitioner as a normative person. Yet, referent and expert power tend to be inconsistent with one another and probably cannot be developed simultaneously. As Raven (1982) has noted, it is very difficult for a patient to ascribe superior knowledge to the physician (the basis of expert power), and also see the physician as like himself in some way (the basis of referent power). Problems like this have not yet been resolved in the literature on social power in the health professional-patient relationship (Rodin & Janis, 1979, 1982; Rodin, 1982).

Finally, some forms of social power might actually be contraindicated in health settings because of their adverse side effects. For example, if threats and intimidation are used (coercive power), patients might rebel in an effort to restore what they feel may be their lost freedom (Brehm, 1966). If an individual makes a commitment to follow a special diet, but this commitment is made merely in response to social pressures or threats from the health professional (or from others such as family), the patient may never internalize the commitment to health action. The individual's feeling of restricted freedom of choice may result in a rebellious effort to regain that freedom (Brehm, 1966). The patient may even search for another, less coercive practitioner (Kasteler et al., 1976). Doing so, however, may involve undermining the special diet. The patient may thus endanger his or her own health. To avoid this rebellious effort, the health professional must facilitate changes in the patient's beliefs and attitudes so that they are in line with behavioral goals (Hertroijs, 1974).

The use of coercive power or reward power might also affect the powerholder's (practitioner's) beliefs about the patient. The more the practitioner uses directive and controlling means to bring about compliance, the more likely he or she is to believe that the patient's behavior is not self-controlled (Kipnis, 1976). Thus, we see that for many reasons the patient's development of an internal commitment may be prevented by the use of some forms of social power.

INTENTION AS ANTECEDENT TO ACTION

This entire chapter has been devoted to understanding the formation of behavioral intentions—the individual's subjective probability that he or she will engage in a particular behavior. We have been concerned with the formation of intentions primarily because *under the appropriate conditions*, intentions are good predictors of overt action. A stated intention to purchase something, for example, is a good predictor of purchasing (Gormeley, 1974). Intention is also a good predictor of drug use (Goldstein, Gleason, & Korn, 1975). Triandis (1977) and Fishbein and Ajzen (1975; also Ajzen & Fishbein, 1980) reviewed considerable empirical and theoretical literature in support of the importance of intentions as antecedents to behavior.

In the prediction of patient cooperation with medical treatment, intentions are quite important. Davis (1968) reviewed research by Korsch which related compliance to mothers' stated intentions to follow a physician's advice regarding care of their children. In this research, mothers of pediatric patients were asked (by an impartial researcher after their visit with the doctor) whether or not they intended to comply with the physician's suggested medical treatment regimen for the child. Mothers who stated that they had no intention of following the advice indeed were later found (on a follow-up home visit) to be noncompliant. Those who stated that they intended to follow the advice were much more likely to be compliant, although other factors did intervene between the intention and the behavior.

It is important for the health professional to elicit his or her patient's statement of an intention to comply. The stated intention is a good indication of the effectiveness of belief-change attempts. The stated intention suggests that, in the absence of barriers, the patient is planning to carry out the health action. An assessment of the patient's intention, then, is necessary in order for the health professional to decide whether to plan further methods of persuasion, or to begin a specific behavioral-change program with the patient.

The patient's stated intention may also work to increase the probability that a behavioral change will be made. A patient's verbally stated intention to comply can serve as a public commitment. "Commitment refers to the pledging or binding of an individual to a particular behavioral act" (Kiesler & Sakamura, 1966, p. 349). Commitment makes the promise to act less changeable, and the degree of an individual's commitment tells how easily he or she might dispense with the promise if necessary. Thus, a verbal statement of intention to carry out a particular behavior—especially a statement of the actual degree of commitment of the individual (measured as an intentional probability)—can increase the chances that the behavior will be carried out.

Studies of the effects of patients' stated intentions have typically shown that one or a combination of the following basic forms of commitment can significantly improve compliance: a simple verbal commitment to the health professional to follow the regimen; a written promise retained by the health professional; and a written contingency contract in which the health professional agrees to deliver some reinforcement (money, tokens, time) in return for patient compliance, within some mutually agreed-upon time frame. (This latter form of commitment involves behavior modification principles, considered in Chapter 7.) As an example of the first and simplest type, Levy, Yamashita, and Pow (1979) have shown that simple verbal commitment increased the likelihood that subjects enrolled in a flu innoculation program would return a postcard reporting the occurrence of flu symptoms. This type of compliance is simple and short term, involving only one action (mailing a postcard). Similarly, studies of both simple verbal commitment and verbal commitment with a written promise to perform a single task have shown that compliance increases significantly in proportion to the amount of commitment elicited (Levy, 1977; Wurtele, Galanos, & Roberts, 1980). More research is presently needed, however, to examine the effects of simple verbal commitment on the performance of multiple-task compliance behaviors.

Becker and Maiman (1980) have reviewed a number of studies in which patient-provider contingency contracts were used to enhance patient compliance. They demonstrated that contingency contracting significantly increases patient adherence (even among previously noncompliant patients). As we noted earlier in considering reward power, however, a problem with most contingency contracting is that long-term, self-reinforcement for behavioral and life-style changes is not likely to result. Indeed, the research on contracts has typically focused on very specific, limited behaviors (such as taking pills or following a specific diet). Typically, however, when the contingent reinforcements are withdrawn, the individual stops performing the health behavior.

So far, the literature shows a paucity of research on the acquisition and self-maintenance of healthy, long-term, self-reinforcing behaviors (Becker & Maiman, 1980). As we have seen in the present chapter, one important requirement for such change is commitment that follows from the individual's perception that he or she is free to act otherwise. The statement of an intention to follow a particular course of health action enhances the individual's feelings of personal responsibility for his or her behavior. The perception of personal responsibility appears to be at the core of true commitment (Kiesler, 1971), and hence is a critical prerequisite to the achievement and maintenance of long-term behavior change.

External commitment—the public statement of an intention—is not likely to come about easily. Most people do not want other peoples' knowledge of their intended behaviors to constrain and limit their freedom to change intentions (Kiesler, 1971). Therefore, the formation of intentions through adjustment of beliefs, attitudes, and subjective norms must be carried out with care, and these antecedents to the formation of intentions must be solidly constructed. A patient's publicly stated commitment demands the careful development of his or her supporting beliefs, attitudes, and subjective norms. Once achieved, the solidly based intention is likely to contribute significantly to the fulfillment of the behavioral goal.

FROM BEHAVIORAL INTENTIONS TO BEHAVIORS

Studies of the relationship between behavioral intentions and the actual performance of behavior suggest that while the relationship between the two may be high, there is no one-to-one correspondence (Ajzen & Fishbein,

1974). The more specific the behavioral intention elicited (e.g., "to eat only at mealtimes" rather than "to lose weight"), the more precisely will behavior correspond to (be predicted from) the intention. Even a stated public (verbal or written) commitment on the part of the patient, however, does not insure behavior change and cooperation with the treatment. Broken New Year's resolutions well illustrate the difficulty of translating intentions into behavior.

For a variety of reasons, an individual may be unable to carry out his or her intended health behaviors. These reasons may involve the physical, social, and/or psychological state of the person (Kirscht, Becker, & Eveland, 1976). Social disapproval and family criticism, as well as deeply ingrained habits, may interfere with following the regimen (Rosenstock & Kirscht, 1979; Triandis, 1977). In fact, a great variety of obstructing or facilitating factors are likely to influence whether the behavioral intentions are carried out (Aday & Andersen, 1974). In the next chapter, we consider these facilitating and inhibiting factors in greater detail, and examine some methods for overcoming barriers to and enhancing supports of the translation of intentions into behaviors.

7

From Intentions to Behaviors: Supports and Barriers in the Accomplishment of Medical Goals

Once the patient has overcome his or her initial skepticism of, or opposition to, a treatment regimen, and has developed attitudes and subjective norms consistent with it, he or she inaugurates the intention to carry out a health behavior. As we saw in Chapter 6, the intention to enact a health behavior—whether to take medication regularly or to adhere to a diet, exercise, or smoking-cessation program—is a joint function of the individual's attitudes and subjective norms. Each of these is weighted by its importance. Health practitioners often consider their efforts successful when the patient is persuaded to change his or her beliefs, attitudes, and subjective norms. The statement of a behavioral intention sees the patient sent home to accomplish the promised behavioral goal. Practitioners typically do not recognize, however, that the adage, "The road to hell is paved with good intentions," probably applies to no issue better than to the development of health behavior. New Year's resolutions, broken soon after they are made, also illustrate the lack of correspondence between intentions and behavior. In fact, it is precisely because the patient is left on his or her own to accomplish behavioral goals—without skill, knowledge, or support—that failure is all but guaranteed.

In this chapter we examine some of the difficulties that accompany the translation of behavioral intentions into behavior change. We investigate some of the typical barriers encountered by well-intentioned patients when they are left to contend with their medical prescriptions. We analyze methods by which practitioners might assess these barriers and the forms of assistance available to patients to overcome them. We also consider factors that, conversely, may support the transition from intentions to behavior. We emphasize throughout that there is no single or simple solution to the problems of translating intentions into behavioral changes. The important factors are manageable in number and character and they are considered within the boundaries of practicality by the practitioner who is caring for patients.

The barriers and supports we consider are, in many instances, related to one another in a reciprocal fashion—such as when the absence of the support is itself a barrier to change. An excellent example of this is family support. The presence of a supportive, helpful kinship network (composed primarily but not exclusively of individuals who live in the patient's home) is extremely useful in enhancing the patient's ability to carry out the treatment regimen. Family members may provide tangible help (such as cooking tasty, salt-free meals for the hypertensive patient) and/or psychological help (such as providing encouragement and emotional support when the patient is discouraged about the regimen). Lack of family support, on the other hand, represents not only the absence of yet another bridge across the gap between intentions and behaviors. Instead, the absence of family support may represent a barrier precisely because family support is expected as a validation of the patient's own worth and the value of his or her health goals. If family members display hostility toward the patient's attempts to follow the regimen (for example, if a husband deliberately tempts his dieting wife with fattening foods and/or disparages her and says that she is destined to be fat), a significant barrier to the fulfillment of the behavioral intention is erected. In this chapter we examine various barriers and supports, and we strive to keep in mind the reciprocal nature of their operation.

SUPPORTS AND BARRIERS TO BEHAVIOR CHANGE

Access to Medical Care

It probably comes as no surprise that certain practical issues in patients' lives may limit (or totally obstruct) their capacity to cooperate with medical recommendations. This is particularly true when the regimen requires keeping referral or follow-up appointments at a medical clinic or private physician's office. The patient's access to medical care (primarily the availability of treatment within the range of the patient's resources) has proven to be among the most important determinants of compliance and preventive health behavior (Cummings, Becker, & Maile, 1980). Access to care is one of six factors common to most models of health behavior (reviewed in Chapter 4). Access is particularly important when patients are recommended for follow-up care after an initial health screening (such as for hypertension), when a preventive-medicine regimen (such as immunization) is recommended, or when treatment for a medical condition requires periodic monitoring during appointed medical visits. In order to understand fully the role of access in compliance, we must examine its many individual aspects as they enhance or hinder health behavior.

Characteristics of clinic scheduling tend to influence compliance with appointment keeping. If a long period of time elapses between the screening detection of a patient's medical problem and the referral appointment, the patient is less likely to keep the appointment (Finnerty, Shaw, & Himmelsbach, 1973; Glogow, 1973; Hoenig & Ragg, 1966). Presumably, the patient has more time to forget about the appointment (or possibly to change beliefs or subjective norms and hence intentions to comply with it). In addition, the longer the waiting time for the patient once he or she has arrived at the clinic for the appointment (in some studies this was documented to be well over an hour), the less likely the patient is to keep the next appointment (Alpert, 1964; Geersten, Gray, & Ward, 1973; Raynes & Warren, 1971).

Factors in patients' lives that interfere with reaching their source of medical care may significantly affect their compliance with appointments. Patients cite the following reasons for not keeping their appointments: a lost appointment slip (Harfouche et al., 1973); confusion over the appointment (Hansen, 1953; Badgley & Furnal, 1961); difficulty getting an appointment (Tuomilehto, Rajala, & Puska, 1976); inability to get a babysitter (Alpert, 1964; Bracken, 1977; Rickels, Anderson, & Howard, 1968); lack of transportation (Abernethy, 1976; Alpert, 1964; Harfouche et al., 1973; Mealey, 1975; Rickels et al., 1968); and weather conditions (Mealey, 1975).

The Cost of Treatment

A related issue is financial need. Many studies report that patients cite their financial needs as explanation for their noncompliance (Alpert, 1964; Caldwell et al., 1970; Davidson, Hudson, & Parry, 1975; Kincey, Bradshaw, & Ley, 1975; Oh, 1974; Weintraub, Au, & Lasagna, 1973). Indeed, some research has found a positive relationship between compliance and income (Brand, Smith, & Brand, 1977; Brand & Smith, 1974; Collette & Ludwig, 1969; Ludy, Gagnon, & Caiola, 1977; Moulding, Onstad, & Sbarbaro, 1970; Suchman, 1967). Two have found a negative relationship, however (Ludwig & Gibson, 1969; Murthy, 1977), and Haynes, Taylor, and Sackett (1979,

Table 6, p. 461) reviewed 20 studies that examined income anu ˎ and found no relationship between them. How do we resolve this que..

First, the financial cost of treatment in comparison to the patient's income should be considered solely as a potential barrier between intentions and behaviors, not as a general determinant of compliance. The finding that providing patients with free medications had no effect on their medication compliance (Cody & Robinson, 1977; Bonnar, Goldberg, & Smith, 1969), for example, suggests that lack of resources and the cost of treatment do not, in general, function as significant impediments to compliance. It is only after beliefs and attitudes have been formed to support intentions that resources operate on behavior. Thus, the removal of resource barriers is likely to be effective only after behavioral intentions have been achieved.

Second, since financial affordability of the regimen is a necessary (though not sufficient) condition for compliance (Alpert, 1964; Brand, Smith, & Brand, 1977; Hemminki & Heikkila, 1975), affordability should be examined by the practitioner whenever an individual patient is assigned a particular treatment regimen. The patient's financial capacity to follow the regimen at the time that it is prescribed requires exploration. In many instances, less expensive generic drugs might be prescribed (Bonnar, Goldberg, & Smith, 1969; Cody & Robinson, 1977; Stamler et al., 1975; Haynes et al., 1977; MacHann, 1976) or an alternative method of treatment might be chosen (Colcher & Bass, 1972; Feinstein et al., 1968; Hudson & Sbarboro, 1973; Onstad, Sbarboro, & Rotenberg, 1970; Romm, Armstron, & Prior, 1975; Russel et al., 1976; Silverstone & Solomon, 1965; Epstein & McCoy, 1975; Haynes et al., 1977) and compliance consequently improved. Of course, as we noted above, other costs must also be taken into account in understanding and attempting to overcome a patient's difficulties in translating his intentions into behavior.

Complexity of the Treatment Regimen

Many studies have sought to examine the relationship between compliance and both characteristics of the disease and the difficulty of the treatment regimen. Some important results have emerged.

Haynes (1979a) has reviewed the literature and concluded that with only a few exceptions that involve psychiatric illness (psychiatric patients, particularly those with schizophrenia, paranoid features, and personality disorders, are less compliant than other psychiatric patients and less compliant than medical patients in following a drug-treatment regimen), disease factors have relatively minimal influence on compliance. Disease severity has not emerged as an important impetus to compliance. Nor has patients' increasing symptom severity been found to improve their cooperation with the treatment regimen. In addition, previous experience with a disease, and even prior hospitalization that resulted from it, did not encourage compliance with treatment. One disease-related factor—the physician's rating of disease prognosis—was associated with higher compliance (Lipman et al., 1965). The more positive the prognosis, the greater the compliance (although the direction of causality here is, of course, not clear). For the most part, however, as Haynes (1979a) concluded, disease features are not important factors in patient compliance: "Since none of these factors offers much of an opportunity for the detection or improvement of compliance, future research in this area must have a relatively low priority" (Haynes, 1979a, p. 53).

The number of medications or treatments prescribed for a patient has a significant and clear effect on his or her compliance. The more treatments or medications prescribed, the lower the compliance rate (Brand, Smith, & Brand, 1977; Clinite & Kabat, 1969; Davis & Eichhorn, 1963; Francis, Korsch, & Morris, 1969; Hemminki & Heikkila, 1975; Hulka et al., 1975; Malahy, 1966; Neely & Patrick, 1968; Parkin et al., 1976; Weintraub, Au, & Lasagna, 1973). Presumably, difficulties arise in coordinating a number of different regimens at once. In addition, resources needed in order to follow one regimen may be consumed by attempts to follow another. The duration of treatment also has a consistent relationship to compliance such that compliance decreases with the amount of time the patient has been assigned to the regimen (Bergman & Werner, 1963; Charney et al., 1967; Glick, 1965; Gordis & Markowitz, 1971; Ireland, 1960; McKenney et al., 1973; Romm, Armstrong, & Prior, 1975; Williams & Duncan, 1976). Over time, it is likely that resources become depleted and/or that motivations to follow the medical recommendations dwindle.

A few popular but erroneous notions about compliance barriers continue to persist among practitioners. The first of these notions is that the number of pills required to be taken per day influences compliance. Contrary to practitioners' beliefs, however, Haynes (1979a) found in a number of studies, that reducing the number of pills *per day* did not enhance patients' accurate adherence to the regimen (Parkin et al., 1976; McInnis, 1970; Lima et al., 1976). A second erroneous notion is a common claim made by practitioners—that treatment-regimen side effects cause noncompliance. This is supported in only two studies reviewed by Haynes (1979a: Rickels, Boren, & Stuart, 1964; Nelson et al., 1975) and both were studies of psychiatric patients. The bulk of evidence for medical patients asserts that this notion is not correct. Two controlled studies found no differences in side effects between compliers and noncompliers (Latiolais & Berry, 1969; Willcox, Gillan, & Hare, 1965) and 13 studies that examined patients' reasons for not following their medication regimens accurately found that side effects generally appeared well down the list, mentioned by only 5 to 10 percent of patients.

Further, Haynes argued that noticeable drug side effects are simply not very common.

Dispensing the Medication

It is interesting that the form in which a drug is dispensed can serve as a barrier to carrying out the required regimen. Lane, Barbarite, Bergner, and Harris (1971) found that the use of safety-lock pill containers (child-proof) resulted in significantly less medication taking among patients than did the use of regular, easy-to-open pill containers. In addition, Mattar, Markello, and Yaffe (1975a, 1975b) found that community pharmacists themselves actually made errors in their dispensing of medication, such that in 15 percent of all prescriptions for ten-day courses of antibiotics, fewer pills were given to the patient than were prescribed. This suggests, incidentally, that researchers who use pill counts to measure compliance should make an effort to determine or control the number of pills that the patient had to begin with. Such action may be necessary if one's assessment of patient compliance with the medication regimen is to be accurate.

The Multiproblem Patient

While nearly every patient faces some barriers to the translation of intentions into behaviors, a few patients, by virtue of their social environment, financial status, or other characteristics, experience an overwhelming number of these barriers. Practitioners sometimes encounter patients whose social functioning is so chaotic that their cooperation with treatment and hence their physical health is seriously impaired. Health professionals are sometimes overwhelmed by the dismal history that such a patient presents. This history is usually characterized by turmoil such as unemployment, poverty, and trouble with the law. Rarely do such patients plan ahead because they lead a "crisis life." They respond to demands on a day-to-day basis. Because of this, following a long-term treatment regimen is difficult or impossible. Although the patient may intend to follow the regimen, and may believe that it is important to do so, the demands of everyday life focus the patient's attention not on "getting ahead" but simply on "getting by" (Golden, 1978).

The multiproblem patient can easily frustrate the practitioner who wants to help but may have no idea where to start. Golden (1978) suggests first allowing the patient to vent (in a limited way) some of his pent-up frustrations, upset, anger, and confusion, and then helping the patient to organize the problems with which he must deal. This organization may aid the patient to examine and cope with one problem at a time. The patient should then be encouraged to make decisions aimed at solving individual problems—with the help of the practitioner. The problems that demand immediate solutions should be solved first, so that the patient's emotions and day-to-day functioning can be brought to a stable equilibrium. Concrete aid in the form of referrals to social agencies may then be very useful.

Like any other patient, the multiproblem patient may either rebel or acquiesce, but never develop internal motivations if decisions about behavioral changes are imposed upon him or her. As with all other patients, the attitudes, beliefs, and social norms of the multiproblem patient must be changed in order to create a behavioral intention. Once the behavioral intention is achieved, the practitioner's role in reducing barriers and enhancing supports to behavior change may be critically important.

Social Support

In an extensive review of factors that influence patient compliance with medical regimens, Becker and Maiman (1980) pointed to growing evidence that social support, particularly from the patient's family, plays an important role in initiating and maintaining compliance behavior. Haynes (1979b) also noted that the influence of family support on behavior change is considerable. There is little doubt that the illness of one individual can profoundly affect members of his or her family and intimate social group. Studies have documented that acute and, sometimes even more so, chronic illness in a child can seriously disrupt the life of the family as a whole (Gordon & Kutner, 1965; Mattsson, 1972). The loss of health in the family breadwinner or in the individual who is primarily responsible for the family's day-to-day needs can have an equally disturbing impact. Family members may experience frustration, anger, guilt, sadness, and remorse in response to their loved one's illness.

As we saw in Chapter 5, the family plays a central role in health and illness. The family is the primary source of health habits, and parents are normally the individual's first teachers about preventive health behaviors. The family also contributes to the individual's self-definition that his symptom condition constitutes illness. In addition, the family (and other sources of support, such as close friends) may enhance the individual's health by serving as "buffers" to life stress (Cassell, 1976). Relatedly, Kaplan, Cassel, and Gore (1977) have noted that persons undergoing stressful life events (such as loss of a job) are often protected from harmful psychological consequences when these events are experienced in the presence of social supports. Social support from family and friends may help individuals to cope with the problems and stresses of both acute and chronic illness. The literature shows some noteworthy correlations between the receipt of social support and patients' actual physical, social, and emotional coping with and recovery from illness. While the findings of this research are not yet clear-cut, the results to date are rather compelling. Further examination of this issue is particularly needed in order to determine the kinds of social support that affect various illness conditions, and the manner in which these effects operate (DiMatteo & Hays, 1981). It has been proposed that one means by which social support may affect recovery from illness is through patient compliance with preventive and rehabilitative regimens (see DiMatteo & Hays, 1981). Indeed, many of the models of preventive and rehabilitative health behavior considered in Chapter 4 (Table 4.1) include a component that reflects social contact, social interaction, or social support. The positive presence of other people seems to be an important contributor to a patient's enactment of his or her required health behaviors. That this factor is one of the few consistently identified as a potential facilitator of patients' health behavior suggests that it merits further exploration (Cummings, Becker, & Maile, 1980).

The notion that behavior change might be facilitated by support from the patient's family and close social network is indeed an appealing one. It suggests the potential value of enlisting individuals who care deeply about the welfare of the patient to prompt, remind, aid, and support him or her to translate intentions into behaviors. In order to determine whether this approach is feasible or worthwhile, of course, the meaning of social support, and the conditions under which a patient's health behavior would be enhanced by the presence of supportive others must be understood clearly.

Social support is not a singular concept. Rather, it involves many different phenomena. Among researchers, the definitions are quite varied, and so comparison of empirical studies is often difficult. Social support might involve, for example, information from others that one is valued and esteemed by them, that one is cared for and loved, and that one is part of a network of mutual obligations (Cobb, 1976). Social support has also been defined even more generally as simply any input that furthers the goals of the receiver of the support (Caplan et al., 1976). Social support is usually seen as consisting of aid in any form from others who help the person meet his particular goals or deal with troublesome or problematic situations (Tolsdorf, 1976). Robert Caplan (1979), a psychologist who has studied many aspects of social support, has specified two dimensions on which to examine this concept: objective-subjective and tangible-psychological. Objective supports are determined by outside observers while subjective supports depend upon the target person's perceptions. Tangible supports consist of physical resources that benefit the receiver psychologically or physically. Psychological supports are behaviors that provide the receiver with cognitions and/or help the receiver to develop affective states engendering physical and psychological well-being. The distinction between subjective and objective support is considered important because in some circumstances a relatively low correlation may exist between the support actually provided by others and the individual's perception of that support. If in an effort to eliminate the bias of self-reporting one examines only objective assessments of the support available to the individual, an important phenomenological issue central to any examination of a patient's available social support would be overlooked. This is the very important consideration that the patient's own point of view is critical. Individuals may differ profoundly among themselves in their needs and expectations. It should therefore be remembered that the number and kind of interpersonal contacts with friends and relatives necessary to achieve some beneficial effects may differ quite impressively among various people (Donald et al., 1978; Kiritz & Moos, 1974; Lipowski, 1969). Thus, in attempting to assess the amount and kind of support available to the individual, both objective and subjective information should be taken into account by the practitioner.

In assisting a patient to translate his or her health intentions into behavior, a family member or friend might be emotionally supportive and exhibit the facilitative conditions of warmth, empathy, and genuineness such as identified by Carl Rogers (1957). The supportive person might also provide information to the recipient, or a new perspective on the problem. Or, he or she might intervene in the problem directly (Gottlieb, 1978). In order to understand fully the impact of social support on any individual's health behavior, it is necessary for a practitioner to understand clearly the form (or forms) of social support available to the patient, and how that support might operate for him or her. A clear understanding of the patient's need for social support and the human resources available to him or her are likely to be quite valuable to the practitioner in aiding the transformation of patients' intentions into well-established, long-term health behaviors. Here we examine some general issues related to the question of how social support actually operates on the patient's ability to translate intentions into behavior change, and how various sources and forms of social support might differ in their effects on health behaviors.

The Family. In times of illness, most people turn first to their families for physical assistance and emotional support (Croog, Lipson, & Levine, 1972). Family members typically help one another, and over the course of many years orchestrate a balanced social exchange (Pilisuk & Froland, 1978). Primarily because of their proximity and/or intimacy, family members provide needed physical and emotional help to one another. Various studies have found that family support enhances behavioral compliance with medical treatments. Carpenter and Davis (1976) found that family support helped arthritis patients carry out their prescribed exercise program. In another study, family support helped children to follow a low-calorie diet (Coplin, Hine, & Gormican, 1976). In yet another study, family support helped middle-aged men to follow a physical fitness program (Heinzelmann & Bagley, 1970). Family support also aided cooperation with home dialysis (Mac-

Elveen, 1972). Finally, the spouse's support enhanced use of a splint by arthritis patients (Oakes et al., 1970). In many of these studies, it was difficult or impossible to separate physical from emotional support and to determine which was most important. In fact, one often implied the other. For example, in a study of hypertensive patients, emotional support from the spouse was found to reduce the patient's depression and psychological strain from engaging in a lifetime regimen of blood-pressure control (Caplan et al., 1976). The support provided by spouses was not purely emotional, however, for spouses also helped tremendously in the day-to-day planning and maintenance of the treatment regimen.

In summary, family support appears to be a promising factor in facilitating the intention-behavior link. In their recent review, for example, Haynes, Taylor, and Sackett (1979, p. 462, Table 7) cited 21 studies to that date that had examined family support. Fifteen of them showed a significant positive effect of family influence on patients' behavioral compliance. In addition, studies of patients' perceptions of barriers to their behavioral compliance show lack of family support cited as extremely important (Davidson, Hudson, & Parry, 1975; Glick, 1965).

The closeness and involvement of the patient's family might also create some detrimental effects. The conditions under which these detrimental effects might occur must therefore be assessed in order to attain a full understanding of the role of the family. In viewing each patient as an individual with various demands on his or her time and energy, we see that for some patients, family involvement may be viewed as stressful. Furthermore, some patients who particularly value independence may experience family involvement as an attempt to limit their autonomy (Caplan et al., 1976). Family closeness and mutual obligation might, under some circumstances, interfere with fulfillment of the treatment regimen. For example, the concurrent illness of a family member was cited by patients as an important reason for their own inability to follow their treatment regimen (Alpert, 1964; Badgley & Furnal, 1961; Hansen, 1953). Family instability may also affect compliance detrimentally (Alpert, 1964; Diamond, Weiss, & Grynbaum, 1968; Elling, Whittemore, & Green, 1960; MacDonald, Hagberg, & Grossman, 1963). Presumably because of the interfering effect of a lack of resources, the larger the family, the lower likelihood exists that the patient will follow the treatment (Alpert, 1964; Becker et al., 1975; Cobb et al., 1954; Gordis, Markowitz & Lilienfeld, 1969; Hurtado, Greenlick, & Columbo, 1973; MacDonald, Hagberg & Grossman, 1963). Finally, Daschner and Marget (1975) found that one family factor cited by patients as a barrier to taking their medication was that a child in the family threw their medication away!

Friends and Social Participation. The family is not the only source of support to affect patients' compliance. In fact, interactions with nonkin have, in some cases, been found to predict health behavior better than kinship or family ties. Although not a strong finding (for it is still somewhat equivocal), social isolation seems to contribute to patient noncompliance (Baekeland, Lundwall, & Shanahan, 1973; Nelson et al., 1975; Schwartz et al., 1962). Further, there is evidence that social participation and integration positively predict compliance (Pam et al., 1973; Vertinsky et al., 1976; Williams & Lee, 1975). Studies of the influence of friends on compliance show a primarily positive relationship (Bewley & Bland, 1977; Gray, Kesler & Moody, 1966; Parkes, Brown, & Monck, 1962). Langlie (1977) reported that a good predictor of preventive health behavior was the frequency with which the individual interacts with people outside his or her kindred social group or family. Presumably the greater diversity of other individuals encountered, the greater the chance that a person might meet others who engage in preventive health behavior after whom he might model himself.

Some important questions remain in the literature regarding the role of friendship networks in compliance and preventive health behavior (Pilisuk & Froland, 1978). One hopes that these questions will be answered in future research on friendship networks and compliance. First of all, we are still unable to define which aspects of friendship networks are important to compliance—the frequency of contacts with friends, the duration of those contacts, the symmetry (balance of control) in the relationships, the accessibility and geographic density of friends, or the intensity and intimacy of friendship. The character of friendship as an enduring network of mutual aid as well as of attitudinal norms and values (as we considered in Chapter 5) is a crucial issue for examination in future research (Sussman, 1965; Litwak & Szelenyi, 1969).

In regard to future research, it should also be noted that the studies reviewed in these last two sections (on family and friends) have not explicitly examined social support as a determinant of postintention behavior change. Rather, these studies have examined the relationship between the social support variable in question and compliance while assuming an implicit intentional commitment on the part of the patient. The role of other people has therefore been considered as a facilitator or inhibitor of enactment of the target behavior. Precisely how the social network operates on intentions (if, in fact, intentions are explicitly spelled out) and how friends and family might modify these intentions by altering patients' beliefs and attitudes are important topics for future research.

Social Support Groups. Reliance on a network of friends or family members for behavioral and emotional support of a health behavior may be somewhat risky. Nonkin may be helpful for instilling health values, but their actual day-to-day involvement in the patient's treatment regimen is likely to be quite limited. Family members as well as friends may have little information about the regimen, and thus may be unable to evaluate the patient's degree of adherence to it accurately. They might also be unable to understand fully the patient's difficulties in following the recommendations. It might then be quite easy for the patient to discount admonitions and recommendations of those he feels do not understand his problems.

Peer-group influence (or peer pressure) has been found to be consistently successful as a strategy for enhancing compliance (Curtis, Simpson, & Steven, 1976; Garb & Stunkard, 1974; Piper, Jones, & Matthews, 1974; Williams & Duncan, 1976; Bebbington, 1976). These successful peer groups, however, tend to be of a special sort. They consist of individuals who are involved in the same (or similar) regimens as the patient. Groups such as the following have been studied and found effective in enhancing compliance: groups of individuals quitting smoking by rapid puffing method involving group discussions (Curtis, Simpson, & Steven, 1976); self-help obesity groups involving group support (Garb & Stunkard, 1974); smoking education/prevention for junior-high-school students (Piper, Jones, & Matthews, 1974); Weight Watchers weight-control groups (outside analysis of results) (Williams & Duncan, 1976); and Alcoholics Anonymous (Bebington, 1976).

Groups such as these offer members more than just support from people who are experiencing the same problems. The groups offer information, behavior-change instruction, and other techniques for achieving the behavioral goal. For example, Weight Watchers provides members with information, menus, and charts on which to record both food intake and weight loss. Thus, we are not suggesting that social support operates alone in these groups. Rather, on the basis of the evidence, we suggest that group support among individuals with similar problems is *one* very important factor (which works along with other factors) in helping to equate behavioral intentions with behaviors. Consideration of the operation of group support illustrates (as Caplan et al., 1976, p. 7, noted) that a direct link between social support and adherence need not necessarily exist. Social support may be a necessary but not sufficient condition for behavior change and adherence to the prescribed regimen. It might operate to encourage a patient (who felt generally competent to undertake the regimen) to go about taking the initial first step. Social support might simply enhance the effects of other factors such as skill at behavioral self-control.

Various group-support formats that have been found to be successful are: (1) weekly group discussions that involve the exchange of tangible support such as ideas and information (e.g., recipes for low-calorie and low-salt foods) and emotional support, such as general encouragement, understanding, and the expression of the value of the goal; (2) a "buddy system" in which individuals are paired off and each member provides the other with moral support in times of temptation to abandon the regimen (Hamilton & Borstein, 1979, found this to be quite successful for patients in a smoking abstinence program); (3) groups from which one or more persons provide a mechanism for communication with each individual concerning the effect of illness and the subsequent treatment regimen on his or her present and future life. Usually the patient receives a supportive, information-giving visit (for example, Reach to Recovery for the new mastectomy patient while she is still hospitalized— Gussow & Tracy, 1978). One purpose of this visit is to put the patient into contact with a model of rehabilitation—someone who has fulfilled the regimen successfully and has experienced a positive outcome. This contact with the patient is usually made when such assurances are most needed—when the patient's anxieties and uncertainties about functioning are the highest.

Gussow and Tracy (1978) noted that the various kinds of social support groups noted above provide one or more of the following factors in facilitating achievement of the goal of rehabilitation: (1) a role model who regularly reinforces the advantages of successfully following the regimen; (2) a reservoir of new, special information and coping techniques (such as concerning physical care, rehabilitation insurance, disability programs, and employment discrimination); (3) an avenue for the expression of strong sentiments which, if continually directed toward the family, would be disruptive of their normal role relationships; (4) training for patients in how to normalize their behavior as much as possible within the confines of the disability; (5) behavioral monitoring done by others in the group (usually discrete, low-level watchful, and protective); and (6) education of medical personnel about the proper care of patients.

A major value of the mutual-help support group is that it supplants the necessarily brief education and limited support available to the patient from the physician or other busy health professional. The support group can incorporate social processes into the dynamics of coping and adjusting to the medical treatment regimen. The group can also help to facilitate the patient's relationship with his or her own social network. Many groups also include the patient's spouse or entire family. These groups are not social clubs with a goal of entertainment, but rather are oriented to supplementing the existing inadequacies in the medical-care system. They are usually used most effectively in combination with traditional ambulatory clinic services (Cole, O'Conner, & Bennett, 1979).

For many types of conditions, *continuing* support is essential in preventing "backsliding," that is, discontinuing compliance after engaging in it for a period of time. Adherence to a regimen for high blood pressure, for example, usually involves taking medication and following a special low-salt diet. It requires a lifelong commitment. Obviously patients cannot be expected to attend classes or group meetings once a week for their entire lives. Furthermore, as Caplan et al. (1976) noted, it might be very difficult for any educational system to provide enough information or material to sustain patients' interest for a particularly long time. How, then, might continuing support be provided, and the patient's involvement in his or her treatment regimen maintained? Caplan et al. (1976) examined the successful operation of informal support groups in which hypertensive patients and their spouses met periodically at one anothers' homes. They brought low-sodium, low-fat snacks and shared their experiences. These meetings boosted their morale because the patients provided one another with social reinforcement for adhering to the regimen. This reinforcement was typically not available in day-to-day life from normotensive friends. Normally, too, support is not available from health-care practitioners. Caplan (1976) suggested that the development of voluntary organizations run by well-motivated people would be a useful method for helping to bring patients the continued support they need for lifelong adherence to medical regimens. Such groups tend to be efficient and effective because they draw their resources and energy from the very people whom they serve.

Epilogue to Social Support

As we saw in Chapters 2 and 3, noncompliance is often a visible manifestation of dysfunctional communication between practitioner and patient. This is true for a number of reasons. When patients receive indifferent reception and feel their practitioners do not understand them, they abandon their obligations and commitments to follow the assigned regimen. When the health care delivered provides the patient with very little individual attention and with very little responsibility for the management of his or her illness, rejection of the regimen is likely to be fostered. As we have seen in this chapter, social variables can likewise play an important role in compliance. A patient may be helped tremendously to comply if he or she has some sense of belonging to a group of individuals to whom his or her compliance is of importance. This group may be family, friends, or a social organization formed for the purpose of dealing with the illness. The practitioner's awareness of the patient's level and kind of social support may be critical to the enhancement of the patient's cooperation with the regimen. The patient's sense of belongingness may be used by the practitioner to promote an obligation to carry out the regimen. The practitioner might also provide direct encouragement for the social network of the patient to continue their important function. Thus, the practitioner's awareness of and involvement in the patient's psychosocial life is central to the practitioner's ability to use the social support available to improve the patient's compliance.

Although never studied longitudinally, social support is potentially very promising in enhancing long-term self-maintenance programs, and in supporting the translation of continually maintained intentions into continued behavioral accomplishment. In popular trade books on self-control (those most notably based on sound research literature are by Farquhar, 1978, and Mahoney & Mahoney, 1976), the patient's attention to his or her own social environment is advocated as a central component in the self-control process. Farquhar (1978) specifically advocates the use of a contract co-signed by the patient and a supportive individual who promises to be a "helper." The patient may list specific behaviors that he will enact, for example: (1) walk for one half-hour each day during lunch, (2) reward himself for reaching two and a half miles on a pedometer (reward being one half-hour of reading a favorite novel), and (3) record in journal the daily activities each night before retiring. The helper's responsibilities are enumerated as well: (1) walk with the patient during lunch hour and support efforts to exercise more; (2) review and evaluate the progress of the patient. The self-directed change is in the hands of the patient; he or she enlists and controls the commitment of another to provide social support. Mahoney and Mahoney (1976) suggest even more extensive involvement of the social network by advocating the patient's own assessment of members of the social environment. This involves making a list of the specific family members and friends with whom the patient interacts, and keeping track of their degree of support for the regimen. Support may involve their specific actions in introducing or removing temptations, and in helping the patient to develop appropriate reactions to those temptations. The Mahoneys suggest that the patient gain control of the support by asking for it and by reinforcing it. They advocate the use of contracts in which the supporter promises to provide particular forms of support to the patient. They also point to the role of groups, and suggest ways for individuals to form supportive groups of persons and to enlist their continued help.

Throughout this section, we have examined the role of supportive others in enhancing the relationship between intentions and behaviors. We have seen that by helping the patient to overcome physical and emotional difficulties associated with the treatment regimen, other people can help to render the behavior change more likely. As we noted a number of times throughout this section, however, social support seems to be a necessary but not a sufficient condition for behavior change and maintenance. In the following sections, we consider various other important determinants of the translation of intentions into health behavior change and maintenance. These include behavioral and cognitive approaches to self-control, and some important issues relating to the role of the health professional.

A BEHAVIORAL APPROACH TO COMPLIANCE

Despite their stated intentions, patients often experience considerable difficulty carrying out specific health-related behaviors largely because of the powerful force of habit. Changes in behavior patterns are often difficult to attain because previously learned behaviors obstruct or supervene in the process of acquiring new behaviors. Behaviors are typically prompted and maintained by environmental characteristics and events rather than freely generated by the individual. This suggests that the enactment of new behaviors and the changing of old ones requires knowledge of the operation of environmental cues and of methods for controlling their influence. Change essentially requires taming of the force of habit. Regarding this, Becker and Maiman (1980) noted that "it appears necessary to train the individual in self-discipline through such means as practice sessions and providing reinforcements" (p. 117). Indeed, it has been demonstrated that supervised practice of the treatment regimen is one of the most important components of the compliance process once a behavioral intention has been achieved (Bowen, Rich, & Schlatfeldt, 1961; McAlister et al., 1976).

In this section, we examine strategies for bridging the gap between behavioral intentions and actual behavior change. These strategies focus on overt behavior and are based on the belief that since health behavior is learned and habitual (Zifferblatt, 1975; Kasl, 1975; Rosenstock & Kirscht, 1979), old behavior patterns can be eliminated and new ones can be developed to take their place. While many of the behavioral techniques we consider here have been examined in the literature as isolated strategies for improving patient compliance, we present them here within a broader picture of a behavioral approach to compliance. The success of these strategies provides evidence that a behavioral approach is among the most fruitful for enhancing patient compliance once an intention has been stated. The value of a behavioral approach is suggested, too, by the recently developing popularity of a field known as "Behavioral Medicine." This approach uses the clinical techniques derived from the experimental analysis of behavior to prevent or manage illness problems (Katz & Zlutnick, 1975).

Advantages of a Behavioral Approach

A behavioral approach to health-behavior change and maintenance has many advantages. It concentrates on future, not past, behaviors. It is an optimistic approach because it suggests that with appropriate learning, a person can change. This approach never labels an individual as hopelessly noncompliant because of defects in his or her personality. Rather, problems in translating intentions into behaviors are seen as stemming from faulty learning history, or from the detrimental operation of environmental cues. Suppose a patient who has emphysema is required to engage in a daily program of walking to build breathing capacity but does not carry out the recommendation despite her stated intention to do so. She may easily be labeled by the health professional as lazy and unmotivated. A behavioral approach, however, would avoid such a label entirely and instead would look to the factors that are presently interfering with the successful enactment of the behavior. A behavioral approach would consider the problems as stemming from the patient's lack of skill at monitoring her own behavior and her neglect or inappropriate use of reinforcements for herself for walking. Knowledge of the behavioral issues relevant to achieving the target behavior can help patient and practitioner to design behavioral contingencies to enhance performance of the behavior.

Another advantage of the behavioral approach is that problems are defined in terms of specific behaviors—exactly what the person does, where he does it, when and with whom he does it, etc. The definition of the problem in specific behavioral terms avoids inaccurate and deprecating generalizations, and focuses attention on accurate assessment using methods developed in and supported by empirical research. For example, a behavioral analysis using detailed records of a patient's behavior might find that he or she overeats only at home, in the evening, standing up in the kitchen. A behavioral change derived from this assessment could be one that restricts the individual's eating to the dining room, sitting down with a carefully prepared, balanced meal. Further, by defining the solution in specific behavioral terms, the gradual process of change can be measured, and the individual's specific behavioral changes can be appropriately rewarded. As we will see in this section, the most effective behavioral program is one that enhances the patient's self-control. A basic principle of behavior therapy is that the reinforcement of a particular behavior will increase its occurrence.Desired behaviors can be maintained throughout an individual's life if he or she can be taught to engage in self-reinforcement for those behaviors. Thus, any behavior can be removed from the control of environmental reinforcements and be brought under control of self-imposed reinforcements. Once behavioral skills are developed by the patient, these skills can be applied in any situation, and (in principle) all health-related behavior problems can be overcome.

Behavioral management of compliance demands a commitment by the practitioner to psychosocial issues in the care of the patient. A focus on the environment of the patient, for example, requires the health professional's understanding of the patient's physical and social environment. Whenever possible, a practitioner working within a behavioral orientation will work with the patient's entire social network, either by involving it directly or by working with the patient's perceptions of how it affects his or her behavior. Such an approach should always emphasize the patient's self-management in dealing with this environment in solving medical compliance problems. This is important because the structure of the health-care system limits the time available for direct contact with patients. Behavioral self-management can be taught to the patient in a relatively short time (by paraprofessionals) and can be followed up in regular, albeit brief, meetings with the patient. Thus, the commitment of the practitioner is not impractical. The behavior program's utility lies in the fact that most of the work is done by the patient at home.

Finally, a behavioral approach to bridging the gap between intentions and behaviors demands that the health professional learn one basic behavioral model—one that comprehensively applies to many different situations. There exists a great deal of evidence that behavioral self-management principles can be effectively applied in a variety of clinical settings to deal with many different clinical problems. Furthermore, a behavioral approach allows the practitioner to specify precisely why and how various self-management techniques and strategies work.

Criticisms of A Behavioral Approach

Despite its many advantages, the behavioral approach to compliance and health-behavior change has met with some criticism. The term "behavior modification" calls up images for many people of "automated behavior control." Some imagine, for example, caged animals who receive painful punishments from experimenters for the sake of "learning" (Packard, 1977). The technique is criticized by some as unethical or inhumane. Such notions are erroneous. Research involving punishments is not very common, particularly since rewards are more effective in shaping behavior. Research is done with animals (primarily rats and pigeons) in order to establish some basic principles of behavior conditioning and modification so that they might be effectively applied to solving human problems (Rimm & Masters, 1974).

Another erroneous belief that tends to give behavior modification a poor "public image" is the common criticism that it deals only with simple, outward behaviors, while the person's "true feelings" remain hidden below the surface and unchanged (Packard, 1977). In fact, behavior therapy (which involves the application of behavior modification principles to solve clinical problems), deals not only with motor responses but also with affect (emotions), sensations, imagination, and cognitions. All of these are viewed as "behaviors." They are intertwined with one another, and behavioral principles can be used to change them. Thoughts, feelings, and sensations can be assessed, evaluated, and subjected to patterns of reinforcement just as can overt motor responses. Behavioral principles can be successfully applied to all these aspects of psychological life (Martin & Poland, 1980).

Relatedly, behavior therapy is sometimes thought to be too simplistic, partly because many behavior modification procedures have been developed from studies on animals. Although the experimental studies have focused on simple, individual behaviors rather than on complex, integrated ones, the findings have important application to complex repertoires of human behavior. Even complex behaviors can be broken down into minute, individual ones, and can be changed by means of behavior modification. In addition, although the reinforcements that are most useful for shaping human behavior are different from those that successfully shape animals (for example, human beings, unlike animals, will be effectively reinforced with social and interpersonal rewards that have symbolic value), the principles of reinforcement operate with humans in the same manner as they do with animal subjects.

Another criticism often leveled against behavior modification is that individual human beings are so variable in their characteristics that a scientific approach to behavior change is too sterile and inflexible to be worthwhile. It is argued that individuals respond to situations and events in different ways, and no two people are likely to follow the same behavioral schedule. In fact, this individuality is precisely the goal of the behavioral approach. The methods are designed with the individual in mind, and the behavioral model is extremely flexible. On the following pages, a number of general methods for behavior change will be presented. Their application to medical regimen compliance and to health-behavior change will be made clear. We will see that methods of self-monitoring, self-assessment, and self-reinforcement can be developed to suit the needs of each individual patient. The key to success is flexibility and responsiveness to the patient's needs.

Finally, it is sometimes argued by critics of the behavioral approach that this method removes the individual's freedom of choice (Packard, 1977). In fact, the behavioral techniques we outline here *enhance* the freedom of the individual, and actually increase the individual's behavioral choices. This approach to self-control and self-regulation places the responsibility for initial and continued change into the hands of the patient.

Behavioral Self-Control

The ultimate goal of the behavioral approach presented here is for the patient to initiate and maintain the translation of his or her intentions into behaviors. In common usage, self-control usually refers to a person's ability to refrain from engaging in certain behaviors such as eating or drinking too much, smoking, or inappropriately expressing emotion. Although our society values self-control, many people relinquish their attempts to achieve self-control because they believe it is something a person naturally "has." In truth, however, self-control is something that a person "does" (Thoresen & Mahoney, 1974). This is an important distinction. The evidence is quite clear that self-control is a skill that can be acquired (Goldstein & Kanfer, 1979).

The health professional's commitment to helping his or her patient learn self-control (or self-management) is critically important for a number of reasons. First, the health professional cannot monitor all of the patient's behaviors 24 hours a day, even if the patient were hospitalized. Second, if the health professional does monitor (albeit sporadically) the patient's behavior, and provides the appropriate responses to shape the behaviors, the patient will never learn self-control. Performance of the desired behavior (e.g., avoiding a cigarette or a hot fudge sundae) under these conditions will only occur if the health professional is continually available to provide reinforcements for it. Third, a more effective program of behavior change will be developed if the patient contributes to it, and if he or she plays a major part in decisions regarding the rewards and punishments to be instituted. Once the patient has stated an intention to make a behavioral change, his or her commitment is assured and so the patient can be relied upon to help alter his or her own environment and control his or her own reinforcements. This can be done, however, only if the patient develops the necessary behavioral skills. The practitioner's goal is to train the individual to control his or her own behavior and to achieve self-directed change (Kanfer, 1980). Here, again, we see the importance of the patient's internalization of medical recommendations and personal responsibility for self-control—a notion that has been a guiding theme throughout this book.

The entire picture of compliance, then, looks something like this: the patient must believe in the importance of the regimen, alter his or her social norms to coincide with it, and state an intention to comply. Once this is done, the patient must monitor and assess his or her own behaviors and the environmental antecedents and consequences attached to them, alter those contingencies, and engage in appropriate self-reinforcement. The patient must ultimately assume responsibility for and control over his or her own health behavior.

A Brief Review of Behavioral Principles

A few basic principles of classical and operant conditioning are critically important to the design of a patient's self-management program. We review these briefly here in order to illustrate the various aspects of the behavioral approach to patient compliance. Further information may be found in reviews of behavioral methods by Bandura (1969), Rimm and Masters (1974), Stuart and Davis (1972), and Mahoney and Thoresen (1974).

Classical Conditioning. Classical or respondent conditioning is a process by which a behavior comes to be evoked by a once-neutral stimulus because that stimulus was paired with one that automatically evoked the behavior. Consider Dana, an overweight 15-year-old who often nibbles on chocolate when she watches television. Eventually, even when there is no chocolate near her and she has not been thinking about it, Dana becomes hungry and craves chocolate as soon as she turns on the television set. Similarly, students who associate smoking with studying may have a great deal of difficulty resisting a cigarette when they sit down to study.

Because classical conditioning can occur so easily (and seemingly inadvertently), a few relatively simple practical interventions may work quite well to help patients control their health behavior. A dieting patient should restrict his or her eating to one (and only one) location in the house because neutral stimuli in various parts of the house can, after being paired with the smell and taste of food, trigger a desire to eat. Control over the location of one's eating is therefore essential. Relatedly, stimulus generalization is relevant to health-behavior control. This is a process by which the conditioned response (the desire for chocolate, in Dana's case) comes to be evoked when a stimulus similar to the one that first elicited the responses is encountered. Thus, when Dana's desire for chocolate is elicited by watching a movie at the theater as well as by watching television at home, stimulus generalization has occurred. Finally, if the stimulus (the television) were encountered by Dana a number of times when it was *not* paired with the chocolate, the conditioned response (her desire for chocolate) would be eliminated. This phenomenon is called extinction (see Wolpe, 1958, for a review of these conditioning principles).

Operant Conditioning. Operant conditioning is based on the principle that behavior is shaped by the consequences that follow it. More precisely, whether or not a particular behavior will be repeated in the future depends upon its consequences in the past. Much of the initial research on this form of conditioning was done by psychologist B. F. Skinner, who concentrated on the study of *operants* (Skinner, 1938). Much research has been done since then on this form of behavior modification (Bandura, 1969; Karoly, 1980). Operants are freely emitted behaviors that "operate" on the environment. They are controlled by their environmental consequences. This led Skinner and others to argue that the individual and his or her environmental context are interdependent. Operant behavior that is *rewarded* by the environment is more likely to be repeated. Behavior that is *punished* is less likely to occur again.

Operant conditioning can be self-imposed through the process of self-regulation—a critical factor in health-behavior change (Kanfer, 1980). Three stages occur in the process of self-regulation: self-monitoring, self-evaluation, and self-reinforcement. Continued compliance with medical treatment demands the development of these three components (Kanfer, 1980).

Self-monitoring or self-observation, involves deliberate and careful attention to one's own behavior. The patient might be encouraged to become aware of precisely what he eats, how often he smokes, etc. Complete details of behavior—the precise activity (e.g., measured portions of food eaten), the time of day of the activity, the antecedent and consequent events and feelings—might be recorded in a diary. The analysis of behavior patterns (for example, the occurrence and the typical consequences of eating, smoking, and exercise) is the critical first step to behavior change. The second stage in self-regulation is *self-evaluation*. It involves evaluating the behavior assessed through self-monitoring against a specific criterion or ideal. Self-evaluation can result in correction of the target behavior if *self-reinforcement* for doing so is administered. Self-reinforcement for behavior that matches or approximates the criterion behavior is likely to enhance the behavior change.

Commitment to behavior change does not guarantee self-regulation. Many people lack awareness of their own present behavior and of ways to modify it. Their performance criteria are vague (for example, how many calories constitute an excessive number, and how many calories are available in various foods). Their knowledge of appropriate rewards, and the timing of such rewards, is often sparse. Indeed, some may be unaware that accepting the reward *before* performing the target behavior will not bring about successful modification! Because of this, patient education and the support of patients' skill development in all aspects of self-regulation can be extremely important to the achievement of health-behavior change.

Related Behavioral Strategies for Modifying Health Behaviors

Prompts and Reminders. What initially brings about the desired health behavior (or approximations of it) so that reinforcements can be administered to increase its future frequency? Generally, a behavioral *prompt* (carried out by the individual himself, or by others in his environment) serves to facilitate the occurrence of the desired behavior by reminding the person to initiate it, or by otherwise making the behavior salient. A prompt can take many forms. It can be a reminder from another (such as a telephone call from the clinic regarding an appointment or a reminder postcard that a medication prescription should be refilled at the pharmacy). A prompt might also take the form of a reminder note from the individual to himself or herself. Commercially available refrigerator signs that present such phrases as "A moment on the lips, forever on the hips" serve as behavioral prompts to avoid snacking. The avoidance of temptation or the enactment of an incompatible behavior might then be reinforced, and its frequency thus increased.

Prompts have been used in a number of studies to increase patients' keeping of their clinic appointments. Mailed reminders for appointments have been found to be effective in pediatric settings (Shepard & Moseley, 1976; Meller & Anderson, 1976) and in a cardiology clinic (Cook, Morch, & Noble, 1976). Telephone reminders have also proven effective (as tested in a pediatric setting by Shepard & Moseley, 1976). In long-term care for chronic illness, written or telephone reminders brought a 13 to 20 percent increase in appointment keeping (Brigg & Mudd, 1968; Nazarian, Mechaber, Charney, & Coulter, 1974). For the most part, when the cost of scheduling the appointment, retrieving the chart, lost revenue, and physician's wasted time as a result of a failed appointment are taken into account, the prevention of last-minute broken or failed appointments is considerably cost effective.

It has also been found that prompts improve medication compliance (Lima et al., 1976). Telephone prompts have been found to help ease patients' anxieties, especially among those who had second thoughts about their prescribed treatment regimen or about returning to the clinic (Brigg & Mudd, 1968). Other behavioral prompts that have been examined in research include pill calendars and special pill packages designed to aid memory. These tend to work relatively well in short-term medication regimens and in regimens of contraceptive pills. Two studies (Dickey, Mattar, & Chudzik, 1975; and Linkewich, Catalano, & Flack, 1974) found that instructions and special pill calendars that helped patients keep track of the medication they were taking helped improve medication compliance. Special packaging in a "unit dose strip" also aided memory (Linkewich et al., 1974). Pill containers with a timed alarm buzzer also helped to remind patients to take their medications. The best system involved an alarm signal that required deactivation by the patient. This was superior to one that shut off automatically (Azrin & Powell, 1969) because patients could not ignore it. Special pill containers had no effect on compliance with long-term chronic illnesses such as hypertension, however (Eshelman & Fitzloff, 1976). This latter finding supports the statement by Haynes (1979) that compliance with long-term regimens is difficult to attain and "the effort required is intensive, often clumsy, and must be maintained as long as compliance is required" (Haynes, 1979b, p. 128). Thus, it is unlikely that one simple intervention such as a special pill container will encourage compliance over a long period of time. More complex behavioral strategies are needed.

A formal behavior modification program for hypertensive patients was developed in an experimental study by Haynes and colleagues (1976). This program included self-monitoring of blood pressure and pill consumption, linking the taking of medication with daily events that were reinforcing, and providing monetary incentives and other forms of reinforcement for compliance. This intervention achieved a 21 percent average improvement in compliance with antihypertensive medications. Behavioral strategies were found by these, as well as other researchers, to be very effective (Dunbar et al., 1979). (While some of the strategies we propose in this chapter may appear at first to be impractical, their effectiveness with a motivated patient—one who has stated a commitment to change—makes the effort required to institute them well worth the investment. In addition, it has been found that a nurse, acting as a family-health-management specialist, can achieve as good results as a physician in instituting programs of self-management with patients [Fink, Malloy et al., 1969; Fink, Martin et al., 1969].)

Tailoring the Regimen. One very effective behavioral technique, employed in the controlled study by Haynes et al. (1976), involves tailoring the treatment regimen to the habits and rituals, times and places in the individual's daily life. One example of tailoring the regimen would involve a b.i.d. (twice a day) hypertension medication that assigned one dosage at dinnertime and one dosage immediately upon arising.

Graduated Regimen Implementation. In behavior modification, desirable behaviors are increased by a process called *shaping*. Shaping requires the provision of reinforcement for successive approximations to the desired behavior. Shaping involves the initial rewarding of any approximation to the desired behavior (for example, when Mr. Mentone praises Mrs. Mentone for walking her first mile, although the ultimate goal of her exercise program is three miles a day). Over the course of time, only progressively closer approximations of the desired behavior are reinforced. (Mr. Mentone eventually praises Mrs. Mentone only when she achieves three miles on a given day, but does not praise her when she walks less than her goal.)

Graduated regimen implementation employs the principle of behavior shaping. The patient is initially rewarded for adhering to some part of the treatment regimen. Then, as the patient achieves the limited version of the treatment regimen, another component is added to it, and the patient is reinforced only for adhering to that. As the patient achieves each successive level of the regimen, he or she more closely approximates the complete regimen and moves in stepwise fashion to build a behavioral repertoire (Matthews & Hingson, 1977). Kanfer and Phillips (1970) note that this is an important technique, but that it needs more investigation, particularly in medical settings.

Contingency Contracting. Contingency contracts are among the best behavioral strategies. They involve contracts (usually between the health professional and patient, or between family members and patient) to provide specific rewards for specifically enacted behaviors. Mahoney and Thoresen (1974) noted that five conditions are necessary for a contingency contract to be successful: (1) it must be fair; (2) the terms must be clear; (3) it must be generally positive (i.e., rewarding good behaviors rather than punishing bad ones); (4) it must identify procedures clearly and these procedures must be carried out consistently and systematically; and (5) at least one other person should participate. The best kind of contract is one in which the person eventually comes to administer his own rewards and another person is merely available for support and perhaps for advice. Initially, however, the contract is likely to be most effective when the positive consequences of action are administered by another person.

Contingency contracts have a number of advantages for patient compliance. With the help of the practitioner, the individual can plan his or her own regimen, and individualize the treatment. Inappropriate expectations can be cleared up. When a written outline of behavioral expectations is drawn up, a formal commitment is made. Finally, there is incentive value in having a self-established goal. Modest success has been achieved with treatments based on contingency contracts, particularly with regimens for dieting (Harris & Bruner, 1971; Dinoff, Rickard, & Colwick, 1972; Mann, 1972) and medication taking (Lewis & Michnich, 1977). One major problem with contingency contracts has been uncovered in the dieting research, however. The weight losses achieved were not maintained after termination of the contingency contract.

Self-Monitoring

As we mentioned earlier, self-monitoring is an important component of self-regulation. Through self-monitoring, the individual collects data on the problem so that decisions can be made regarding the regimen and specific changes required to achieve it (Johnson & White, 1971; Maletzky, 1974; Nelson, Lipinski, & Black, 1976). There is some evidence (Kanfer, 1970) that self-monitoring may automatically lead to alterations in behavior. The conditions under which this occurs may be quite specific, however. Monitoring the physical outcome alone (for example, blood pressure—Carnahan & Nugent, 1975; or weight—Rimanczyk, 1974) did not help the patient to gain control over the behavior. However, self-monitoring of the specific behavior (for example, food intake in the Rimanczyk, 1974 study) did enhance compliance with the weight-loss regimen. One study (Bellak, Rozensky, & Schwartz, 1974) found that it was best to record the food about to be eaten, rather than what was already eaten, in attempting to control food intake. Whether self-monitoring alone is generally worth the trouble is questionable, however, for Mahoney, Moura, and Wade (1973) found that the effects of self-monitoring alone were very weak. This is still a somewhat controversial issue, however, and deserves further investigation.

Reinforcement

Any consequence that follows a behavior and increases the future likelihood of the behavior is called *positive reinforcement* (or reward). Positive reinforcement is not a quality of the consequence because the same consequence can serve to increase the performance of the behavior by one person, but not affect its performance by another. A consequence, therefore, is a positive reinforcement only if it increases the target behavior. A positive reinforcement can take any form. It can be material (such as a dish of ice cream or spinach, or a new suit), social (such as receiving attention, praise, compliments, or a whack from another person), or emotional (feeling happy, or upset, or self-satisfied). If a behavior is desirable, and one wants to increase its performance, it should be followed by something that is a positive reinforcement for the performer of the behavior.

Negative reinforcement, on the other hand, increases the performance of the desired behavior when the behavior causes its removal. A relevant example involves hunger pangs and eating. A person will repeat the behavior of eating if eating removes hunger pangs. People may also eat to remove or reduce the unpleasant feeling of depression. Likewise, they may smoke cigarettes to remove or reduce anxiety; they may drink to alleviate boredom. The concept of negative reinforcement helps to explain why apparently self-destructive behaviors sometimes persist even though they do not obviously appear to be followed by positive consequences. When self-destructive behaviors "serve a need" (for example, when they remove some negative state), they continue because of negative reinforcement.

Many studies have documented the value of reinforcement in achieving behavior changes (e.g., Mann, 1972; Bigelow et al., 1976). These studies have found that rewards need not be tangible. Social rewards (e.g., attention from family, friends, or the clinician) serve as excellent reinforcers for behavior (Alderman & Schoenbaum, 1975; Oakes et al., 1970; Becker & Green, 1975; Alderman, 1976, 1977; Fass, Green, & Deeds, 1977). The long-term maintenance of behavior by rewards from others is unlikely, however. Rather, self-reward—reinforcement that is self-generated—is needed in order to bring about continued behavior (Bellack, Rozensky, & Schwartz, 1974; Mahoney, 1974; Mahoney, Moura, & Wade, 1973).

Research has shown that it is particularly important for behavior to be modified by reinforcements rather than by punishments. Reinforcement for engaging in an alternative behavior that interferes with one that is proscribed is preferable to punishment for engaging in the proscribed behavior. In addition, the best reinforcements are those that are intrinsic to the goal behavior itself (for example, reduced muscle tension as a result of exercise; greater ability to breathe and loss of chronic cough from avoiding cigarette smoking) (Bandura, 1977). The health professional's role in helping the patient to identify the intrinsic rewards of adherence to a behavior that is initially very difficult can be critically important.

The acquisition and maintenance of new behaviors require skills, and often it is the deficit of these skills and the anxiety caused by that deficit that prevent patients from initiating new health behaviors. Anxiety, fear of failure, and fear of embarrassment may cause the person to avoid any contact with the new activity, thus further preventing the development of new skills. An example is the older person who fears looking foolish or experiencing discomfort upon beginning an exercise program after many years of avoiding exercise completely. The practitioner may need to work with such a patient in order to identify an acceptable initial form of the desired activity (for example, walking around the neighborhood slowly after dinner, as opposed to running, or beginning a tennis class). This initial form must be one that does not bring about anxiety or fear of embarrassment for the patient. Shaping of the behavior to approach the goal can then take place. In this way, the practitioner can demonstrate respect for the patient, and in helping him or her to overcome fear and embarrassment, can encourage the patient's development of a new set of skills.

In the behavioral framework we present here, anxiety signals the deficit of skills. The health professional might encourage the patient to use anxiety to signal the need for *new learning* (Martin & Poland, 1980; Goldiamond, 1974). A focus on building new skills is important in encouraging both the patient's and health professional's positive expectations. An excellent example of the use of such skill training is a study by Atkins (1981) in which a health counselor worked individually with patients with chronic obstructive pulmonary disease to improve their compliance with an exercise prescription designed to improve their lung capacity. During a home visit, the health counselor reviewed each patient's daily schedule in order to identify, along with the patient, the most appropriate times during which he or she might walk. Other barriers to compliance were also uncovered and dealt with—barriers such as not having a safe place to walk and not having comfortable shoes to wear. Questions about how to walk, at what pace to walk, etc., were answered precisely, and patients were given instructions in behavioral self-monitoring, evaluation, and reinforcement. The results strongly supported the importance of a very clear specification of the regimen in the establishment of patient compliance.

COGNITIVE FACTORS AND THE ROLE OF SELF-INSTRUCTION

Behavioral intervention alone may not be sufficient. What people think tends to influence their achievement and maintenance of behavior change. Cognitive factors are therefore very important to health behavior. In fact, research has recently begun to suggest that the most effective methods for health-behavior change involve a combination of cognitive and behavior modification.

Cognitive factors are themselves quite important for a number of reasons. The degree to which the patient attributes his health-behavior change to himself versus an external agent such as the health professional may influence the likelihood of his maintenance of the behavior change (Davison & Valins, 1969; Davison, Tsujimoto, & Galros, 1973). Feelings of self-efficacy and expectations for one's own ability play a decisive role in the maintenance of behavior change (Wilson, 1980). Strategies for maintaining health behaviors often rely on symbolic operations such as rehearsing coping reactions to high-risk situations. These are situations that provoke temptation to engage in behaviors that are incompatible with the health regimen. Stress "inoculation" training using self-instruction (e.g., "Okay self, you can avoid that piece of cake. Just keep trying."), guided imagery (e.g., picturing oneself avoiding the cake at a party), and relaxation can be extremely effective in preparing patients to maintain their particular health regimen under temptation (Goldfried & Goldfried, 1975; Meichenbaum, 1977).

Understanding and control of cognitive factors are also important because a perfectly good behavioral change program can easily be ruined by the patient's use of negative self-statements. While an adaptive reaction to a dietary indiscretion might involve a self-statement like, "Well, that's my indiscretion for the month. I'll write that in my diet log and go on eating healthful meals again," some patients engage in maladaptive self-talk. They may say to themselves: "See, I really am a pig. I can't stick to a diet no matter what. I guess I am doomed to be fat." At this prompting, they abandon the regimen entirely. Likewise, after a day or two of careful self-management and control, one dieter might focus reinforcingly on thoughts of health and self-control while another focuses self-punishingly on discomfort and deprivation—making continued maintenance unpleasant.

There is an important interplay between a patient's behavioral repertoire and what he says to himself. Because of this, any practitioner who is involved in helping patients to achieve behavioral changes must be aware of the role of cognitive factors. The practitioner must also aid patients to become more aware of their own thoughts, encourage their collection of data to refute their negative self-statements, and encourage their production of self-instructions incompatible with failure. The practitioner may also successfully use behavioral methods (and teach patients to use behavioral self-control) to reinforce the production of patients' positive self-statements.

While operant methods can be used successfully to enhance behavioral compliance with medical regimens (Zifferblatt, 1975), the addition of cognitive interventions (producing a cognitive-behavior modification approach; Meichenbaum, 1977; Meichenbaum & Genest, 1980) has the power to increase that success substantially. Strictly behavioral approaches may work when patients' internal dialogues do not undermine their behavioral changes. However, when patients' internal dialogues must be changed in order that they may support and not interfere with the process of behavioral self-control, a cognitive-behavioral approach may be successfully applied. Behavior modification of those internal dialogues may be designed in order to modify what patients say to themselves, and with techniques of self-control of their cognitions, patients may learn to enhance their enactment of health-related behaviors further.

SUPPORTS AND BARRIERS FROM THE HEALTH PROFESSIONAL

As we have seen throughout this book, the health professional—physician, nurse, nurse practitioner, or physician's assistant—plays a key role in the development, enhancement, and maintenance of the patient's cooperation with treatment. Health practitioners are likely to be the first source of information about the required regimen. Because of their primary contact, practitioners can strongly affect the patient's commitment to a correct regimen—particularly by means of clear communication about the regimen. In Chapter 2, we examined the many problems that may arise in practitioner-patient communication, and considered ways in which these problems might be overcome so that the patient may know precisely what the practitioner expects him or her to do. Likewise, in Chapter 3 we examined the central role played by the health professional's rapport with the patient in motivating patient cooperation. The strength of this role was found to depend upon the quality of the relationship between practitioner and patient, and upon the trust that characterizes it. In addition, after considering patients' beliefs, attitudes, and social norms (in Chapters 4 and 5), we examined (in Chapter 6) the central role of the practitioner in changing those beliefs, attitudes, and norms through persuasion and social influence. We have emphasized throughout this book the vital importance and potential impact of the health practitioner.

In order to understand fully how the practitioner might enhance his or her role in patient cooperation with treatment, we must examine the factors that limit the practitioner's commitment to and involvement with patients. Limitations may be subtle, such as when the practitioner who tries to help the multiproblem patient finds the difficulties too overwhelming to expect any positive changes. These limitations may be even more obvious, such as when the practitioner himself or herself is unable to engage in self-control, but instead practices the very behaviors (overeating, smoking, excessive drinking) that are prohibited to the patient. Needless to say, lack of self-control on the part of the practitioner can devalue the credibility of the practitioner's message, and can significantly reduce the patient's acceptance of the regimen. So, too, might the practitioner's poor knowledge of or disinterest in psychosocial issues in patient care. Inattention to patients' attitudes, beliefs, norms, knowledge, thoughts, and behavioral schedules—as a result of time constraints, lack of understanding, or lack of caring and interest on the part of the practitioner—is likely to form a barrier to patient compliance.

The constraints under which practitioners must operate are very real and are usually fully understood only by those who are privy to the workings of the health-care system. Physically punishing, emotionally wrenching duties often challenge (seemingly beyond reasonable limits) the capacity of the practitioner to educate, support, and reinforce the patient. The stresses and demands of medical practice and training, embedded deeply within an unresponsive health-care system, can often serve to thwart the best-intentioned practitioner and his or her plans for total patient care. If the practitioner's efforts to deliver reinforcement, understanding, support, and education to patients remain wholly unacknowledged by superiors, and also cost the practitioner energy and time, the continued provision of such care for patients is unlikely.

In this section, we identify and examine some of the barriers to patient compliance that stem directly from the health professional. We do *not* believe that practitioners are inherently at fault for these barriers to patient compliance. Thus, we seek to identify the constraints on health professionals that may bring about and exacerbate their erection of these barriers. In our attempts to understand the constraints and limitations that health care professionals experience, we hope to learn something about how they might be alleviated.

Practitioners' Pessimism

Just as practitioners' positive expectations about their patients' capacity to change attitudes, beliefs, and behavior may be communicated to patients and thus serve to enhance their capabilities, so too might practitioners' pessimism about patients' abilities to change be translated into barriers to patient compliance. As we have noted in Chapter 3, practitioners' negative expectations, manifested in angry or hostile references to their patients, may bring about a severe breakdown in patient motivation to comply (Salzman et al., 1970; Milmoe et al., 1967).

With no group is this more clearly manifested than with patients who are economically poor. Surveys and other methods of assessment have shown that attitudes of professional helpers (both physical and mental-health practitioners) toward poor patients are uniformly pessimistic (Pratt, 1970; Wills, 1978). Either because of experience or stereotype (or more likely from a combination of both), practitioners tend to view poor patients as unlikely to make behavioral changes to enhance their health. Because of this expectation, these patients are less likely to be given explanations or information about their treatment and they are ignored as individuals and given little personal consideration (Duff & Hollingshead, 1968).

Practitioners' attitudes about the "hopelessness" of preventive action with poor patients may, in fact, be based upon some very real barriers in the care of poor patients. Patients of lower socioeconomic class rarely have a private physician of their own to whom they might turn as a source of medical care and preventive health education. Instead, poor patients usually enter the health-care system through the "emergency room" and are usually at that time considerably sicker than are those patients who have enjoyed regular care. They may have also delayed treatment because of their lack of medical information (Antonovsky, Zola, & Kosa, 1969). Poor people who are ill usually delay expressing their symptoms until illness has become totally disruptive to the conduct of their daily lives. Patients in poor surroundings typically fear the high technology of academic medical centers (Norman, 1969). Not suprisingly, communication gaps result when physicians conclude that patients who have delayed seeking care for a developing illness condition have done so because they are not concerned enough about their health.

As we will see below, practitioners often tend to attribute noncompliance to the personal characteristics of the patient rather than to his or her situational constraints. This is a common social-psychological phenomenon known both as a personalistic tendency (Wills, 1978) and the actor-observer effect (Jones & Nisbett, 1971). It is not peculiar to practitioners of medicine, nor does it apply only to the observation of the behavior of poor patients. It can have some important implications for many aspects of medical care.

Personalistic Tendency

As we noted in Chapter 4, it has often been assumed by health professionals that the best explanation for patients' poor cooperation with health regimens is that they possess "uncooperative personalities" (Davis, 1966). Many health professionals believe this to be true despite their inability to specify precisely what an uncooperative personality is. It is important to understand this phenomenon because it points to a number of issues that are relevant to motivating patients to assume responsibility for their care. It is possible, for example, that attributing patient noncompliance to patient personality represents the health professional's attempt to shift the sole blame for noncompliance onto the patient. This orientation may result from frustrated attempts to promote patient adherence to the therapeutic regimens or to preventive health behavior. The assumption that patient personality is an important determinant of noncompliance might also develop from health professionals' observations of consistency in patient behavior. This consistency may lead to the attribution of unchangeable traits to patients. Of course, as we noted in Chapter 4, no set of enduring personal traits has been found to render an individual noncompliant.

An important social-psychological phenomenon suggests another explanation for the health professional's focus on patient personality as a determinant of noncompliant behavior. This phenomenon also helps to explain some of the difficulties that arise in practitioner-patient communication. Studies of attribution processes (decisions about the causes of behavior) point to differences between actors and observers in the explanations they offer for behavior. Individuals performing the behaviors (the actors; for example, patients who do not take their medication or follow a diet regimen) tend to attribute the cause of their behavior to situational factors. A patient may say, for example, that he or she did not follow a diet regimen because of family pressure to eat during the holidays or because of the inability to find appropriate foods at a restaurant. On the other hand, observers of the behavior (for example, health professionals) are likely to attribute the cause of the behavior (failing to follow the diet regimen) to characteristics of the person. Thus, the health professional may say that the patient is uncooperative, lazy, or lacking in self-control (Jones, 1977; Jones & Nisbett, 1971). One reason for this bias stems from differences in information available to the actor and to the observer. The actor is able to see the factors that constrain his or her behavior, while the observer is aware of only the behavior itself. A second reason is that an actor is more likely to recognize that his or her behavior has been different in other situations and has varied according to the constraints of those situations, whereas the observer may evaluate the actor's behavior only in contrast with that of other persons. The health professional may fail to see what the patient can see—that although the patient has been able to follow other regimens or engage in self-control in the past, during that particular period, or because of difficulties arising from the environment or some problematic social situation, he or she is unable to carry out the behavioral goal. Interestingly, actors and observers can be induced to exchange perspectives when the information available to each is exchanged. In one study, this was done with videotape replay (Storms, 1973). When the actor saw himself as others saw him, he tended to make dispositional attributions to his behavior. When shown the perspective of the actor, the observer was able to see the situational constraints and as a result made more situational attributions about the actor's behavior.

It is important for health professionals to understand this personalistic tendency (or actor/observer effect), and to recognize the situational problems that patients experience in their attempts to care for themselves and to take responsibility for their health care. If differences in perspective are not understood, health professionals are likely to be easily frustrated with what they believe is the patient's unwillingness or inherent incapacity to follow recommendations for his or her health. Practitioners are also likely to blame or become derogatory toward patients who do not take responsibility for their own care. Practitioners may come to believe that patients *cannot* change and hence may relinquish their attempts to influence patients' behavior. Thus, methods for enhancing practitioners' awareness of patients' situational constraints (and perhaps even enhancing patients' awareness of practitioners' constraints) may help to promote their mutual understanding and may enhance practitioners' willingness and ability to help patients overcome the barriers to their compliance.

Practitioners' Decisions about Their Patients

The processes of medical diagnosis and treatment can be affected by psychological and sociological factors involving practitioners' attitudes toward their patients. Practitioners' decisions regarding psychiatric diagnoses, for example, are influencd by the patient's social class. Lower-class patients are more likely to be judged aberrant in their behaviors (Hollingshead & Redlich, 1958; Lee & Tenerlin, 1970). They are given psychiatric treatment for less time and with less intensity if they are of the lower class (Shader et al., 1969), although patients' expectations for psychiatric treatment do not differ among the social classes (Frank, Eisenthal, & Lazare, 1978). Decisions about the use of heroic measures, about the institution of long-term, difficult treatments, and about considerations of a cost-benefit nature in the allocation of medical resources tend to be biased toward the provision of better care for middle- and upper-class patients than for lower-class patients (Crane, 1973, 1975a, 1975b; Sudnow, 1967; Cornish & Miller, 1976; Haney, 1975; and Tischler, 1966).

Other Perceptions of Clients by Professional Helpers

In addition to the personalistic tendency in attributions considered above, Wills (1978) has found that professional helpers in general are influenced by interpersonal attraction, such that the more similar the patient's social class, values, and interests are to those of the practitioner, the more positive the outcome of care is likely to be. Nordholm (1980) found that physically attractive patients were believed to be good patients as well. Baekeland and Lundwall (1975) examined a number of variables that affected patients' dropping out of treatment (both medical and psychiatric) and concluded that the patient's perceived similarity to and liking by the therapist were important in preventing drop-out from treatment. Dissimilarity to and dislike for the patient were associated with patient dropout. The implications of this research are intriguing, for all these studies suggest that health professionals' preferences for and expectations about patients can have a profound effect on patients' achievement of healthful outcomes.

Wills (1978) reviewed many studies that demonstrated that medical practitioners held negative attitudes toward client resistance or noncompliance. In a study of physicians' responses to various issues in patient care, for example, Ort, Ford, and Liske (1964) found that physicians were very positive toward patients who accepted their control and followed orders but were profoundly dissatisfied with and rejecting of patients who were difficult to manage or who were uncooperative or rebellious. Studies of hospitalization (Lorber, 1975; Taylor, 1979) also demonstrate that socially assertive patients tend to make poor adjustments to the hospital, and are treated in a negative fashion by the staff. It is probably not surprising to find that after devoting considerable effort to helping their clients, practitioners dislike those who obstruct their efforts. This dislike may have some very important implications, however, since it may function as a serious impediment to patient cooperation.

Physician Characteristics

Practitioners' professional identities tend to influence their attitudes toward and treatment of patients, a point demonstrated clearly in studies of physicians' career specialization. Physicians in the different specialities tend to vary in their attribution of a psychological origin to patients' complaints (Zola, 1963). Dickinson and Pearson (1979) found in a study of graduates over four years from five different medical schools that those with a low probability of encountering dying patients (e.g., OB-GYN specialists) tended to be less open about and accepting of death and dying than physicians in specialties that have a high probability of encountering death. We see in these examples that physicians in various specialties have differing ways of dealing with psychosocial issues in the care of their patients.

Physicians can also be characterized as either interventionist or health-maintenance oriented (Haney, 1975). Linn and Lewis (1979), for example, demonstrated that physicians in practice vary considerably in their acceptance of patients' self-care. (In this study, self-care referred to patients' general reliance on their own knowledge and abilities to diagnose and treat minor health problems.) Physicians who expressed the most favorable attitudes toward self-care were younger (under 46), of Jewish background, and in group or clinic practice, and had an internal health locus of control (see Chapter 4). This latter finding indicates that physicians who believed health is largely a matter of one's own efforts (rather than dependent upon luck or powerful others) were more positive toward patients' self-control and responsibility for their own health. Physicians in this survey who were against self-care were older than 46, Protestant, and in private solo practice, and had an external health locus of control. Thus, physicians' attitudes toward the locus of control and responsibility for health were related to their estimates of the worth and appropriateness of patient self-care. The research on this question is still sparse, although a complete understanding of practitioners' attitudes toward patients' responsibility for their own health would be valuable. Since their attitudes may indeed influence patient cooperation with preventive and rehabilitative regimens, the study of individual differences among practitioners is an important issue to pursue in further research.

From Practitioner Attitudes to Practitioner Behaviors

Practitioners' attitudes and emotional reactions to patients are not irrelevant to clinical performance. In fact, practitioners' feelings (both negative and positive) have been shown in some studies to influence their behaviors toward patients. A study by Linn (1979), for example, demonstrated that first-year residents in internal medicine who held more positive attitudes of benevolence and caring toward patients as people (as measured by a validated questionnaire) were judged by their attending physicians to be clinically most competent. The attitudes of these physicians were likely translated into behaviors toward patients. Similarly, in a study by Staudenmayer and Lefkowitz (1981), 234 adult asthma patients were treated by 28 internists in a fellowship program in allergy. Each of the study physicians was rated by two staff supervising physicians according to his or her sensitivity to the "whole patient" and concern with the welfare of the patient as more than just a clinical case. The physicians were then classified into two categories on the basis of these ratings (high sensitivity and low sensitivity). Physicians who were rated as highly sensitive tended to keep hospitalized (and continue to care for) those patients who had very low levels of concern about their illness or very high levels of fear. The low-sensitivity physicians, on the other hand, discharged this type of patient from the hospital early, and prescribed steroid medication. High levels of fear were suggestive of a possible need for continued support, and very low levels of patient concern pointed to possible denial on the part of the patient. The highly sensitive physicians noted these as potential problems, and kept these patients hospitalized in order to observe them carefully and care for them. Thus, again we see that practitioner attitudes and awareness may be reflected in the care they deliver to patients. While further research on this issue is needed, the evidence so far suggests that practitioners' attitudes toward patients may be translated into behaviors toward those patients. Consequences for the patients' health outcomes and compliance behavior may result. The practitioner's poor expectations, lack of consistent feedback, ignorance of the patient's psychosocial condition, and ignorance of various behavior-change techniques may indeed contribute to poor outcomes, despite strong behavior-change intentions on the part of the patient.

All that we have considered so far may seem to suggest that practitioners alone are at fault who knowingly or unknowingly slight a patient's concerns or hold negative expectations. This is far from our intent. In fact, we argue below that the atmosphere in which medicine is typically practiced invites and supports many of the difficulties that practitioners experience in their attempts to enhance patients' behavior change. In the next section we examine some characteristics of medical training and practice that may intervene between practitioners' initial desires to serve patients and the attitudes and behaviors they subsequently develop toward them. These attitudes and behaviors develop with significant influence from the medical-care system. Indeed, to understand the practitioner's role in compliance fully we need to consider the practitioner in the context of medical training and practice.

THE PRACTITIONER IN CONTEXT

Training

Any attempt to understand the role of the practitioner in patient compliance must take into account the process of training and consider the perspectives of health-care educators and students. Many aspects of the education of health professionals are relevant to their care of patients. Since considerably more research has been done on the training of physicians than on the training of any other health practitioners, here we will examine the results of the research on medical education. This research reflects the many issues and problems that are common to all the health professions.

In medical training, social concerns are often difficult to maintain. Rezler (1974) has concluded that in the typical medical school, efforts to teach humanistic or holistic attitudes to medical students are inadequate and short lived. The goal of courses in behavioral science is often simply to pass the National Board Examination in Behavioral Science. What may be even more important, however, is that the character of medical training may seriously *hinder* the development of physicians' ability to consider the many issues related to patient compliance with treatment. Research on medical education (see Rosenberg, 1979) suggests that the typical medical-school atmosphere in this country (particularly its clinical phase of training) is cold and hostile in its approach, doing violence to the self-image of the medical student and undermining his or her self-concept and idealism (Becker & Geer, 1958; Becker et al., 1961; Rogoff, 1957). Furthermore, faculty were trained, for the most part, during the era of medicine (Funkenstein, 1978) when intellectual and scientific research values were emphasized (the 1940s and 1950s). These were placed high above community and human-service values. Although "community" and "human service" are recognized as the watchwords of the present era in medicine, students are not reinforced for putting concern for the patient above scientific pursuit (Eichna, 1980; Christie & Merton, 1958). Many students remain disillusioned and confused as a result. They are without role models. Moreover, the conduct of medical education fosters a high degree of compulsivity in students. This is certainly a useful trait, considering the exacting nature of medical work, but it is dangerous nonetheless. The reason is that the intellectualization required may cause many students to cope with the demands made on them by compartmentalizing and even denying their emotions in their care of patients (Cartwright, 1979).

The environment within which student physicians work and learn may even profoundly affect their behavior toward their patients. The effects of the hospital atmosphere and educational program environment have been studied by sociologists who analyzed the profession and its values exemplified in practice and in training (Becker & Geer, 1958; Freidson, 1970). Structural variables such as the type of hospital in which residency training takes place (university versus community), for example, can strongly influence the approach to patient care that is developed by the physician (Mumford, 1970). The degree of stratification on teaching wards operates in a similar manner. In regard to the latter issue, Seeman and Evans (1961a, 1961b), found that interns who trained on wards in which status differences between them and senior staff were minimized tended to spend more time with their patients and tended to offer them more psychological support than did interns from wards that emphasized status differences. On low-stratification wards, interns felt their staff physicians were more willing to share time with them, and so they in turn shared time with their patients. In addition, the interns on the low-stratification wards rated the teaching they received as better than did the interns on wards with high stratification.

Some established methods of medical training, then, tend to foster physicians' communication and rapport with patients, and focus attention on the patient as a whole person. Certain factors are likely to facilitate patients' fulfillment of their behavioral regimens. These involve lower stratification and greater faculty contact in physicians' training, and a hospital orientation that emphasizes holistic care of patients and places value on community service. Research suggests, not surprisingly, that physicians tend to treat patients much as they themselves are treated. For example, emotionally abused, misunderstood, alienated, anxious interns and residents are unlikely to have much energy or motivation for providing emotional support, understanding, and reassurance to their patients. Clearly, the medical system affects the caregiver.

Practitioners' Stress and the Care of Patients

Of all the professions, medicine is among the highest in income, prestige, and diversification, with numerous opportunities for exposure to a wide range of human experiences. Intellectual and emotional challenges are many, but the emotional challenges in particular can often serve also as liabilities. Emotional stress can indeed be a serious occupational hazard for many physicians. The result is a greater probability of suicide, heart disease, alcoholism, and drug abuse among physicians than in the general population (King, 1970; Rose & Rosow, 1973; Modlin & Montes, 1964). Not surprisingly, such stress may also interfere with patient communication and rapport, and the efforts required to influence their health beliefs, norms, and behaviors (Cartwright, 1979).

Nurses, too, are often stressed and emotionally frustrated in medical practice. They tend to experience a large discrepancy between what they have been taught in nursing school regarding the importance of the psychosocial care of patients and the expectations of their jobs as providers of technical ministrations who are allowed little time for psychosocial issues (Kramer, 1974).

The sources of anxiety and tension for the practitioner lie partly in problems and contradictions inherent in the role of the health professional. For example, practitioners often cope with the overwhelming distress of death and suffering by intellectualizing. They solve their inherent emotional dilemmas by becoming detached from their patients and by isolating their emotional reactions from their instrumental reactions (the behaviors necessary to take physical care of the patient). Indeed, this way of coping is often encouraged in the professional world of patient care. Evidence is accumulating, however, that while they may be advantageous for the practitioner in solving the short-run anxiety problem, intellectualization and detachment are likely, in the long-run, to encourage practitioners' emotional exhaustion, cynicism, and dehumanization of patients. The phenomenon is known in the literature as "burn out" (Maslach, 1976) and it affects a wide variety of human-service workers, not only physicians and nurses.

A more effective solution, studies have found, is for the practitioner to face the emotion, possibly by sharing it with other health professionals. Caregivers must *receive* emotional support if they are to provide it to their patients. In addition, institutional sanctions for attention to psychosocial aspects of the care of patients are necessary. Without incentives for physicians and other health professionals to talk with patients, to deal with them empathically, sensitively, and supportively, and to encourage their behavior change and maintenance, such care is unlikely to be provided. Economic incentives are not always feasible, but interpersonal incentives may be quite effective. Most important is the health professional's feeling that he or she is valued in some way for bothering to attend to and deal with the whole patient openly and empathically. The health-care system must reinforce the practitioner for facilitating patients' cooperation with their medical-care regimens.

A related issue involves the frustration experienced by physicians and other health-care practitioners who are asked by their patients to remedy health problems and physical damage brought on primarily by patients' neglect of their own health. While some patients may believe that heart valves can be replaced as easily as valves on an automobile, practitioners recognize the limitations of medical care. The prevalence of "self-destructive behavior" (Knowles, 1977) often places the practitioner in a position that makes salient questions relating to the philosophy, ethics, and legality of care. The extent to which patients accept personal responsibility for their health may profoundly affect the practitioner-patient relationship.

Finally, the structure and functioning of the health-care delivery system must be understood if some basic supports to the development of effective practitioner-patient relationships are to be available. One major obstacle to the development of optimal, compliance-enhancing medical care is the shortage of time. First, practitioners, especially physicians, usually have very little time to pursue humanizing aspects of their own lives such as family, friends, hobbies, exercise, and other relaxations. Such limitation is legendary. It can directly affect the practitioners' behavior in their one-to-one interactions with patients. The problem stems, however, from an issue that is far removed from the one-to-one practitioner-patient interaction. Instead the problem is rooted in social, economic, and political factors related to the shortage and maldistribution of health-care practitioners. Second, time is important because although within certain limits the quality, not the quantity, of time is the key to interactional success in the practitioner-patient relationship, the fact remains that stringent restrictions on the length of the practitioner-patient interaction (for example, ten minutes in some health-maintenance organizations) can seriously hamper efforts to pursue anything but the most perfunctory, task-oriented communication.

Stresses on health practitioners are very real, and the effects of these stresses on the treatment of patients can be documented. In understanding these stresses, their effects might be overcome. As a result, barriers that impede the translation of patients' intentions into behaviors might be lessened or altogether removed.

In this chapter, we have examined many barriers to and supports for the translation of patients' intentions into health behaviors. Some factors considered were well documented empirically, such as the positive effects of skill in behavioral self-control. Other factors, as we pointed out, require considerably more research in order to understand fully their implications for patients' health behavior. The barriers and supports considered in this chapter point out the importance of using patients' stated intentions as stepping stones to behavior change. Intentions, however, are not the final goal in the process of enhancing patient compliance. Rather, the enhancement of supports and minimization of barriers is necessary to translate behavioral intentions into health behaviors.

8

Implications of a Social-Psychological Approach to Compliance

Noncompliance is, without doubt, a value-laden concept. The term itself calls forth a certain degree of controversy. An important manifestation of this controversy may be found in the widespread criticism of the term "noncompliance" in medicine on the basis of its authoritative connotations. In the traditional model of medical practice, the authority (read practitioner) is imbued with a legitimate right to exact obedience. The patient is expected to follow orders that it is understood are in the interest of the patient's own good. It follows, then, that the practitioner is held to know what is best for the patient. By ignoring the practitioner's advice or by rebelling against it, the patient demonstrates himself or herself to be unwise, irresponsible, or (worse yet) morally culpable (Stone, 1979). On the other hand, noncompliance might be viewed as a type of patient triumph if it is seen to represent the adult patient's overthrow of the practitioner's inappropriately exerted authority (Marshall, 1981). By exhibiting noncompliance, the patient is seen to reassert his or her right to self-determination. Thus, the values that surround the concept of noncompliance may be quite disparate in character. Any book that seeks to understand patient compliance with medical regimens should address these disparate views in some manner. Of necessity, such a book must present a philosophical, moral, and/or ethical position with regard to noncompliance and to the practitioner-patient relationship from which it derives.

BASIC ASSUMPTIONS

Theories of compliance behavior, like theories of influence in general, implicitly spell out (intentionally or not) the specific obligations of both parties and the conditions under which particular behaviors are expected to emerge. In this chapter, we attempt to clarify and render explicit the many implicit assumptions that have guided the arguments in this book. We do so in order that these assumptions may be examined. From them we shall derive and propose a set of ethical principles to govern the practice of modern medicine as it is directed toward eliciting patient compliance.

We have empirically derived the following assertions that we hold as basic assumptions:

1. Modern medical science *is* efficacious and therefore the recommendations made by a medical practitioner (in collaboration with the patient) will, if adhered to, benefit the patient. (Although debates have raged in the popular and professional literature regarding the "actual" efficacy of modern medicine, we cannot adequately address this issue here. Other writers have considered this topic in some depth; see Ingelfinger, 1978; Dubos, 1959; Carlson, 1975; Starr, 1981; Thomas, 1979; McKeown, 1976; and Illich, 1976, for discussions.)
2. The practitioner is an expert on matters of health and illness by virtue of his or her special command over medical knowledge.
3. Present rates of patient compliance with both long- and short-term regimens are wholly inadequate (see Chapter 1).
4. The clinical prescription (i.e., the medical recommendation) is bound to be incorrect if its formulation is not based on a negotiated consideration of the patient's beliefs, values, norms, resources, and constraints.
5. The patient is an expert on matters pertaining to his or her own beliefs, values, norms, resources, and constraints.
6. The patient retains both the right and the responsibility to determine the course of his or her own life in medical matters that affect him or her directly. (Here we omit the cases in which the individual represents a public health hazard, such as the carrier of typhoid or the violent psychotic, who have the potential, respectively, to infect an entire population or to bludgeon a good proportion of it.)

A QUESTION OF ETHICS

Any discussion of rights and responsibilities involves a consideration of ethical issues. In our consideration here, we adopt a convention proposed by ethicist Albert Jonsen (1979). According to Jonsen, ethics can be understood in two ways: (1) as principles that govern the behavior expected of a person (health professional) in the ordinary course of his or her daily action; and (2) as principles that govern correct action under extraordinary conditions in which acceptable standards are not applicable or in which the problem at issue is ill-defined. According to Jonsen, "In current medical ethics, so much attention is paid to ethics in the second sense that the fundamental truths of the patient-physician relationship are sadly neglected" (Jonsen, 1979, p. 115). In considering the ethics of the practitioner-patient relationship as they relate to compliance, we address these former, often neglected issues. Specifically, in this chapter we review the nature of current social opinion and consider evidence supporting the importance of the following ethical principles as they relate to the practitioner's role in eliciting patient compliance. (We state these here because we believe, as does Haynes, 1979, that ethical issues belong "up front" where they can be examined explicitly.) After considering the evidence, we shall conclude that:

1. The practitioner carries the greater responsibility for effective practitioner-patient communication.
2. The practitioner has a duty to encourage patients to make considered decisions regarding their own health care (whenever it is possible for them to do so).
3. The practitioner has a duty to believe in the efficacy of his or her own prescriptions, and to attempt to bring about the patient's belief as well.
4. The practitioner, as an expert on matters of health, should follow ethical guidelines (examined later) regarding truthfulness and non-coercive action in attempting to educate and persuade his or her patients. The practitioner's approach should allow for a full range of patient self-determination.
5. The practitioner has a duty to assist the patient in complying with the recommendations generated in the clinical encounter.

It is important to keep in mind that there are "various types of *noncompliance by physicians*; for example, failure to report test results to patients, followup on symptoms brought to their attention by patients, schedule tests and appointments within the medically indicated time limits, or contact patients regarding new evidence of a risk in their current therapy or the availability of an improved therapy." (Pratt, 1978, p. 209). Such actions are of as much importance in patient care as patients' noncompliance. Here, we are assuming that practitioners *can* be counted on to fulfill the basic responsibilities of their role.

A SOCIAL-PSYCHOLOGICAL APPROACH

What is a social-psychological approach to patient compliance? In essence, such an approach holds that at the determinant core of the compliance phenomenon lies the structure and nature of the interpersonal relationship from which the request to comply is derived. Examinations and considerations of noncompliance are held in this view to be most accurate when they include the interpersonal context in which compliance may (or may not) occur.

In keeping with a social-psychological approach, we note that compliance involves a process of social influence wherein the real, imagined, or implied presence of one person (the practitioner) affects the behavior of another (the patient) (Harvey & Smith, 1977). Any process of influence is invariably reciprocal in nature. Each participant can and does influence the other. Therefore, although it is true that patients influence their practitioners, our book has been concerned primarily with the social psychology of the *practitioner's* role—the influence that the practitioner has on the patient's beliefs, values, norms, expectations, constraints, and resources. Further, we have argued throughout that the medical practitioner exerts his or her social influence by means of the interpersonal relationship established with the patient. While the interpersonal influence may be strongest when their interaction is face to face, the practitioner's influence can be exerted at any time through the thoughts, memories, and expectations of the patient. We hold that the ultimate goal of a social-psychological approach to patient compliance is the patient's eventual internalization of the medical recommendation, internalization being "the propensity to perform a recommended behavior when one is removed in time and/or place from the source of influence" (Rodin, 1982, p. 62).

The Process of Negotiation

Another of our important basic assumptions is that in seeking medical care, people attempt to gain information about attaining health and overcoming illness. Here we are using the word "information" in a very broad sense to constitute any "medical advice." As such, it may involve simple reassurance, an instant cure, a long-term course of therapy, or the satisfaction of queries about the medical problem, among other things. We view the precise actions in which patients ultimately engage as the subject of an inevitable process of negotiation that occurs in the practitioner-patient encounter. We agree with Stimson and Webb's (1978) view that:

> People do not hand over all control and decision-making to the doctor merely by becoming patients. . . . Both patient and doctor . . . attempt to control and

> direct the consultation along their own desired lines, to persuade the other to recognize or accept a particular perspective on, and orientation to, the problem that has been brought. . . . Seeing the consultation in terms of each actor trying to influence the other brings in the concept of negotiation. . . . Negotiation is a process. That patient and doctor both use strategies to influence each other does not mean that one or the other is going to be successful. But the concept of negotiation means that we see the outcome as the result of their interaction and the strategies they have each adopted, rather than as determined solely by the facts that are brought and the application of the skills that the doctor has. [pp. 144-145]

The participants to the clinical encounter bring with them their own systems of beliefs, values, goals, expectations, and so on. These factors are seen to enter into and occasionally to direct the process of negotiation, which itself may be neither explicit nor recognized and consciously intended as such by the participants (Roth, 1963). It occurs nonetheless.

The Conditions of Negotiation

As we have seen throughout, compliance is most likely to occur when certain conditions are met in the practitioner-patient exchange. Information must be communicated effectively (Chapter 2) and a relationship of mutual trust must be developed (Chapter 3). Once a therapeutic atmosphere of openness, trust, and hope is established, the patient is likely to be willing to disclose to the practitioner the beliefs, expectations, and social-normative constraints that affect his or her health-behavior intentions. These factors can then enter into the negotiation between the practitioner and the patient. The practitioner, by exerting social influence, can attempt to assist the patient in building a behavioral commitment on the basis of the patient's beliefs and social norms. It is only then that interventions can be put into operation most effectively (Chapter 7). In practice, interventions such as a special diet, or a convenient pill regimen or (for the adventurous) a pill box sporting an alarm buzzer are often undertaken without the appropriate prerequisites. As we have seen, however, no convenient regimen, no special diet, no gimmicky pill container is likely to be adequate to the task of enhancing a patient's compliance if a behavioral commitment has not first been made. Further, no patient will maintain a commitment or follow a treatment regimen that he or she does not believe will work, toward a goal he or she does not particularly value, against the wishes of his or her family and friends, or for a practitioner he or she does not particularly like or respect. On the other hand, if trust and open communication are developed in the practitioner-patient relationship, if the patient's beliefs are taken into consideration, and if a regimen is chosen that is consistent with the patient's social values and normative constraints, the patient's commitment to the regimen is likely to be deepened. Only after a commitment is established is patient compliance likely to be enhanced with techniques such as those that seek to improve the patient's memory or render the regimen easier to follow.

The Content of Negotiation

Throughout this book we have argued that patient commitment will be most likely brought about through a process of negotiation over information, beliefs, and values. In order to optimize the chances of success, this negotiation approach favors a particular style of interaction in which the practitioner strives to hear and understand the patient's request (Eisenthal et al., 1979). The practitioner uses this request as the central component in the process of negotiation over treatment. The process of negotiation is not biased in the patient's favor, and the patient does not always obtain precisely what he or she wants. Instead, negotiation serves primarily to legitimize the patient's ideas about treatment and to involve the patient in both the planning and the implementation of therapeutic maneuvers. Neither does this approach give tremendous import to the practitioner's recommendations merely by virtue of their origin. As we shall see later, the modern-day practitioner can no longer rely on his or her "legitimate right" to give orders. Therefore, a burden of persuasion and interpersonal influence falls squarely on his or her shoulders.

The many and varied issues presented in this book have had as their primary objective the examination and subsequent enhancement of the capacity of the practitioner to influence his or her patients. Persuasion is geared toward the combined goals of: (1) enhancing patient cooperation with medical recommendations; (2) enhancing the efficacy of medicine by means of enhancing compliance and by encouraging the application of "nonspecific factors" to the healing process, see Chapter 3; and (3) enhancing the satisfaction of all participants to the health transaction. The issues we have presented in this book are intended not simply as techniques for achieving these goals—not a mere *modus operandi* in the practitioner's bag of tricks. Rather, we have presented a *scheme* that can be used (in the light of the specific goals and resources of each patient) as a *guideline* in creating an appropriate plan of action for enhancing compliance. This scheme may be used to guide the assessment and alteration (if necessary) of the conduct of communication, the interpersonal relationship, the beliefs, the social norms, and the behavioral and cognitive skills of the patient.

The Consequences of Negotiation

The compliance issues examined here should be viewed as comprising a new and more timely approach to both medical care and the practitioner-patient relationship—one in which the patient maintains his or her right and responsibility to be self-determining. Personal responsibility on the part of the patient is at the core of this approach. In this scheme, the goal of the medical practitioner is to explore the beliefs, sociocultural values, and norms of each patient, and in the context of a relationship characterized by trust and clear communication, to negotiate a mutually satisfactory treatment. The patient's contribution to this process of collaboration should insure that the regimen is one that is best suited to him or her as an individual. The obligation of the practitioner as an expert is then *not* merely to insure that the patient follows orders, but to work with the patient in addressing the many issues relevant to the fulfillment of the clinical prescription. The practitioner's social influence is aimed at insuring the patient's *internalization of the medical recommendation that he or she has had an active part in formulating*. We have presented evidence that an orientation characterized by negotiation and mutual participation of practitioner and patient is the most likely to bring about the patient's compliance with medical recommendations.

THE ROLE OF PRACTITIONER AND PATIENT

In Chapter 2 we considered Talcott Parson's theory of the sick role, according to which the social roles of both practitioner and patient are explicitly delineated (Parsons, 1951, 1975). Parsons claims to have formulated these roles "in the light of American values and social structure" (Parsons, 1958). Briefly in review, the medical practitioner functions as the gate-keeper to the sick role and as such is expected to be affectively neutral, technically knowledgeable, and oriented solely toward the good of the patient. The practitioner and the patient are separated by the "competence gap," in which the practitioner has more medical expertise than the patient and possesses information to which the patient has limited access. In part because of this competence gap, and in part because of the advantages that accompany the patient's adoption of the sick role (for example, exemption from usual obligations of work, and exemption from blame for the condition), the patient is obliged to cooperate with the practitioner's treatment recommendations.

As we saw also in Chapter 2, some theorists (notably Freidson, 1961) have criticized Parsons for presenting a theory of practitioner-patient interaction with little or no basis in social reality. The sick-role conceptualization, in Freidson's view, merely depicts the *normative prescriptions* of the practitioner and patient—the way that each *should* behave given the particular expectations and values of our society. Freidson has argued that Parsons' theory does not describe the manner in which the practitioner and patient actually do behave, nor does it reflect the transactions that empirical study has shown actually occur between them. Freidson has suggested that the virtue of Parsons' "analysis is that it provides us with a definition of (philosophically) the 'essence' of the relationship" (Freidson, 1961, p. 190).

American Values and Social Structure

Despite the obvious limitations of Parsons' approach for predicting the nature of ongoing doctor-patient interaction, we believe that his normative prescriptions are very useful in developing an understanding of the ethical issues in patient compliance. Parsons' prescriptions reflect in an important way many critical issues relevant to the ethics of the practitioner's role. Of course, discussions of ethical issues are, to a significant degree, bound by the cultural values and social structure of the particular society under consideration (Callahan, 1980). Hence, Parsons' normative prescriptions can be viewed as pointing to what is most acceptable in our society—a society that holds certain values sacred. As Wilson (1970) has pointed out, Parsons' approach was based primarily upon an American middle-class pattern of values in which an emphasis is placed on the merits of "individual responsibility, deliberate striving and grooming of the self toward health and mastery, and activism in the carrying out of normal social roles, particularly in the occupational sphere" (Wilson, 1970, p. 24). The entirely voluntary approach of both the patient and the practitioner to the therapeutic encounter was also emphasized by Parsons. The practitioner and the patient were seen to act as essentially free agents who willingly chose to interact with one another. "The decision by the patient to seek care and the selection of whom he would consult were a matter of individual choice. This was seen as a direct consequence of our culture, reflecting several of its major value orientations: individualism, orientation toward the future" (Bloom & Summey, 1976, p. 36), as well as self-determination and freedom of choice.

These values of individualism, future orientation, freedom of choice, and self-determination have been partly responsible for our society's recent entertainment of the notion that a major component of the etiology of many diseases (particularly those chronic conditions most prevalent in America today) is the self-destructive behavior of the persons afflicted. In different cultures, however, different considerations hold sway. In Italy, for example, the national health service law refers only to structural and environmental conditions as causes of disease and human suffering, never to the individual. In America, though, it is accepted that people become sick in part because of their behavior. They eat too much, drive wrecklessly, fail to exercise, smoke cigarettes, and resort to alcohol in order to relax and cope with the stresses of their daily lives. Despite the social and interpersonal danger inherent in "blaming the victim" of serious disease, many people—health professionals and lay persons alike—are beginning to place an ever greater emphasis on the origins of disease as lying primarily in personal misbehavior (Knowles,

1977). Hence, while many of the Parsonian prescriptions for doctor and patient remain, the sick-role prescription that the patient is not held responsible for his or her illness is beginning to change. Such an orientation is understandable in terms of the basic values of our society, as noted above. It also reflects the recent developing societal unwillingness to finance further the high cost of health care (Crawford, 1981). Thus, while it motivates some inherently positive developments, the ideology of personal responsibility also presents some dangers.

Personal Responsibility: The Pros and Cons

At the psychological level, it has been asserted that therapeutic modes of thought that place responsibility for people's physical conditions *outside* themselves (in the environment, or in the social or cultural milieu) tend to exempt them from making critical judgments and relieve them of moral responsibility for personal action. If sickness is defined in terms of an invasion of the person by forces outside of his or her own conscious control, then the patient's recognition of his or her own responsibility for recovery is circumvented. It follows that the individual must then passively accept the diseased and helpless condition. Lasch (1979) has argued that this orientation encourages a permanent suspension of the moral sense of the patient and inappropriately relieves the individual of personal responsibility. The erosion of moral responsibility for health and illness results in a waning of the capacity for self-help (Lasch, 1979). In this view, if culpability is eliminated, then so is competence. Any patient who is held "not guilty" with respect to his or her health and recovery from illness (either in the sense of having control over the etiology of the disease, or in having control over its course through the enactment of specific regimen) is rendered essentially unable to help him/herself. This argument is extended further: by delivering oneself into the hands of the specialist and adopting a submissive orientation, one becomes essentially dependent upon medical authority (Illich, 1976). Hence, the recent emphasis on self-control and personal responsibility (in overcoming illness and in attaining and maintaining health) in effect forces the patient to demonstrate an active orientation toward his or her own health. Such an orientation should serve to foster *collaboration* with the practitioner, rather than submission to his or her control.

Two important problems arise from this emphasis on personal responsibility for health and illness, however. The first is the extreme view sometimes taken in which people totally reject the medical establishment. They assume that since they are solely responsible for and in control of their own health, medical professionals have *no* expertise of any particular value to them. A strong belief in the importance of self-help in medical care may even prompt some people to reject the medical profession altogether (Cobb, 1954). As a result, they may ignore the onset and progression of serious disease (caused by factors quite beyond their immediate or personal control). They may also insist upon nonmedical treatments, which may be dangerous in themselves or simply as they preclude effective medical treatment (Kronenfeld, 1979).

The second problem that arises in focusing too closely on personal responsibility involves a neglect of the powerful impact of both social and environmental factors on health. Dangerous workplaces, pollution, and poverty are all factors known to promote disease and interfere with the attainment and maintenance of health. Also, as we have seen in Chapter 7, environmental issues are of great importance and may interfere with the patient's compliance with medical regimens. If patients are to conform to their treatment regimens, resources must be available and barriers must be overcome. A myopic focus on individual habits without some attention to the social and physical environment is likely to be misconceived, since in fact the social and cultural environment of the patient may ultimately dictate what he or she can and cannot do.

As an example, consider the patient who has made a personal commitment to undertake a medical regimen. Despite this commitment, his cooperation is likely to be preempted if the regimen is hotly opposed by his social group or culture. To label the patient who passes up a socially or culturally condemned regimen as irresponsible about his health most certainly represents insensitivity to the patient as a person and undermines the goal of helping the patient to internalize the health regimen. Further, the political and economic situations that support social and environmental causes of disease and impediments to health should not be ignored, for without some attention by practitioners and lay persons alike, these factors may never be improved or their negative impact lessened. Hence, factors outside the control of the patient should not be ignored when the patient's individual responsibility is emphasized.

Overemphasis of either approach—of habits and personal culpability on the one hand, or of environmental and social factors on the other—is both inappropriate and dangerous. An emphasis on habits can be taken too far, to the extent that for every disease that befalls a patient, the search for why he or she "deserves" the disease might be undertaken (Sontag, 1978; Lerner, 1975). Likewise, an emphasis on social and environmental factors can be overdone to the point where pain and suffering are assumed to have their roots in flawed institutions and environments alone and thus are immune to personal control. For example, the argument that toxic chemicals, noise, and environmental stress lead people to seek relief through unhealthy means (such as alcohol, cigarettes, and licit or illicit mood-altering drugs) (Conrad & Kern, 1981) paints a picture of human beings as helpless, passive, and ignorant. Self-destruction is condoned as a method of coping with environmental threat. Thus, we see that in attempting to understand the origins of health and illness, the truism holds that regardless of their direction, extreme positions are likely to be destructive.

If we remain aware of the potential dangers of its overemphasis, the concept of personal responsibility can be very important and useful in health care. Inherent in this concept of personal responsibility is the patient's self-control over what he or she should and will do in order to maintain or regain health. Patient responsibility is, in essence, a cultural belief set within the symbolic framework of health as a basic human value. It has been argued that American society has always been in favor of notions of self-help and of avoiding reliance on experts (Hofstadter, 1962). The recent emphasis on rejection of what is described as "the medicalization of everyday life" (Fox, 1977; Illich, 1976) can be viewed as a reflection of traditional American values but also as part of a broader new social ideology characterized by frugality, economic striving, and self-help. (Medicalization involves an expansion of medical expertise to encompass social and psychological phenomena, and hence the removal of personal responsibility and control via the overapplication of medical methods and technology.) It is manifested not only in self-help medicine, but also in such individual pursuits as do-it-yourself plumbing, home improvement, income tax, and law. Experts (physicians, plumbers, accountants, lawyers) are consulted only when self-help is not possible or has failed (Kronenfeld, 1979).

How might the encouragement of the patient's acceptance of personal responsibility for matters of health actually benefit the patient? As we have seen, many psychological and motivational advantages accompany patients' feelings of self-control and self-determination. Researchers in the field of social psychology have demonstrated time and again that individuals are more likely to maintain changes in their beliefs and their behaviors when they perceive that those changes result from their own free will (Festinger, 1957; Deci, 1975), and when they feel that they have an opportunity to act otherwise (Kiesler, 1971). Researchers have similarly found that feelings of self-determination (as opposed to coercion) are in and of themselves powerful motivating forces (De Charms, 1968). Many studies of the psychology of commitment, as it operates in various settings including health care, have demonstrated that feelings of self-determination and personal responsibility regarding the enactment of particular behaviors increase the individual's behavioral commitment as well as his or her actual adherence to the behavioral task (Collins & Hoyt, 1972; Pranulis, Dabbs, & Johnson, 1975; Rodin, 1982). Kiesler (1971) goes so far as to suggest that commitment itself can be defined as the perception that one is responsible for one's own behavior.

Implications of an Ethic of Personal Responsibility

Social ideologies do not arise *de novo* or from within the mysterious confines of social vacuums. Social policy (health policy included) is biased in favor of politically and economically dominant groups. The ideology of personal or individual responsibility reflects, as we have noted, traditional Western values. Some argue that it is also totally inattentive to the social causes of disease. The ideology of personal responsibility therefore supports the political and economic status quo, and it obviates the necessity for social-welfare programs designed to eliminate environmental dangers to the health of the unassuming masses. Vincente Navarro (1976) has argued that the basic discrepancy between the orientations of practitioners and patients—a conflict that necessitates negotiation and resolution—obscures rather than clarifies the structure of power in our society. The ultimate societal power, according to Navarro, rests in the hands of the ruling corporate class and the financial institutions. Any restructuring of the practitioner-patient relationship to include effective bargaining and negotiation would leave untouched the powers *behind* medicine that are the real factors determining the health of the people. We feel that such an argument renders both practitioner and patient impotent and implies that nothing they can do short of revolution will aid them in improving their health. Such views exist, and they must be acknowledged. We do not accept them in their entirety, however, because they leave untouched the important issues of the locus of human frailty and the socially sanctioned nature of irresponsibility. In fact, we consider the practitioner and patient themselves to be the two most important factors in determining the patient's ultimate health behavior and compliance.

Andre De Vries (1980), in discussing the health-care responsibilities of the individual as a citizen, holds that while the individual cannot always be held solely responsible for his or her *state* of health (since health, as we have seen, is not totally amenable to personal control), the individual is responsible "for the *care* of his health, and that in three respects: self-care, choice of and interaction with the health professional, and determination of the forms of health care system in his society" (DeVries, 1980, p. 100). In this view, the ultimate responsibility for the structure of institutions in a society (in the case of our study, medical institutions) rests in the hands of the people.

Arluke (1978) refuted Navarro's assertion that the basic conflict between lay persons and professionals actually obscures the structure of power. Arluke argued that this conflict between the practitioner and patient may, in fact, have very little to do with social-class considerations or economics. Rather, this conflict arises from the control of medical knowledge (Freidson, 1970). Arluke has suggested that because of their virtual monopoly over medical knowledge, physicians are able to exercise a great deal of power over the judgments of government decision makers regarding public health, health care, and related factors. Decisions about government spending on health care—the forms it will take and the philosophies that will govern it—are made on the basis of information controlled by medical practitioners (for example, through the American Medical Association). "Through their control over knowledge, providers play an active role in forming the judgments of decision makers. Navarro underestimates the consequences of the social organization of knowledge which class by itself does not allow us to predict" (Arluke, 1978, p. 438). Here we return once again to the issue of conflict over control of medical knowledge—the very same control that is at the heart of the professional-patient relationship. We contend that *the major issue* related to health and patient compliance at the societal level is the same as that at the level of interpersonal interaction—control over medical knowledge.

SHARED KNOWLEDGE AND POWER: A TIMELY MODEL OF MEDICAL CARE

Physicians and other medical practitioners are often charged with concealing medical information from their patients (see Chapter 2). Explanations advanced by practitioners to account for this practice include: information takes too long to convey; some information overly concerns patients; patients seldom understand anyway; patients often misunderstand and become needlessly worried; oftentimes the changing nature of the medical condition makes communication difficult and so information conveyed prematurely may jeopardize the patient's trust in the practitioner; patients don't really want to know; and patients don't listen in any case. Practitioners often feel, too, that patients approach them under conditions of such distress and disorientation that they are not, all in all, capable of making responsible decisions concerning their own care, even if they have the information to do so. "A patient is weak and overwhelmed by his illness, lacks medical knowledge and skill, lacks objectivity about his predicament, comes seeking help, and is dependent, passive, and obedient. This image has been proffered not only as an accurate version of how people behave with physicians, but also as a venerable posture for the client" (Pratt, 1978, p. 211). Recall, however, that Stimson and Webb (1975) (see Chapter 3) argued that the patient actually does *not* relinquish control and decision-making power to the clinician but only uses the *illusion* of dependency on the practitioner as a self-presentation strategy in order to fulfill the practitioner's expectations and manipulate his or her sentiments and behaviors.

These expectations promote the role of the "good patient" (in contrast to the problem patient). The good patient is one who is "conforming, cooperative, generally uncomplaining, not demanding, and who does not interrupt medical routines" (Pratt, 1978, p. 212; see also Lorber, 1975; Taylor, 1979). Practitioners encourage good patient behavior because it is largely self-serving for them to do so. Furthermore, under conditions of information deprivation, a patient is left with little choice but to become a passive recipient of medical care. Under such conditions, the patient's "case" becomes much easier to manage, for knowledge in this sense is power. Lack of knowledge precludes responsibility, however. "There is one right which is a primary requisite for the realization of any individual health care responsibility system. That is the right to information. *No responsibility is possible without knowlege on which to base one's judgment*" (DeVries, 1980, p. 102, emphasis added).

In recent years, medicine's traditional authority and secrecy have been severely challenged. One such challenge focuses on medicine's traditional ethic of practitioner control and patient-centered action. "Medicine is nine-tenths a professionally perpetuated mystery, self-aggrandisement of a sect, a bureaucracy like most bureaucracies interested primarily in its own survival, not the welfare of its clientele; today its goal is self-preservation" (Silver, 1977, p. 10). While this view is extreme, such sentiments have no doubt contributed to our society's recent reemphasis on personal responsibility, self-care, and self-determination regarding matters of health. Evidence is beginning to mount in support of the need for a new model of medical care.

This new model of health care is different from traditional medical care because it is based on a contract that assumes an underlying equality between the practitioner and the patient. Any "physician-patient relationship is contractual . . . both in a legal sense and an ethical sense" (Marsh, 1979, p. 133). The type of contract traditionally adhered to in medicine is referred to in the law as "fiduciary." A fiduciary contract reflects the paternalistic or Hippocratic model of medical care. In this type of arrangement, the patient contracts for services from the professional by entrusting himself or herself to the practitioner's care. The traditional practitioner is in total control and is held to know what is best for the patient. The practitioner's responsibility to the patient derives from the patient's request for care. It is assumed, of course, that the practitioner will not exploit, manipulate, or take undue advantage of the patient. Veatch (1972), however, has proposed that there may also exist a very different type of practitioner-patient relationship involving the "contractual model" of medical care. At the very basis of the contractual model is the equality or balance of power between the contracting parties. The contract represents a totally autonomous decision on the part of each person to be committed to the provisions of the contract. The contract requires also that the parties be rational, that they possess enough information to serve their own interests, and that they have enough independence of judgment to make a free and rational choice. In contrast to the traditional, paternalistic model of medical care, a contractual arrangement between practitioner and patient places on the patient (and hence removes from the practitioner) a good deal of the responsibility for decision making and for a positive health outcome (Masters, 1975; MacIntyre, 1977).

In the negotiated mutual contract (explicitly written or verbally agreed to) between the practitioner and patient, both have given their informed consent to the regimen. There is a no-fault attitude toward noncompliant behavior, and the responsibility for the outcome of treatment is mutual. This ideal practitioner-patient relationship encourages, indeed expects, compliance behavior. The contract preserves the ideals of freedom for both parties, mutual understanding, and mutual responsibility. The contractual model also represents a practical ideal, for it is attainable given certain operational principles. These principles are, in essence, the ones presented in detail throughout this book. In the contractual relationship, neither party "loses." Rather, both "win" when compliance occurs because compliance is a mutually satisfactory outcome.

The contractual model of the practitioner-patient relationship is by no means new. It was first described in 1956 by Szasz and Hollender. They called it the "mutual participation model" (reviewed in Chapter 3). In the mutual participation model, patients participate in major decisions regarding their own health care and they contribute crucial information for the development of the most appropriate format for their care. Szasz and Hollender (1956) proposed this model as most effective for the care of the chronically ill patient. Although the extent and seriousness of the problem of noncompliance was hardly recognized at the time, these authors noted the usefulness of this model for enhancing patient compliance. They noted also that the mutual participation approach was rarely used in medicine, and that many physicians (at least at that time) would probably reject it out of hand. According to Szasz and Hollender (1956), the mutual participation orientation (like the contractual model noted above) requires that "the participants (1) have approximately equal power, (2) be mutually interdependent (i.e., need each other), and (3) engage in activity that will be in some ways satisfying to both" (p. 587). In sum, the goal of the mutual participation model is for the practitioner to "help the patient help himself."

A contractual (or mutual participation) model is likely to be more acceptable to practitioners and patients today than it has ever been before. At present, our society places very little value on manifestations of omnipotence (Maddison, 1980). Certainly in medicine, both patients and practitioners are ready and willing to abandon the notion of the "doctor as God." Patients are no longer eager to ascribe to practitioners knowledge and skill beyond what they actually possess. Nor are practitioners content to take on the burden of that role (which would require that they be continually available to the demands of their dependent patients, and that they take responsibility for decisions that should be the patients' own). Our society is witnessing a general decline in the old-fashioned kind of professionalism that placed all power in the hands of the professional and required that the patient merely submit to and follow orders. Whereas in the past any practitioner who "helped his client help himself" was considered vaguely suspect (perhaps even thought to be incompetent), now the opposite seems to be true (Maddison, 1980). Patients are presently better educated and more highly informed on matters of health and illness than ever before in history. They are also, for the most part, unwilling simply to entrust themselves to an authoritative, paternalistic practitioner.

Criticisms of Contractual Medicine

Arguments have been levied against the contractual model of medicine. According to Kass (1980) and Siegler (1980), the contractual model views medicine not as a profession but rather as a technical service, delivered or provided in much the same manner as auto repair or plumbing. The focus on equality in the contractual model is seen to orient the medical practitioner to "selling" and the patient to "buying," and to defy age-old notions of medicine as an art and a profession. Relatedly, Siegler (1980) has argued against what he perceives to be a recent tendency to view medicine as a trade. He has proposed that within a contractual model, the mysterious process of healing is circumvented and the crucially important interpersonal bond between the practitioner and his patient is lost. The contract, he posits, destroys the nonspecific aspects of treatment that are manifested in such phenomena as the placebo effect. Kass and Siegler further argue (albeit without empirical support) that the contractual model presupposes and exacerbates an *absence* of trust in the practitioner. The contractual model, which requires negotiation, is said to destroy the essence of the healing activity which is based upon the patient's investment of hope, trust, and confidence in the practitioner. It is argued that the contractual model is untenable because of the vicissitudes of chance inherent in medicine and the inequality of knowledge and expertise between practitioner and patient. Siegler argued that contractual medicine would bring about an impoverished practitioner-patient relationship, would reduce practitioners' commitment to their patients, and would encourage defensive medicine.

Resolving Criticisms of Contractual Medicine

The contractual model of medical care is based on negotiation, the communication of information, and shared power between practitioner and patient. As we have seen throughout this book, a great deal of empirical evidence supports these factors as central to the enhancement of patient compliance. We examine in detail below the strong evidence that refutes arguments levied against the contractual model and supports the potential value and appropriateness of a mutual participation model of health care.

We have argued that the practitioner-patient relationship is characterized by a process of mutual exchange of information, and we have emphasized that the knowledge differential between practitioner and patient in the therapeutic relationship is two-sided. That is, while the practitioner has more knowledge than the patient about medical issues in general, the patient has more knowledge than the practitioner about the many psychological, social, and environmental factors that ultimately affect his or her own compliance with the medical regimen. Knowledge of these factors is critically important, for they must be carefully considered in order that an appropriate regimen may be designed for the patient. If compliance is accepted as a primary goal of the health-care transaction, both parties must be equal in this knowledge. Further, no evidence exists that trust is destroyed in a relationship in which both parties explicitly spell out their respective obligations and expectations. In fact, as we saw in Chapter 3, the reverse is true. The more open and honest the practitioner and patient are with one another regarding their expectations, desires, and beliefs, the more likely it is that trust will be developed. Trust is enhanced when knowledge and competence are possessed. On the other hand, the more secretive the practitioner, the more likely the patient is to conclude that he or she has something to hide. In addition, the contention that the contractual model leads to poor practitioner commitment has no supporting evidence. In fact, it may be true that practitioners are *more* committed to patients who take an active part in their care and maintain personal responsibility for their health—behavior that is more likely than abdication of control to be in keeping with the practitioner's values.

Finally, the practice of defensive medicine by practitioners results not from a contractual approach but rather from the tendency of dissatisfied patients to litigate. Defensive medicine is likely to be exacerbated, not eliminated, by mysterious, secretive, and authoritative practitioners. Vaccarino (1977), a malpractice lawyer, has linked patient litigiousness to their dissatisfaction with the practitioner-patient relationship—particularly to the withholding of information from the patient and the lack of consideration for the patient as a human being with needs for respect and support. Patients who are prohibited from participating in their medical care are more (not less) likely to litigate, thus causing practitioners to be more (not less) concerned with defensive medicine. When patients are fully involved in their treatment (via mutual participation and contracting), they automatically share with the practitioner in the responsibility for its outcome.

The present trend toward increased recognition of patients' rights (Kass, 1980) and increased patient autonomy is acknowledged even by critics of this ideology to be "in part in response to excessive authoritarianism and mystification—and even arrogance—on the part of physicians" (p. 1815). In fact, it may be true that even in the "good old days" when paternalistic medicine was most prevalent, medical practitioners showed little respect for the patient as a person, and so their patients failed to trust them. Despite some nostalgic reminiscences about the "good old doc" of which we are now reminded again (see Eisenberg, 1977), evidence exists to suggest that medical practitioners were in fact not held in particularly high esteem in the good old days. "Again I hear the voices indignantly muttering old phrases about the high character of a noble profession and the honor and conscience of its members. I must reply that the medical profession has not a high character; it has an infamous character. I do not know a single thoughtful and well-informed person who does not feel that the tragedy of illness at present is that it delivers you helplessly into the hands of a profession which you deeply mistrust (Shaw, 1911, p. 8). Similar distrusting sentiments have been echoed through the ages. We cite selected quotations from Strauss (1968) as evidence that throughout history, medicine has in fact always been held in ill repute. One medical historian has asserted that "literary men do less to mold than they do to mirror the public's point of view" (Corcoran, 1961, p. 150). Therefore, consider these passages:

> The doctors are not content with having control over the sickness; they make health itself sick, in order to prevent people from being able at any time to escape their authority. [Michel de Montaigne, 1533-1592]

> I find [medicine] . . . one of the greatest follies of mankind; and if I look at it from a philosophical point of view, I've never seen a sillier lot of humbuggery. I don't think there is anything more ridiculous than that one man should undertake to cure another. [Molière, 1622-1673]

> It is so hard that one cannot really have confidence in doctors and yet cannot do without them. [Johann von Goethe, 1749-1832]

> Indeed, the medical profession is not different from any other; its members are for the most part, ordinary empty-headed dolts, ready to see what is not there and to deny the obvious. [Thomas Mann, 1875-1955]

Without the controls imposed by a negotiated approach to the practitioner-patient relationship within a contractual model of medicine, it may be relatively easy for medical practitioners to destroy rather than enhance their patients' trust.

Yet another reason why patients are likely to be unwilling to trust the paternalistic practitioner fully involves the fact that physicians' values and patients' values are quite often at odds. For the practitioner, curing or controlling the disease is usually the most important goal (within the confines of a busy practice). For the patient, many multifaceted and complexly intertwined goals must be achieved. The patient is preoccupied with issues related to his or her personal well-being. As we have noted in Chapter 5, for example, the diabetes patient, Mrs. Tomasetti, perceived her restricted diet in far more complex ways than did her physicians. Mrs. Tomasetti tried to maintain both her restricted diet *and* her place of central importance in her family who, because of her Italian heritage, highly valued cooking and eating high-calorie foods. To her physicians, the problem was simply to get Mrs. Tomasetti to follow her diet. Her physicians did not consider (nor did they value) the personal ramifications that accompanied the diet. They did not recognize or attend to the possibility of ridicule from Mrs. Tomasetti's friends and family, loss of love, alienation from her social network, and loss of her meaning and sense of worth. We are often made aware of such value discrepancies between practitioner and patient when we are faced with more dramatic issues. For example, a patient may desire to be allowed to die from his debilitating terminal illness although his physicians employ sophisticated and expensive technology in order to keep him alive for as long as possible. Practitioners may decide to remove a patient's cancerous limb when the patient would prefer to be spared the trauma of amputation despite the solemn prognosis of a shorter life that accompanies less aggressive therapy. Under conditions of life and death drama, these differences in values become very obvious. Such differences are *always* present, however, because of the very different cultural and social backgrounds and experiences of medical practitioners (particularly physicians) compared to most of their patients. These value differences may concern issues as central to patient compliance as willingness to delay gratification and to plan and sacrifice for the future (Davis, 1946), or relatedly, a general awareness of the passage of time (Horton, 1967). These perceptual differences are very likely to operate even under the most ideal circumstances of health care, unless specific actions (such as contracting and negotiating) are taken to deal with them.

The stereotype of the medical practitioner as a "miracle worker" has faded in recent years and is all but gone from the present era of medicine (Maddison, 1980). The medical technology presently available to the practitioner is more highly developed than ever before and has the potential to exert a very significant impact on the patient's life. In the past, few drugs or surgical procedures were available to the practitioner and so "trust" often meant little more than knowing the physician would be at one's bedside or would prescribe an obnoxious-tasting tonic. Today, however, the potential for an undesirable outcome as a result of the application of modern technology is frightening indeed. The potency of many drugs creates the possibility for distressing temporary or even permanent side effects (for example, impotence or tardive dyskinesia). Surgeries are accompanied by the risk of disfiguration and disability. The power of medicine has affected the image of the medical practitioner.

The nostalgia for the old-time physician that many people seem to have today (see Eisenberg, 1977) may be in part related to the very power of today's medical technology. It is not likely that this nostalgia stems from patients' desires to return to the authoritative manner of the old-time practitioner. Rather, the lure of the old-time physician is probably related to people's yearning for care as individuals and not as mere medical cases. In earlier times, physicians are reported to have known their patients well, having had a long acquaintance with them and their families. Typically, a practitioner lived and practiced in one town or county all his life, and his patients and their families were likewise geographically stable. These physicians usually knew the answers to questions regarding the potential effect of a particular regimen on the patient's family life. These physicians knew how any regimen would fit in with their patients' beliefs, resources, and hopes for the future. Regimens and treatments were never "standard," but were chosen after consideration of the issues relevant to each patient as an individual. Because of the limited time spent by today's practitioners with their patients, and because of their limited knowledge of and involvement with patients' families, modern-day practitioners have greater difficulty obtaining the information they need in order to design medical treatments that are individually appropriate for each of their patients. Thus, the methods presented in this book arc especially important. These methods enhance the capacity of the present-day practitioner to gather and act upon the information needed in order to design treatments that will optimize patients' participation, satisfaction, and subsequent compliance.

In sum, the contractual model of health care is the most timely approach to the practitioner-patient relationship: "The notion of the physician as benevolent and paternalistic figure who decides all for the patient is inconsistent with today's educated public. It is surely incongruous in a democratic society in which the rights of self-determination are being assured by law. In a day when the remote effects of individual medical acts are so consequential, we cannot be satisfied with an ethic which is so inexplicit about social responsibilities" (Pellegrino, 1973, p. 135).

It should not be expected that the benevolent intentions of the practitioner will be accepted outright by patients. "The doctor can never, Parsons not withstanding, be solely concerned . . . with the patient's self-interest. The doctor must keep one eye out for his or her own welfare. . . . The doctor always has commitments to other patients, to his or her other roles [e.g., father, husband], to norms relating to not being taken in or exploited [e.g., by malingerers]" (Antonovsky, 1979, p. 203). Thus, there are practical limitations to the practitioner's other-directedness, and these limitations are obvious even to patients.

We believe that, for the most part, medical practitioners continue to act in what they believe to be the best interest of their patients. However, in the absence of information from the patient about his or her culture, beliefs, family expectations, and resources (that is, in the absence of the patient's participation), the practitioner is forced to make decisions based solely on his or her own point of view. The practitioner's point of view will very likely be different from that of the patient. Any decision made without the patient's full participation is likely to be much less than optimal.

ETHICAL ISSUES CONFRONTING PRACTITIONER AND PATIENT IN A MODERN ERA

In modern times, there has surfaced an observable decline in the level of respect for persons in positions of authority and a noticeable increase in the level of criticism of professionals in general, particularly by younger persons (Maddison, 1980). Haug (1976) and Haug and Lavin (1981) have marshalled considerable evidence that the young (under 40) are in fact the most likely to question the physician's authority and to be skeptical of the physician's service orientation. They are also the most likely to be convinced of their own right to make health decisions, with or without the participation of their medical practitioners. People no longer trust experts unquestioningly, for they recall evidence (often made prominent by the media) of instances in which experts (of all kinds) have been seriously wrong regarding the very issues about which they are trusted to have expert knowledge.

Some contemporary-minded medical practitioners recognize and accept this state of affairs. Edmund Pellegrino, a medical philosopher and ethicist, stated in a commencement address to medical students in 1973:

> For centuries, physicians have spoken of their relationships with their patients as something sacred—something not to be profaned by change and immune even in the convulsed world of the twentieth century. To question that traditional relationship is to threaten young and old physicians alike. Yet, *it is precisely that traditional image that will be profoundly transformed in the years immediately ahead, and that transformation will constitute a major ethical challenge your generation of physicians is likely to encounter.* [Pellegrino, 1975, p. 398, emphasis added]

According to Pellegrino (1975), the essence of the patient's belief in the trustworthiness of the practitioner comes not from unspoken issues, but rather from the specification of ideals and the exchange of information. The sharing of values is necessary for optimal decision making in the best interest of the patient.

> It is the failure to recognize this emergent right [to self-determination] that is a major source of patient discontent, anxiety, and litigation. Indeed, this right is so fundamental in a free society that to limit it in the medical transaction is a transgression of justice. The educated and responsible patient wants to base his trust in a firm conviction that the physician's capabilities are being used with full respect for the integrity of his own intellect and will. He wants to understand what the doctor is doing, why he is doing it, what the alternatives may be, and what the future will mean for the things he values most. In a democratic society, every person will want the greatest protection of his rights to self-determination, and the medical situation involves some of the most significant spheres for self-determination. [Pellegrino, 1975, p. 399]

We feel that any practitioner who is willing to behave according to a set of ethical principles based on patient self-determination has the right to expect from his or her patients the information necessary to fulfill the mutual participation model of health care. As we have seen, patients and practitioners must exchange information in order to come to a mutually satisfactory agreement regarding the course of care. The patient, then, also has an ethical responsibility—to make known to his or her medical practitioner the expectations and preferences that he or she has regarding care and all the relevant information necessary to make correct decisions. We argue that it is the practitioner's responsibility to help the patient to do just this. The patient and practitioner must be willing to participate actively in the design of a negotiated regimen. Thus, just as the new model of medical care binds the practitioner, so it binds the patient too. Patients are of necessity somewhat dependent upon practitioners in dealing with their illnesses. Patients should remember (or be reminded), however, that practitioners are limited to their specialty (i.e., medicine) and "in this limitation lies the patient's independence, the seed of his ultimate recovery of full autonomy. He alone can really direct and evaluate his treatment as a whole, for he is the only element of real continuity in it. There is no one who can 'take care of him' totally, as a parent might take care of a child. He is forced to be an adult, to hold on to his power to act and his responsibility for his actions" (Newton, 1979, p. 65). This is true, of course, only if the patient is not totally incapacitated, unconscious, a child, or mentally unfit.

Ethical Issues and Interpersonal Exchanges

If they are to have any effect on the conduct of health care, ethical issues must be translated into precise recommendations for the interpersonal exchange between practitioner and patient. Psychologist George Stone (1979) has outlined some very important ethical questions that arise for *both parties* to the therapeutic relationship when a mutual participation (or contractual) model of health care guides the transaction:

> Am I pursuing goals that have not been acknowledged? Is the other party doing so? Do I know what goals the other party is trying to achieve? Do we have before us a reasonable set of alternatives? Do we agree on the likelihood of the outcomes associated with each, and the values that we assign to those outcomes? Issues of responsibility can then be raised in the context of these specific questions: Is the patient *able* to comprehend the hazards of noncompliance? (Or, is the physician able to present the hazards in such a way that the patient will comprehend?) Do there exist some goals of the patient which are incompatible with the recommended regimen? Do there remain some unreconciled differences in the values assigned to associated outcomes? [Stone, 1979, p. 52]

In examining the ethical responsibilities of the expert (medical practitioner) when working within a mutual participation model, Stone (1979) proposed the need for the practitioner's systematic pursuit of the patient's situation and the implications thereof for the patient's health behavior. In order to accomplish this goal, the practitioner must have the capacity to communicate clearly and effectively with the patient. Three requirements for the practical implementation of these pursuits have been outlined by Stone (1979) and have been examined throughout this book: "First, experts should explore fully the particular situation of each client, not only with regard to the presenting difficulties for which consultation is being sought, but also for factors that will affect the clients' ability and inclination to receive the recommendation and to follow through with the treatment selected" (p. 53). These issues were considered in detail in Chapters 4, 5, and 7, where patients' beliefs, culture, and resources, respectively, were considered.

"The second aspect of responsibility of the expert involves having sufficient knowledge of human behavior and its variations to anticipate patients' difficulties in utilizing the information given. These barriers may be grouped into four broad categories: (1) impediments of language, vocabulary, and conceptual understanding of messages given; (2) differences in expectations regarding desirable or possible outcomes of treatment; (3) differences in role expectations, that is, in expectations regarding rights, duties, and responsibilities; and (4) failures of reception induced by emotional states that result from the stresses of illness, frustrations arising in the course of the expert-client interaction, or insults to the self-esteem of the client" (p. 53). These issues were considered in detail in Chapters 2 and 3 of this book on communication and rapport in the practitioner-patient relationship.

"The third complementary aspect of the responsibility of the expert involves understanding the processes of communication and developing the necessary skills to ensure that the client (or a responsible guardian) hears and comprehends what is to be done" (p. 53). Chapters 2 and 6 (on communication and on influence) examined these aspects of the practitioner-patient relationship.

Communication as an Ethical Responsibility

The many issues we have considered above suggest that the practitioner's capacity to communicate effectively is at the very heart of his or her ethical responsibility to the patient. This capacity to communicate involves not only the skills of communication *process* but a knowledge of *content* as well (see Chapter 1). In essence, the practitioner must know how to go about gathering information from and delivering information to the patient. This involves both verbal and nonverbal communication skills (see Chapters 2 and

3). Communication should be carried out in a manner that (as much as possible) both emphasizes the patient's personal responsibility and reduces his or her anxieties, confusions, and dissatisfactions. The practitioner must also know the appropriate content with which to deal in communicating with the patient—content such as the patient's beliefs, values, perceptions of social norms, and barriers and supports to compliance. "The question is *what is the function of information in medical care*. Communication is the basic tool of medical practice—in this era no diagnosis, treatment, explanation, or prescription, to say nothing of reassurance, occurs without it" (Cassell, 1978, p. 318). Therefore, we hold that a breach of ethics results when communication process and content are inadequate as to the particular requirements of the individual patient.

We have emphasized throughout this book the responsibility of the medical practitioner and have generally downplayed the ethical responsibility of the patient. The reason for presenting such a one-sided argument is that while we hold that the practitioner and patient ultimately *share* in the responsibility for the quality to their interaction and the medical recommendations that result from it, we believe that for a number of reasons the practitioner must shoulder more of the burden for effective interaction. One good reason for this is structural or institutional. At bottom, practitioners have control over the dispensing of most medical resources (such as drugs) and are held legally responsible of the welfare of their patients. Regarding this, recall Hippocrates' warning, quoted in Chapter 1, that the physician is held accountable when patients do not recover, even when they have been noncompliant. Other practical reasons stem from the very conduct of day-to-day medical practice. Practitioners are accustomed to dealing with illness and injury—an atypical and highly distressing event for a patient. Practitioners' anxiety and distress are likely to be quite low in contrast to that of their patients, and so practitioners are able to monitor the communication requirements for successful interaction much more effectively than their patients. In addition, while there has been an adequate amount of research on practitioners' communication to their patients, there has been almost none on the ways in which patients might most effectively communicate with their practitioners. For these reasons, we have focused on the practitioner's role in communication with the patient rather than vice versa. We feel that while it may not be the only way to approach practitioner-patient interaction, patient compliance is likely to be enhanced by the practitioner's acceptance of the responsibility to apply effective communication skills even if the patient fails to disclose information or for whatever reason distorts it. The practitioner himself or herself may thus be able to reduce significantly the probability of undesired medical outcomes that may result from problematic communication. The practitioner need not simply regret and passively accept the communication inadequacies of his or her patients. The practitioner has both the capacity and the responsibility, in our view, to compensate for patients' communication shortcomings.

The dimensions on which the practitioner is ethically responsible in his or her communication with patients have been identified by Haney and Colson (1980). These issues are similar in many ways to those considered above by George Stone (1979) although they tend to focus more on the *content* of communication. Like Stone's analysis, these factors have been considered in depth throughout the previous chapters. The quality of the therapeutic relationship and the practitioner's ethical responsibility to the patient are, according to Haney and Colson, dependent upon four major variables: cultural, social, psychological, and situational. *Cultural factors* involve the practitioner's sharing or understanding of the patient's symbols, values, and rules of behavior. While these factors are not always apparent, as was considered in Chapter 5, they often have an important bearing on the patient's health behavior, acceptance of medical regimens, responses to illness and pain, and feelings about the practitioner. *Social factors* include the influence of social-class identity (and resultant beliefs and values) on patients' reactions to prescriptions for (or proscriptions against) their behavior. An important key to the practitioner's success in overcoming the social differences that typically separate practitioners and patients (and therefore interfere with compliance) is the clear understanding (as we considered in Chapters 2 and 5) of the manner in which social factors can impede communication with the patient. *Psychological factors* are perhaps the most obvious and yet they are typically ignored. Patients' attitudes and beliefs about the treatment and the illness, their modes of communication, and their emotions will significantly affect their health behavior. As we have noted in Chapters 2, 3, and 4, facility in dealing with these factors is an important component of the health practitioner's role. Finally, it is also crucial that *situational factors* relevant to effective communication and to the fulfillment of medical recommendations be recognized and acted upon. As we noted in Chapter 7, such factors are often ignored, yet they may be among the most important pieces of information in eliciting patient compliance. A complete understanding of situational factors is critical if patients are to be helped to translate commitment into actual behavior change.

Issues of communication are relevant not only to the initial contact between practitioners and patients. The factors considered throughout this book remain continually important throughout the course of patient care and must be repeatedly checked and modified. Thus, the practitioner's ethical responsibility to the patient involves not simply a one-time consideration of these issues, but rather the incorporation of them into the everyday practice of medical care. Hence, two objectives must pervade all of medical practice: (1) the establishment of open and effective communication with patients in order to deal with the social, psychological, cultural, and situational factors that affect their compliance; and (2) the encouragement (whenever possible) of a therapeutic relationship based upon mutual responsibility and mutually informed consent of practitioner and patient.

Ethics, Compliance, and the Goal of Medical Care

We hold that these ethical goals are consonant with and actually supportive of the most fundamental goal of medicine—the practitioner's duty to protect the welfare of the patient. The encouragement of compliance demands that the practitioner offer a correct diagnosis and a therapy that will do more good than harm (Sackett, 1979). In the practice of medicine, these requirements are often rather difficult to fulfill because of the inherently probabilistic and uncertain nature of medical diagnosis and care. We hold that because of the psychosocial complexities of patient care, the accomplishment of the ethical goals outlined above—the enhancement of practitioner-patient communication and the establishment of a mutual participation model of care—is also very likely to enhance the fulfillment of the goals of a correct diagnosis and effective treatment.

Jonsen (1979) has examined a number of ethical issues related to compliance with medical regimens. He has asserted that the practitioner possesses considerable legitimate power over the patient on the basis of his or her professional identity and extensive medical knowledge. This knowledge may serve as the practitioner's ethical downfall, however. As part of his or her claim to medical knowledge, the practitioner is expected to be extremely careful in his or her assessment of information about the patient in order that, for example, medications that are more detrimental than beneficial to the patient are not prescribed. Jonsen has noted that a "careless physician" is not only one who fails to collect such physically pertinent information as drug allergies, but also one who fails to make a reasonable inquiry into the patient's social setting and who fails to exert a reasonable effort to educate and motivate the patient as well. According to Jonsen, a practitioner is morally culpable not only when he or she works to achieve compliance with a regimen that is known to be ineffective (perhaps simply in an attempt to appease the patient), but also when the practitioner is paternalistic or authoritative. Such a practitioner gives orders without preparing patients for their acceptance and without supporting patients in their observance. The authoritative practitioner will, in all probability, be guilty of the earlier two breaches of ethics as well, for he or she is very unlikely to be accepting of the patient's input. While it may be initially important to exert firmness and benevolence toward patients, the eventual achievement of a partnership should remain the ultimate goal.

The establishment of an appropriate diagnosis and treatment requires that the patient be persuaded both of the practitioner's good intentions and medical competence and of the need to adopt certain health behaviors. This goal is likely, of course, to be enhanced by nonauthoritative, open communication with the patient. An emphasis on persuasion may seem incongruous amid arguments that patients have a right to self-determination. We believe, however, that *all* human interaction of necessity involves persuasion, and that patients attempt to persuade practitioners just as practitioners attempt to persuade patients. In fact, persuasion is the goal of healers everywhere (Frank, 1977). Persuasion by the practitioner demands effective assessment of the patient's attitudes, beliefs, and social norms, as well as clear and effective communication and interpersonal rapport. Persuasion implies an egalitarian relationship and one of mutual participation, since the practitioner cannot rely on his or her legitimate authority to change the patient's beliefs and behaviors. Of course, we believe that certain basic ethical principles govern the practice of persuasion. The practitioner should not falsify or fabricate evidence; he or she should not distort evidence; specious reasoning should not consciously be used, and the patient should never be deceived about the intent of the communication (Minnick, 1968). Within certain guidelines, then, persuasion promotes patient self-determination.

Some critically important ethical problems reside in the very methods that are most effective in improving patient compliance. The most effective interpersonal strategies for enhancing compliance—education (or persuasion) and behavior modification (in its many forms)—carry with them inner ethical constraints (Jonsen, 1979). Education should be truthful (as noted above) and behavior modification should be free of coercion. These requirements insure the patient's self-determined choices. As we argued in Chapter 6, the goal of compliance-enhancing strategies is the patient's internalization of the health-care regimen. Internalization is, however, very likely to be impeded by falsification or coercion for, as we have noted, people must feel that they have made their own decisions if internalization is to occur (Rodin, 1982). An important ethical issue is also involved, however. A practitioner may feel that the goal of attaining health justifies some distortion of the truth or some application of coercion toward the patient. A physician who wishes his patient to take medication, for example, may conceal its possible long-term side effects, exaggerate the dangers of not following the treatment, or promise more from the medication than it is able to deliver. The goal of compliance may be noble, but the patient deserves, *and ethical considerations demand*, the communication of accurate and realistic information. As we have shown, enthusiastic conveyance of that information toward the goal of persuasion may be in the better interest of the patient. Distortion of information and the use of coercive techniques are not, for they reduce the patient's freedom and rob him or her of the right to make a decision regarding care. These practices are unethical. As Jonsen (1979) has summarized: "First, as a matter or principle, it should be maintained that the object of information, presented in whatever manner, is insight; and the object of training [behavior modification], however automatized, is freedom. All strategies aimed at improving compliance must provide the patient with insight into his or her own situation and self, as well as with the ability of doing otherwise than conforming when he or she judges it best" (p. 117).

In a related manner:

> [C]ertain considerations seem reasonable. First, health should not be considered a unique or singular goal. It should be, for patient and physician alike, one element within the overall goal of attaining a human, free, and dignified manner of life. The drive to obtain health should not compromise other valid human goals. Secondly, information can be conveyed in ways that match the needs of time, situation, and "right to know," yet still be truthful within the whole picture. Persons are sometimes not ready to hear a truth and will, if it is forced upon them, refuse, repress, or fail to comprehend. Such a truth, which will not be incorporated into comprehension and decision, is useless. Still, any strategy for unfolding the truth must aim at the ultimate revelation of the whole picture and the ultimate opportunity for the patient to decide for himself or herself. . . . The sin or failure in the ethics of training [modifying behavior] is *coercion*, the application of physical or psychological pressure to the extent that the patient's own deliberation about his or her situation is impaired. The sin in the ethics of information is the *lie*, the concealment of those facts that will lead a person away from a decision which, even though it may not be in his interests as others define it, is a decision which is truly his or her own. [Jonsen, 1979, pp. 117-118]

Finally, the ethics of compliance enhancement itself is an issue of concern. Sackett has astutely summarized this problematic topic: "The issue is not whether we should attempt to 'bend minds,' for to prohibit this attempt is to prohibit the practice of medicine (and the practices of education and religion); the issue is one of guaranteeing that both the compliance-improving strategy and the regimen to which it is applied have been shown to do more good than harm, and that they are only applied to informed, consenting patients" (Sackett, 1978, p. 9). A truly ethical approach to compliance enhancement, then, demands the full participation of the patient in both decisions about and implementation of medical treatment.

References

CHAPTER 1: THE COMPLIANCE PROBLEM: AN INTRODUCTION

Appelbaum, S. A. The refusal to take one's medicine. *Bulletin of the Menninger Clinic*, 1977, **41**, 511–521.

Baekeland, F. & Lundwall, L. Dropping out of treatment: A critical review. *Psychological Bulletin*, 1975, **82**, 738–783.

Barnlund, D. C. The mystification of meaning: Doctor-patient encounters. *Journal of Medical Education*, 1976, **51**, 716–725.

Barofsky, I. Compliance, adherence, and the therapeutic alliance: Steps in the development of self-care. *Social Science and Medicine*, 1978, **12**, 369–376.

Baron, R. A. & Byrne, D. *Social psychology: Understanding human interaction*. 3rd ed. Boston: Allyn and Bacon, 1981.

Becker, M. H. (Ed.) *The health belief model and personal health behavior*. Thorofare, N.J.: Charles B. Slack, Inc., 1974.

Belloc, N. Relationship of health practices and mortality. *Preventive Medicine*, 1973, **2**, 67–81.

Blane, H. T. *The personality of the alcoholic: Guises of dependency*. New York: Harper & Row, 1968.

Brehm, J. W. *A theory of psychological reactance*. New York: Academic Press, 1966.

Cannell, C. F., Oksenberg, L. & Converse, J. M. (Eds.) *Experiments in interviewing techniques: Field experiments in health reporting, 1971-1977*. Ann Arbor, Mich.: Survey Research Center Institute for Social Research, 1977.

Carlson, L. A. & Bollinger, L. E. Ischaemic heart disease in relation to fasting values of plasma triglycerides and cholesterol: Stockholm Prospective Study. *Lancet*, 1972, **1**, 865–868.

Caron, H. S. & Roth, H. P. Patients' cooperation with a medical regimen. *Journal of the American Medical Association*, 1968, **203**, 922–926.

Caron, H. S. & Roth, H. P. Objective assessment of cooperation with an ulcer diet: Relation to antacid intake and to assigned physician. *American Journal of Medical Science*, 1971, **261**, 61–66.

Cobb, B. Why do people detour to quacks? *The Psychiatric Bulletin*, 1954, **3**, 66–69.

Cummings, K. M., Becker, M. H., & Maile, M. C. Bringing the models together: An empirical approach to combining variables used to explain health actions. *Journal of Behavioral Medicine*, 1980, **3**, 123–145.

Davis, M. S. Variations in patients' compliance with doctors' orders: Analysis of congruence between survey responses and results of empirical investigations. *Journal of Medical Education*, 1966, **41**, 1037–1048.

DiMatteo, M. R. & Friedman, H. S. *Social Psychology and Medicine*. Cambridge, Mass.: Oelgeschlager, Gunn, and Hain, 1982.

DiMatteo, M. R., Prince, L. M., & Taranta, A. Patient's perceptions of physicians' behavior: Determinants of patient commitment to the therapeutic relationship. *Journal of Community Health*, 1979, **4**, 280–290.

Dubos, R. *Mirage of health.* New York: Harper & Row, 1959.

Dunbar, J. M. & Stunkard, A. J. Adherence to diet and drug regimen. In R. Levy, B. Rifkind, B. Dennis, & N. Ernst (Eds.), *Nutrition, lipids, and coronary heart disease*. New York: Raven Press, 1979.

Feinstein, A. R., Wood, H. F., Epstein, J. A., Taranta, A., Simpson, R., & Tursky, E. A controlled study of 3 methods of prophylaxis against streptococcal infection in a population of rheumatic children, ii) Results of the first 3 yrs. of the study, including methods for evaluating the maintenance of oral prophylaxis. *New England Journal of Medicine*, 1959, **260**, 697–702.

Festinger, L. *A theory of cognitive dissonance*. Evanston, Ill.: Row, Peterson, 1957.

Francis, V., Korsch, B. M., & Morris, M. J. Gaps in doctor-patient communication. *New England Journal of Medicine*, 1969, **280**, 535–540.

Frank, J. D. *Persuasion and healing*. Baltimore: Johns Hopkins University Press, 1961.

Freidson, E. *Profession of medicine*. New York: Dodd, Mead, 1970.

Fuchs, V. *Who shall live*? New York: Basic Books, 1975.

Gillum, R. F. & Barsky, A. J. Diagnosis and management of patient noncompliance. *Journal of the American Medical Association*, 1974, **228**, 1563–1567.

Gordis, L., Markowitz, M., & Lilienfeld, A. M. The inaccuracy in using interviews to estimate patient reliability in taking medications at home. *Medical Care*, 1969, **7**, 49–54.

Hayes-Bautista, D. E. Termination of the patient-practitioner relationship: Divorce, patient style. *Journal of Health and Social Behavior*, 1976, **17**, 12–21.

Haynes, R. B. Introduction. In R. B. Haynes, D. W. Taylor, & D. L. Sackett (Eds.), *Compliance in health care*. Baltimore: Johns Hopkins University Press, 1979, pp. 1–7.

Henderson, L. Physician and patient as a social system. *New England Journal of Medicine*, 1935, **212**, 819–823.

Henderson, J. B., Hall, S. M., & Lipton, H. L. Changing self-destructive behaviors. In G. C. Stone, F. Cohen, & N. E. Adler (Eds.), *Health psychology*. San Francisco: Jossey-Bass, 1979, Chap. 6, pp. 141–160.

Hippocrates. *Volume II: On Decorum* (with English translation) by W. H. S. Jones. London: William Heinemann, 1923.

Ingelfinger, F. J. Medicine: Meritorious or meritricious? *Science*, 1978, **200**, 942–946.

Inui, J. F., Yourtee, E. L., & Williamson, J. W. Improved outcomes in hypertension after physician tutorials. *Annals of Internal Medicine*, 1976, **84**, 649–651.

Kasteler, J., Kane, R. L., Olsen, D. M., & Thetford, C. Issues underlying prevalence of "doctor-shopping" behavior. *Journal of Health and Social Behavior*, 1976, **17**, 328–339.

Knowles, J. H. The responsibility of the individual. *Daedalus*, 1977, **106**, 57–80.

Korsch, B. M., Gozzi, E. K., & Francis, V. Gaps in doctor-patient communication. I: Doctor-patient interaction and patient satisfaction. *Pediatrics*, 1968, **42**, 855–871.

Langlie, J. K. Social networks, health beliefs, and preventive health behavior. *Journal of Health and Social Behavior*, 1977, **18**, 244–260.

Luntz, G. & Austin, R. New stick test for P.A.S. in urine: Report on use of "Phenistix" and problems of long-term chemotherapy for tuberculosis. *British Medical Journal*, 1960 (June 4), **1**, 1679–1684.

Marquis, K. H. Effects of social reinforcement on health reporting in the household interview. *Sociometry*, 1970, **33**, 203–215.

McClellan, T. A. & Cowan, G. Use of antipsychotic and antidepressant drugs by chronically ill patients. *American Journal of Psychiatry*, 1970, **126**, 113–115.

McKeown, G. *The role of medicine: Dream, mirage, or nemesis*. London: Blackwell, 1976.

Mechanic, D. *Medical sociology: A selective view*. New York: The Free Press, 1968.

Moulding, T. S., Onstad, G. D., & Sbarbaro, J. A. Supervision of outpatient drug therapy with the medication monitor. *Annals of Internal Medicine*, 1970, **73**, 559–564.

Mumford, E. The responses of patients to medical advice. In R. C. Simons & H. Pardes (Eds.), *Understanding human behavior in health and illness*. Baltimore: Williams and Wilkins Co., 1977.

Mushlin, A. I. & Appel, F. A. Diagnosing patient noncompliance. *Archives of Internal Medicine*, 1977, **137**, 318–321.

Norell, S. E. Accuracy of patient interviews and estimates by clinical staff in determining medication compliance. *Social Science and Medicine*, 1981, **15E**, 57–61.

Park, L. D. & Lipman, R. S. A comparison of patient dosage deviation reports with pill counts. *Psychopharmacologia*, 1964, **6**, 299–302.

Parsons, T. *The social system*. Glencoe, Ill.: The Free Press, 1951, pp. 428–479.

———. Definitions of health and illness in the light of American values and social structure. In E. G. Jaco (Ed.), *Patients, physicians and illness*. New York: The Free Press, 1958, pp. 165–187.

Pelletier, K. R. *Holistic medicine*. Delacorte Press/Seymour Lawrence, 1979.

Plaja, A. O., Cohen, L. M., & Samora, J. Communication between physicians and patients in outpatient clinics, social and cultural factors. *Milbank Memorial Fund Quarterly*, 1968, **46**, 161–214.

Podell, R. *Physician's guide to compliance in hypertension*. Summit, N.J.: Merck, 1975.

Preston, D. F. & Miller, F. L. The tuberculosis outpatient's defection from therapy. *American Journal of Medical Science*, 1964, **247**, 21–25.

Rickels, K. & Briscoe, E. Assessment of dosage deviation in outpatient drug research. *Journal of Clinical Pharmacology*, 1970, **10**, 153–160.

Robbins, S. L. & Cotran, R. S. *Pathological basis of disease*. 2nd ed. Philadelphia: W. B. Saunders Co., 1979, pp. 598–602.

Rodin, J. & Janis, I. L. The social power of health care practitioners as agents of change. *Journal of Social Issues*, 1979, **35**(1), 60–81.

Rogers, C. R. The necessary and sufficient conditions of therapeutic personality change. *Journal of Consulting Psychology*, 1957, **21**, 95–103.

Rotter, J. B. *Social learning and clinical psychology*. Englewood Cliffs, N.J.: Prentice-Hall, 1954.

Sackett, D. L. A compliance practicum for the busy practitioner. In R. B. Haynes, D. W. Taylor, & D. L. Sackett (Eds.), *Compliance in Health Care*, Baltimore: Johns Hopkins University Press, 1979, chap. 18.

Sackett, D. L. & Haynes, R. B. (Eds.) *Compliance with Therapeutic Regimens*. Baltimore: Johns Hopkins University Press, 1976.

Sackett, D. L. & Snow, J. C. The magnitude and measurement of compliance. In R. B. Haynes, D. W. Taylor, & D. L. Sackett (Eds.), *Compliance in health care*. Baltimore: Johns Hopkins University Press, 1979.

Samora, J., Saunders, L., & Larson, R. F. Medical vocabularly knowledge among hospital patients. *Journal of Health and Human Behavior*, 1961, **2**, 83–89.

Shapiro, A. K. A contribution to a history of the placebo effect. *Behavioral Science*, 1960, **5**, 109–135.

Sheiner, L., Rosenberg, B., Marathe, V. & Peck, C. Differences in serum digoxin concentrations between outpatients and inpatients: An effect of compliance? *Clinical Pharmacology and Therapeutics*, 1974, **15**, 239–246.

Stimson, G. V. Obeying doctors' orders: A view from the other side. *Social Science and Medicine*, 1974, **8**, 97–104.

Stone, G. C. Patient compliance and the role of the expert. *Journal of Social Issues*, 1979, **35**(1), 34–59.

Surgeon General. *Healthy people: The Surgeon General's report on health promotion and disease prevention, 1979*. Washington, D.C.: USDHEW Public Health Services, Office of Asst. Sec. Health & Surgeon General, 1979.

Surgeon General's Report. *Smoking and Health.* Washington, D.C.: Public Health Services publication no. 1103, DHEW, 1964.

Svarstad, B. Physician-patient communication and patient conformity with medical advice. In D. Mechanic (Ed.), *The growth of bureaucratic medicine*. New York: Wiley, 1976.

Thomas, L. *The medusa and the snail.* New York: Viking Press, 1979.

Torrens, P. R. *The American health care system.* St. Louis: C. V. Mosby, 1978.

Waitzkin, H. & Stoeckle, J. D. The communication of information about illness. Clinical, sociological, and methodological considerations. *Advances in Psychosomatic Medicine*, 1972, **8**, 180–215.

CHAPTER 2: PRACTITIONER-PATIENT RELATIONSHIPS: THE COMMUNICATION OF INFORMATION

Anderson, W. T. & Helm, D. T. The physician-patient encounter: A process of reality negotiation. Paper presented at the meeting of the *American Sociological Association*, September, 1977.

Baekeland, F. & Lundwall, L. Dropping out of treatment: A critical review. *Psychological Bulletin*, 1975, **82**(5), 738–783.

Bain, D.J.G. Doctor-patient communication in general practice consultations. *Medical Education*, 1976, **10**, 125–131.

Balint, M. *The doctor, his patient, and the illness.* New York: International Universities Press, 1957.

Barnes, E. *People in hospitals.* London: Macmillan, 1961.

Barnlund, D. C. The mystification of meaning: Doctor-patient encounters. *Journal of Medical Education*, 1976, **51**, 716–725.

Bartlett, E. E. The contributions of consumer health education to primary care practice: A review. *Medical Care*, 1980, **18**, 862–871.

Becker, M. H. & Maiman, L. A. Strategies for enhancing patient compliance. *Journal of Community Health*, 1980, **6**(2), 113–135.

Beecher, H. K. *Measurement of subjective responses: Quantitative effects of drugs.* New York: Oxford University Press, 1959.

Bertakis, K. D. A method of increasing patient retention and satisfaction. *The Journal of Family Practice*, 1977, **5**(2), 217–222.

Blane, H. T. *The personality of the alcoholic: Guises of dependency.* New York: Harper and Row, 1968.

Bloom, S. W. *The doctor and his patient: A sociological interpretation.* New York: Russell Sage Foundation, 1963.

Brant, C. S. & Kutner, B. Physician-patient relations in a teaching hospital. *Journal of Medical Education*, 1957, **32**(10), 703–707.

Brown, S. W. Consumer attitudes toward physicians and health care. *Arizona Medicine*, 1980, **37**(1), 33–36.

Cartwright, A. *Human relations and hospital care.* London: Routledge & Kegan Paul, 1964.

Cassata, D. M. Health communication theory and research: An overview of the communication specialist interface. In D. Nimmo (Ed.), *Communication Yearbook II*, ICA, 1978.

Christy, N. P. English is our second language. *New England Journal of Medicine*, 1979, **300**(17), 979–981.

Cobb, B. Why do people detour to quacks? *The Psychiatric Bulletin*, 1954, **3**, 66–69.

Coe, R. M. *Sociology of Medicine.* 1st ed. New York: McGraw-Hill, 1970.

Cousins, N. *Anatomy of an illness as perceived by the patient.* New York: W. W. Norton, 1979.

Currie, B. F. & Renner, J. H. Patient education: Developing a health care partnership. *Postgraduate Medicine*, 1979, **65**(1), 177–182.

Dangott, L., Thornton, B. C., & Page, P. Communication and pain. *Journal of Communication*, Winter 1978, pp. 30–35.

Daniels, M. J. Affect and its control in the medical intern. *American Journal of Sociology*, 1960, **66**, 259–267.

David, A. K. & Boldt, J. S. A study of preventive health attitudes and behaviors in a family practice setting. *Journal of Family Practice*, 1980, **11**(1), 77–84.

Davis, F. Uncertainty in medical prognosis: Clinical and functional. *American Journal of Sociology*, 1960, **66**, 41–47.

Davis, M. S. Variations in patients' compliance with doctors' advice. An empirical analysis of patterns of communication. *American Journal of Public Health*, 1968, **58**(2), 274–288.

Davis, M. S. Variations in patients' compliance with doctors' orders: Medical practice and doctor-patient interaction. *Psychiatry in Medicine*, 1971, **2**, 31–54.

De Fleur, M. *Theories of mass communication*. New York: David McKay, 1966.

DiMatteo, M. R., Prince, L. M., & Taranta, A. Patients' perceptions of physicians' behavior: Determinants of patient commitment to the therapeutic relationship. *Journal of Community Health*, 1979, **4**, 280–290.

DiMatteo, M. R. & DiNicola, D. D. Sources of assessment of physician performance: a study of comparative reliability and patterns of intercorrelation. *Medical Care*, 1981, **19**, 829–842.

Duff, R. S. & Hollingshead, A. B. *Sickness and society*. New York: Harper and Row, 1968.

Duncan, O. D. Socioeconomic index for occupations in the detailed classification of the Bureau of the Census, 1950 (transformed to NORC scale). In A. J. Reiss, O. D. Duncan, P. K. Hatt, & C. C. North (Eds.), *Occupation and social status*. Glencoe, Ill.: The Free Press, 1961, Appendix B, pp. 263–275.

Egbert, L. D., Battit, G. E., Turndorf, H. & Beecher, H. K. Value of preoperative visit by anesthetist: Study of doctor-patient rapport. *Journal of the American Medical Association*, 1963, **185**, 553–555.

Egbert, L. D., Battit, G. E., Welch, C. E. & Bartlett, M. K. Reduction of postoperative pain by encouragement and instruction of patients: A study of doctor-patient rapport. *New England Journal of Medicine*, 1964, **270**(16), 825–827.

Eisenberg, L. The search for care. *Daedalus*, 1977, **106**, 235–246.

Elstein, A. S. Clinical judgment: Psychological research and medical practice. *Science*, 1976, **194**, 696–700.

Engel, G. L. The care of the patient: Art or science? *The Johns Hopkins Medical Journal*, 1977, **140**, 222–232.

Engel, G. L. & Morgan, W. L. *Interviewing the patient*. Philadelphia: Saunders, 1973.

Feldman, J. J. *The dissemination of health information*. Chicago: Aldine, 1966.

Feller, B. A. *Characteristics of general internists and the content of care of their patients*. Washington, D.C.: U.S. Department of Health, Education, and Welfare, HRA-79-652, 1979.

Fischbach, R. L., Sionelo-Bayog, A., Needle, A., & Delbanco, T. L. The patient and practitioner as co-authors of the medical record. *Patient Counselling and Health Education*, 1980, **2**(1), 1–5.

Fox, R. C. *Experiment perilous: Physicians and patients facing the unknown*. Glencoe, Ill.: The Free Press, 1959.

Francis, V., Korsch, B., & Morris, M. Gaps in doctor-patient communication: Patients' response to medical advice. *New England Journal of Medicine*, 1969, **280**(10), 535–540.

Freemon, B., Negrete, V. F., Davis, M., & Korsch, B. M. Gaps in doctor-patient communication: Doctor-patient interaction analysis. *Pediatric Research*, 1971, **5**, 298–311.

Freidson, E. *Patients' views of medical practice*. New York: Russell Sage Foundation, 1961, pp. 171–191.

———. *Profession of medicine*. New York: Dodd, Mead, 1970.

Freud, S. The dynamics of transference. In *Collected Papers*, Vol. 2. London: Institute of Psychoanalysis and Hogarth Press, 1924.

Friedman, H. S. Nonverbal communication between patients and medical practitioners. *Journal of Social Issues*, 1979, **35**, 82–99.

Fuller, S. S., Endress, M. P., & Johnson, J. E. The effects of cognitive and behavioral control on coping with an aversive health examination. *Journal of Human Stress*, 1978, **4**(4), 18–25.

Gallagher, E. B. (Ed.) *The doctor-patient relationship in the changing health scene*. Washington, D.C.: DHEW (#NIH 78-183), 1978.

Goffman, E. *Asylums*. Garden City, N.Y.: Doubleday, 1961.

Golden, J. S. & Johnston, G. D. Problems of distortion in doctor-patient communications. *Psychiatry in Medicine*, 1970, **1**, 127–149.

Gray, P. G. & Cartwright, A. Choosing and changing doctors. *Lancet*, December 19, 1953, pp. 1308–1309.

Green, L. W. Education strategies to improve compliance with therapeutic and preventive regimens: The recent evidence. In R. B. Haynes, D. W. Taylor, & D. L. Sackett (Eds.), *Compliance in Health Care*. Baltimore: Johns Hopkins University Press, 1979.

Haley, J. *Strategies of psychotherapy*. New York: Grune and Stratton, 1963.

———. *Uncommon therapy: The psychiatric techniques of Milton H. Erickson, M.D.* New York: W. W. Norton, 1973.

Haug, M. R. & Lavin, B. Practitioner or patient—who's in charge? *Journal of Health and Social Behavior*, 1981, **22**, 212–228.

Hayes-Bautista, D. E. Modifying the treatment: Patient compliance, patient control, and medical care. *Social Science and Medicine*, 1976, **10**, 233–238. (a)

———. Termination of the patient-practitioner relationship: Divorce, patient style. *Journal of Health and Social Behavior*, 1976, **17**, 12–21. (b)

Hellmuth, G. A., Johannsen, W. J., & Sorauf, T. Psychological factors in cardiac patients: Distortions of clinical recommendations. *Archives of Environment of Health*, 1966, **12**, 771–775.

Henderson, L. J. Physician and patient as a social system. *New England Journal of Medicine*, 1935, **212**, 819–823.

Hingson, R., Scotch, N. A., Sorenson, J. & Swazey, J. P. *In sickness and in health: Social dimensions of medical care*. St. Louis: C. V. Mosby, 1981.

Houston, B. K. & Holmes, D. S. Effect of avoidant thinking and reappraisal for coping with threat involving temporal uncertainty. *Journal of Personality and Social Psychology*, 1973, **27**, 261–275.

Houston, C. S. & Pasanen, W. E. Patients' perceptions of hospital care. *Hospitals*, 1972, **46**, 70–74.

Hulka, B. S., Cassel, J. C., Kupper, L. L., & Burdette, J. A. Communication compliance and concordance between physicians and patients with prescribed medications. *American Journal of Public Health*, 1976, **66**(9), 847–853.

Illich, I. *Medical nemesis*. New York: Pantheon, 1976.

Janis, I. L. *Psychological stress: Psychoanalytic and behavioral studies of surgical patients*. New York: Wiley, 1958.

Jeffreys, M. The doctor's dilemma—A sociological viewpoint. *Social and Economic Administration*, 1970, **4**, 37–44.

Jellinek, M. Referrals from a psychiatric emergency room: Relationship of compliance to demographic and interview variables. *American Journal of Psychiatry*, 1978, **135**(2), 209–213.

Johnson, J. E. & Leventhal, H. Effects of accurate expectations and behavioral instructions on reactions during a noxious medical examination. *Journal of Personality and Social Psychology*, 1974, **29**(5), 710–718.

Kane, R. L. & Deuschle, K. W. Problems in patient-doctor communications. *Medical Care*, 1967, **5**(4), 260–271.

Kaplan, R. M. Coping with stressful medical exams. In H. S. Friedman & M. R. DiMatteo (Eds.), *Interpersonal issues in health care.* New York: Academic Press, 1982.

Katz, J. L., Weiner, H., Gallagher, T. F., & Hellman, L. Stress, distress, and ego defenses. Psychoendocrine response to impending breast tumor biopsy. *Archives of General Psychiatry*, 1970, **23**, 131–142.

Kelley, A. B. A media role for public health compliance? In R. B. Haynes, D. W. Taylor, & D. L. Sackett (Eds.), *Compliance in health care.* Baltimore: Johns Hopkins University Press, 1979, pp. 193–201.

King, S. H. *Perceptions of illness and medical practice.* New York: Russell Sage Foundation, 1962.

Klapper, J. T. *The effects of mass communication.* Glencoe, Ill.: The Free Press, 1960.

Koos, E. *The health of Regionville.* New York: Columbia University Press, 1954.

Korsch, B. M., Gozzi, E. K., & Francis, V. Gaps in doctor-patient communication. I. Doctor-patient interaction and patient satisfaction. *Pediatrics*, 1968, **42**, 855–871.

Langer, E. J., Janis, I. L., & Wolfer, J. A. Reduction of psychological stress in surgical patients. *Journal of Experimental Social Psychology*, 1975, **11**, 155–165.

Larson, R. & Sutker, S. Value differences and value consensus by socioeconomic levels. *Social Forces*, 1966, **44**, 563–569.

Lebow, J. L. Consumer's assessments of the quality of health care. *Medical Care*, 1974, **12**, 328–337.

Lederer, H. D. How the sick view their world. *Journal of Social Issues*, 1952, **8**, 4–16.

Ley, P. & Spelman, M. S. Communication in an outpatient setting. *British Journal of Social and Clinical Psychology*, 1965, **4**, 114–116.

Lief, H. I. & Fox, R. C. Training for "detached concern" in medical students. In H. I. Lief, V. F. Lief, & N. L. Lief (Eds.), *The psychological basis of medical practice.* New York: Harper and Row, Hoeber Medical Books, 1963, pp. 12–35.

Liptak, G. S., Hulka, B. S., & Cassel, J. C. Effectiveness of physician-mother interactions during infancy. *Pediatrics*, 1977, **60**(2), 186–192.

Lorber, J. Good patients and problem patients: Conformity and deviance in a general hospital. *Journal of Health and Social Behavior*, 1975, **16**, 213–225.

Martin, M. Healthy respect for the word. *Journal of the American Medical Association*, 1978, **239** (26), 2776–2777.

Mazullo, J. M., Lasagna, L., & Griner, P. F. Variations in interpretation of prescription instructions. *Journal of the American Medical Association*, 1974, **227**(8), 929–930.

McIntosh, J. Processes of communication, information seeking and control associated with cancer: A selective review of the literature. *Social Science and Medicine*, 1974, **8**, 167–187.

Mechanic, D. *Medical sociology: A selective view.* New York: The Free Press, 1968.

Melzack, R. Psychological concept and methods for the control of pain. In J. Bonica (Ed.), *Advances in neurology, 4.* New York: Raven Press, 1974.

Mills, R. T. & Krantz, D. S. Information, choice, and reactions to stress: A field experiment in a blood bank with laboratory analogue. *Journal of Personality and Social Psychology*, 1979, **37**(4), 608–620.

Mumford, E. The responses of patients to medical advice. In R. C. Simons & H. Pardes (Eds.), *Understanding human behavior in health and illness.* Baltimore: Williams & Wilkins, 1977.

Newton, J. R. & Reading, A. E. The effect of psychological preparation for pain at intrauterine device insertion. *Contraception*, 1977, **16**, 523.

Osler, Sir William. Lecture to medical students. *Albany Medical Annals*, 1899, **20**, 307.

Parsons, T. *The social system.* Glencoe, Ill.: The Free Press, 1951, pp. 428–479.

———. Definitions of health and illness in the light of American values and social structure. In E. G. Jaco (Ed.), *Patients, physicians, and illness.* New York: The Free Press, 1958, pp. 165–187.

———. The sick role and the role of the physician reconsidered. *Milbank Memorial Fund Quarterly/Health and Society*, 1975, **53**, 257–278.

Power, P. W. & Sax, D. S. The communication of information to the neurological patient: Some implications for family coping. *Journal of Chronic Diseases*, 1978, **31**, 57–65.

Pratt, L., Seligmann, A., & Reader, G. Physicians' views on the level of medical information among patients. *American Journal of Public Health*, 1957, **47**, 1277–1283.

Reading, A. E. The short term effects of psychological preparation for surgery. *Social Science and Medicine*, 1979, **13A**, 641–654.

Roghmann, K. J., Hengst, A., & Zastowny, T. R. Satisfaction with medical care: Its measurement and relation to utilization. *Medical Care*, 1979, **17**, 461–477.

Roter, D. L. Patient participation in the patient-provider interaction: The effects of patient question asking on the quality of interaction satisfaction and compliance. *Health Education Monographs*, Winter 1977, pp. 281–315.

Roter, D. L. The relationship between the content of questions patients ask during the medical visit and patient satisfaction with care and appointment-keeping. Johns Hopkins University School of Hygiene and Public Health, 1981, prepublication draft.

Roth, J. A. *Timetables*. Indianapolis: Bobbs-Merrill, 1963.

Sackett, D. L., Haynes, R. B., Gibson, E. S., Hackett, B. C., Taylor, D. W., Roberts, R. S., & Johnson, A. L. Randomized clinical trial of strategies for improving medication compliance in primary hypertension. *The Lancet*, May 31, 1975, pp. 1205–1212.

Samora, J., Saunders, L., & Larson, R. F. Medical vocabulary knowledge among hospital patients. *Journal of Health and Human Behavior*, 1961, **2**, 83–89.

Schmitt, F. E. & Wooldridge, P. J. Psychological preparation of surgical patients. *Nursing Research*, 1973, **22**, 108–111.

Schulman, B. A. Active patient orientation and outcomes in hypertensive treatment: Application of a socio-organizational perspective. *Medical Care*, 1979, **17**(3), 267–280.

Seeman, M. & Evans, J. Alienation and learning in a hospital setting. *American Sociological Review*, 1962, **27**, 772–782.

Segall, A. & Roberts, L. W. A comparative analysis of physician estimates and levels of medical knowledge among patients. *Sociology of Health and Illness*, 1980, **2**(3), 317–334.

Seligmann, A. W., McGrath, N. E., & Pratt, L. Level of medical information among clinic patients. *Journal of Chronic Diseases*, 1957, **6**, 497.

Shapiro, M. *Getting doctored: Critical reflections on becoming a physician*. Ontario, Canada: Between the Lines, 1978.

Shipley, R. H., Butt, J. H., Horwitz, B., & Farby, J. E. Preparation for a stressful medical procedure: Effect of amount of stimulus pre-exposure and coping style. *Journal of Consulting and Clinical Psychology*, 1978, **46**(3), 499–507.

Skipper, J. & Leonard, R. (Eds.) *Social interaction and patient care*. Philadelphia and Toronto: J. B. Lippincott, 1965.

———. Children, stress, and hospitalization: A field experiment. *Journal of Health and Social Behavior*, 1968, **9**, 275–287.

Skipper, J. K., Tagliacozzo, D., & Mauksch, H. Some possible consequences of limited communication between patients and hospital functionaries. *Journal of Health and Human Behavior*, 1964, **5**, 34–39.

Smith, C. K., Polis, E., & Hadac, R. R. Characteristics of the initial medical interview associated with patient satisfaction and understanding. *The Journal of Family Practice*, 1981, **12**(2), 283–288.

Snyder, D., Lynch, J. J., & Gruss, L. Doctor-patient communications in a private family practice. *Journal of Family Practice*, 1976, **3**, 271–276.

Spelman, M. S., Ley, P., & Jones, C. How do we improve doctor-patient communications in our hospitals? *World Hospitals*, 1966, **2**, 126–134.

Stevens, D. P., Stagg, R., & Mackay, I. R. What happens when hospitalized patients see their own records. *Annals of Internal Medicine*, 1977, **86**, 474–477.

Stiles, W. B., Putnam, S. M., Wolf, M. H., & James, S. A. Verbal response mode profiles of patients and physicians in medical screening interviews. *Journal of Medical Education*, 1979, **54**, 81–89. (a)

———. Interaction exchange structure and patient satisfaction with medical interviews. *Medical Care*, 1979, **17**(6), 667–679. (b)

Stone, G. C. Patient compliance and the role of the expert. *Journal of Social Issues*, 1979, **35**, 34–59.

Strauss, M. B. *Familiar medical quotations*. Boston: Little-Brown, 1968.

Surgeon General. *Healthy people: The Surgeon General's Report on health promotion and disease prevention, 1979*. Washington, D.C.: Office of Assistant Secretary of Health, USDHEW Public Health Service, 1979.

Svarstad, B. *The doctor-patient encounter: An observational study of communication and outcome*. Unpublished doctoral dissertation, University of Wisconsin, 1974.

———. Physician-patient communication and patient conformity with medical advice. In D. Mechanic (Ed.), *The growth of bureaucratic medicine*. New York: John Wiley and Sons, 1976.

Szasz, T. S. & Hollender, M. H. A contribution to the philosophy of medicine. The basic models of the doctor-patient relationship. *Archives of Internal Medicine*, 1956, **97**, 585–592.

Taylor, S. E. Hospital patient behavior: Reactance, helplessness, or control? *Journal of Social Issues*, 1979, **35**, 156–184.

Taylor, R. B., Burdette, J. A., Camp, L., & Edwards, J. Purpose of the medical encounter: Identification and influence on process and outcome in 200 encounters in a model family practice center. *The Journal of Family Practice*, 1980, **10**(3), 495–500.

Thurlow, R. M. Malpractice: A growing threat to doctor-patient relations. *Medical Economics*, 1969, **46**, 212.

Vaccarino, J. M. Malpractice: The problem in perspective. *The Journal of the American Medical Association*, 1977, **238**, 861–863.

Vernon, D. T. A. Information seeking in a natural stress situation. *Journal of Applied Psychology*, 1971, **55**(4), 359–363.

Vertinsky, I. B., Thompson, W. A., & Uyero, D. Measuring consumer desire for participation in clinical decision making. *Health Services Research*, 1974, **9**(2), 121–134.

Waitzkin, H. & Stoeckle, J. D. The communication of information about illness. Clinical, sociological and methodological considerations. *Advances in Psychosomatic Medicine*, 1972, **8**, 180–215.

———. Information control and the micropolitics of health care: Summary of an ongoing research project. *Social Science and Medicine*, 1976, **10**, 263–276.

Waitzkin, H. & Waterman, B. *The exploitation of illness in capitalist society*. Indianapolis: Bobbs-Merrill, 1974.

Ware, J. E., Davies-Avery, A., & Stewart, A. L. The measurement and meaning of patient satisfaction. *Health and Medical Care Services Review*, 1978, **1**, 1–14.

West, C. When the doctor is a "lady": Power, status, and gender in physician-patient conversations. In A. Stromberg (Ed.), *Women, health, and medicine*. Palo Alto, Calif.: Mayfield, 1981.

White, A. The patient sits down. *Psychosomatic Medicine*, 1953, **15**, 256–257.

Wilson, R. N. & Bloom, S. W. Patient-practitioner relationships. In H. E. Freeman, S. Levine, & L. G. Reeder (Eds.), *Handbook of medical sociology*. Englewood Cliffs, N.J.: Prentice-Hall, 1972, pp. 315–339.

Wolinsky, F. D. & Wolinsky, S. R. Expecting sick-role legitimation and getting it. *Journal of Health and Social Behavior*, 1981, **22**, 229–242.

Zimbardo, P., Ebbesen, E., & Maslach, C. *Influencing attitudes and changing behavior*. 2nd ed. Reading, Mass.: Addison-Wesley, 1977.

Zola, I. K. In the name of health and illness. *Social Science and Medicine*, 1975, **9**, 83–87.

CHAPTER 3: PRACTITIONER-PATIENT RELATIONSHIPS: RAPPORT AND THE ART OF MEDICINE

Aday, L. A. & Andersen, R. *Access to medical care.* Ann Arbor, Mich.: Health Administration Press, 1975.

Alpert, J. J. Broken appointments. *Pediatrics*, 1964, **34**, 127–132.

Asch, S. E. Forming impressions of personality. *Journal of Abnormal and Social Psychology*, 1946, **41**, 258–290.

Baekeland, F. & Lundwall, L. Dropping out of treatment: A critical review. *Psychological Bulletin*, 1975, **82**, 738–783.

Baker, R. M. & Cassatta, D. M. The physician-patient relationship. In R. B. Taylor (Ed.), *Family medicine: Principles and practice.* New York: Springer-Verlag, 1978, pp. 143–148.

Balint, M. *The doctor, his patient, and the illness.* New York: International Universities Press, 1957.

Barnlund, D. C. The mystification of meaning: Doctor-patient encounters. *Journal of Medical Education*, 1976, **51**, 716–725.

Barro, A. R. Survey and evaluation of approaches to physician performance measurement. *Journal of Medical Education*, 1973, **48**, 1051–1093.

Becker, M. H., Drachman, R. H., & Kirscht, J. P. Motivations as predictors of health behavior. *Health Services Reports*, 1972, **87**, 852–861.

Becker, M. H. & Maiman, L. A. Strategies for enhancing patient compliance. *Journal of Community Health*, 1980, **6**(2), 113–135.

Beecher, H. K. The powerful placebo. *Journal of the American Medical Association*, December 24, 1955, pp. 1602–1606.

———. *Measurement of subjective responses.* New York: Oxford University Press, 1959.

Ben-Sira, Z. The function of the professional's affective behavior in client satisfaction: A revised approach to social interaction theory. *Journal of Health and Social Behavior*, 1976, **17**, 3–11.

———. Affective and instrumental components in the physician-patient relationship: an additional dimension of interaction theory. *Journal of Health and Social Behavior*, 1980, **21**, 170–180.

Bernstein, L. & Bernstein, R. S. *Interviewing: A guide for health professionals.* 3rd ed. New York: Appleton-Century-Crofts, 1980.

Bidwell, C. E. Students and schools: Some observations on client trust in client-serving organizations. In W. R. Rosengren & M. Lefton (Eds.), *Organizations and clients.* Columbus, Ohio: Merrill, 1970, pp. 37–69.

Birdwhistell, R. L. *Kinesics and context.* Philadelphia: University of Pennsylvania Press, 1970.

Blondis, M. N. & Jackson, B. E. *Nonverbal communication with patients.* New York: John Wiley and Sons, 1977.

Bloom, S. W. *The doctor and his patient: A sociological interpretation.* New York: Russell Sage Foundation, 1963.

Blum, R. H. *The psychology of malpractice suits.* San Francisco: The California Medical Association, 1957.

———. *The management of the doctor-patient relationship.* New York: McGraw-Hill, 1960.

Brammer, L. M. *The helping relationship: Process and skills.* 2nd ed. Englewood Cliffs, N.J.: Prentice-Hall, 1979.

Brown, S. W. Consumer attitudes toward physicians and health care. *Arizona Medicine*, 1980, **37**(1), 33–36.

Caplan, E. & Sussman, M. Rank-order of important variables for patient and staff satisfaction. *Journal of Health and Human Behavior*, 1966, **7**, 133–138.

Carkhuff, R. R. *Helping and human relations.* New York: Holt, Rinehart & Winston, 1969.

Cash, T. F. & Salzbach, R. F. The beauty of counseling: Effects of counselor physical attractiveness and self-disclosures on perceptions of counselor behavior. *Journal of Counseling Psychology*, 1978, **25**(4), 283–291.

Cassell, E. J. *The healer's art: A new approach to the doctor-patient relationship.* New York: Penguin Books, 1976.

Caterinicchio, R. P. Testing plausible path models of interpersonal trust in patient-physician treatment relationships. *Social Science and Medicine*, 1979, **13A**, 81–99.

Cobb, B. Why do people detour to quacks? *The Psychiatric Bulletin*, 1954, **3**, 66–69.

Conant, L. H. What helps mothers to speak out. *American Journal of Nursing*, 1969, **69**, 2650–2653.

Cousins, N. *Anatomy of an illness as perceived by the patient.* New York: W. W. Norton, 1979.

Davis, M. S. Physiologic, psychological and demographic factors in patients' compliance with doctors' orders. *Medical Care*, 1968, **6**, 115–122.

———. Variations in patients' compliance with doctors' orders: Medical practice and doctor patient interaction. *Psychiatry in Medicine*, 1971, **2**, 31–54.

Davis, M. S. & Eichhorn, R. Compliance with medical regimens: A panel study. *Journal of Health and Human Behavior*, 1963, **4**, 240–250.

DeGowin, E. J. & DeGowin, R. L. *Bedside diagnostic examination.* 3rd ed. New York: Macmillan, 1976.

Derlega, V. J., Lovell, R., & Chaikin, A. L. Effects of therapist disclosure and its perceived appropriateness on client self-disclosure. *Journal of Consulting and Clinical Psychology*, 1976, **44**, 866.

Deutsch, M. Cooperation and trust: Some theoretical notes. In M. R. Jones (Ed.), *Nebraska Symposium on Motivation.* Lincoln: University of Nebraska Press, 1962, pp. 275–319.

Dies, R. R. Group therapist self-disclosure: An evaluation by clients. *Journal of Counseling Psychology*, 1973, **20**, 344–348.

DiMatteo, M. R. A social-psychological analysis of physician patient rapport: Toward a science of the art of medicine. *Journal of Social Issues*, 1979, **35**(1), 12–33.

DiMatteo, M. R. & DiNicola, D. D. Sources of assessment of physician performance: A study of comparative reliability and patterns of intercorrelation. *Medical Care*, 1981, **19**, 829–842.

———. Social science and the art of medicine: From Hippocrates to holism. In H. S. Friedman & M. R. DiMatteo (Eds.), *Interpersonal issues in health care.* New York: Academic Press, 1982.

DiMatteo, M. R. & Friedman, H. S. (Eds.) Interpersonal relations in health care. *Journal of Social Issues*, 1979, **35**, whole issue 1.

DiMatteo, M. R. & Friedman, H. S. *Social psychology and medicine.* Cambridge, Mass.: Oelgeschlager, Gunn, and Hain, 1982.

DiMatteo, M. R., Friedman, H. S., & Taranta, A. Sensitivity to bodily nonverbal communication as a factor in practitioner-patient rapport. *Journal of Nonverbal Behavior*, 1979, **4**, 18–26.

DiMatteo, M. R. & Hays, R. The significance of patients' perceptions of physician conduct: A study of patient satisfaction in a family practice center. *Journal of Community Health*, 1980, **6**(1), 18–34.

DiMatteo, M. R., Prince, L. M., & Taranta, A. Patients' perceptions of physicians' behavior: Determinants of patient commitment to the therapeutic relationship. *Journal of Community Health*, 1979, **4**, 280–290.

DiMatteo, M. R., Taranta, A., Friedman, H. S., & Prince, L. M. Predicting patient satisfaction from physicians' nonverbal communication skills. *Medical Care*, 1980, **18**, 376–387.

Doyle, B. J. & Ware, J. E. Physician conduct and other factors that affect consumer satisfaction with medical care. *Journal of Medical Education*, 1977, **52**, 793–801.

Duncan, S. Some signals and rules for taking speaking turns in conversations. *Journal of Personality and Social Psychology*, 1972, **23**(2), 283–292.

Easterbrook, J. A. *The determinants of free will: A psychological analysis of responsible, adjustive behavior*. New York: Academic Press, 1978.

Ebert, R. H. Medical education in the United States. *Daedalus*, 1977, **106**(1), 171–184.

Egbert, L. D., Battit, G. E., Turndorf, H., & Beecher, H. K. Value of preoperative visit by anesthetist: Study of doctor-patient rapport. *Journal of the American Medical Association*, 1963, **185**, 553–555.

Egbert, L. D., Battit, G. E., Welch, C. E., & Bartlett, M. K. Reduction of postoperative pain by encouragement and instruction of patients: A study of doctor-patient rapport. *New England Journal of Medicine*, 1964, **270**, 825–827.

Eichna, L. W. Medical education, 1975–1979: A student's perspective. *New England Journal of Medicine*, 1980, **303**, 727–734.

Eisenberg, L. The search for care. *Daedalus*, 1977, **106**, 235–246.

Ekman, P. & Friesen, W. V. Nonverbal leakage and clues to deception. *Psychiatry*, 1969, **32**, 88–106.

———. Detecting deception from the body or face. *Journal of Personality and Social Psychology*, 1974, **29**, 288–298.

Ellsworth, P. Direct gaze as a social stimulus: The example of aggression. In P. Pliner, L. Krames, & T. Alloway (Eds.), *Nonverbal communication of aggression*. New York: Plenum, 1975.

Ellsworth, P., Friedman, H., Perlick, D., & Hoyt, M. Some effects of gaze on subjects motivated to seek or to avoid social comparison. *Journal of Experimental Social Psychology*, 1978, **14**, 69–87.

Elstein, A. S. Clinical judgment: Psychological research and medical practice. *Science*, 1976, **194**, 696–700.

Engel, G. L. The care of the patient: Art or science? *The Johns Hopkins Medical Journal*, 1977, **140**, 222–232. (a)

———. The need for a new medical model: A challenge for biomedicine. *Science*, 1977 (April 8), **196**, 129–136. (b)

Flexner, A. *Medical education in the United States and Canada. Bulletin #4*. New York: Carnegie Foundation for the Advancement of Teaching, 1910.

Flom, P. Performance in the medical internship. *Dissertation Abstracts International*, 1971, **32**(2-B): 1188 (unpublished doctoral dissertation: University of California at Berkeley, 1970).

Francis, V., Korsch, B. M., & Morris, M. J. Gaps in doctor-patient communication. *New England Journal of Medicine*, 1969, **280**, 535–540.

Frank, J. D. Mind-body relationships in illness and healing. *Journal of the International Academy of Preventive Medicine*, 1977, **2**, (3).

———. *Persuasion and healing: A comparative study of psychotherapy*. Rev. ed. Baltimore: Johns Hopkins University Press, 1973.

Freemon, B., Negrete, V., Davis, M., & Korsch, B. Gaps in doctor-patient communication: Doctor-patient interaction analysis. *Pediatric Research*, 1971, **5**, 298–311.

Freidson, E. *Patients' views of medical practice*. New York: Russell Sage Foundation, 1961.

———. *Profession of medicine*. New York: Dodd, Mead, 1970.

Freud, S. Recommendations to physicians practicing psycho-analysis. In J. Strachey (Ed.), *The complete psychological works of Sigmund Freud*. London: Hogarth Press, 1912.

Friedman, H. S. Nonverbal communication between patients and medical practitioners. *Journal of Social Issues*, 1979, **35**, 82–99. (a)

———. The interactive effects of facial expressions of emotion and verbal messages on perceptions of affective meaning. *Journal of Experimental Social Psychology*, 1979, **15**, 453–469. (b)

———. Nonverbal communication in medical interaction. In H. S. Friedman & M. R. DiMatteo (Eds.), *Interpersonal issues in health care*. New York: Academic Press, 1982.

Friedman, H. S. & DiMatteo, M. R. Health care as an interpersonal process. *Journal of Social Issues*, 1979, **35**(1), 1–11.

———. (Eds.) *Interpersonal issues in health care*. New York: Academic Press, 1982.

Giannandrea, V. & Murphy, K. C. Similarity self-disclosure and return for a second interview. *Journal of Counseling Psychology*, 1973, **20**, 545–548.

Gillis, J. S. Social influence therapy: The therapist as manipulator. *Psychology Today*, 1974, **8**, 91–95.

Goffman, E. *The presentation of self in everyday life*. Garden City, N.Y.: Doubleday, 1959.

Goldstein, A. P. *Psychotherapeutic attraction*. Elmsford, N.Y.: Pergamon Press, 1971.

Goodwin, J. S., Goodwin, J. M., & Vogel, A. V. Knowledge and use of placebos by house officers and nurses. *Annals of Internal Medicine*, 1979, **91**, 106–110.

Gough, H., Hall, W., & Harris, R. Admissions procedures as forecasters of performance in medical training. *Journal of Medical Education*, 1963, **38**, 983–998.

———. Evaluation of performance in medical training. *Journal of Medical Education*, 1964, **39**, 679–692.

Gray, P. G. & Cartwright, A. Choosing and changing doctors. *The Lancet*, 1953, December 19, p. 1308.

Greeson, R. R. Beyond transference and interpretation. *International Journal of Psychoanalysis*, 1972, **53**, 213–217.

Haase, R. F. & Tepper, D. T. Nonverbal components of empathic communication. *Journal of Counseling Psychology*, 1972, **19**, 417–424.

Hall, J. A., Roter, D. L., & Rand, C. S. Communication of affect between patient and physician. *Journal of Health and Social Behavior*, 1981, **22**, 18–30.

Harvey, J. H. & Smith, W. P. *Social psychology: An attributional approach*. St. Louis: C. V. Mosby, 1977.

Haug, M. R. Issues of patient acceptance of physician authority in Great Britain. In E. B. Gallagher (Ed.), *The doctor-patient relationship in the changing health scene*. Washington, D. C.: DHEW Pub # (NIH) 78-183, 1978, pp. 239–254.

Henderson, L. Physician and patient as a social system. *New England Journal of Medicine*, 1935, **212**, 819–823.

Henley, N. M. *Body politics*. Englewood Cliffs, N.J.: Prentice-Hall, 1977.

Hewitt, J. P. *Self and society: A symbolic interactionist social psychology*. 2nd ed. Boston: Allyn and Bacon, 1979.

Hippocrates. *Volume II: On Decorum and The Physician*, with English translation by W.H.S. Jones. London: William Heinemann, 1923.

Houston, W. The doctor himself as therapeutic agent. *Annals of Internal Medicine*, 1938, **11**, 1416–1425.

Hulka, B. S. Patient-clinician interactions and compliance. In R. B. Haynes, D. W. Taylor, & D. L. Sackett (Eds.), *Compliance in Health Care*. Baltimore: Johns Hopkins University Press, 1979, pp. 63–77.

Hurtado, A., Greenlick, M., & Columbo, T. Determinants of medical care utilization: Failure to keep appointments. *Medical Care*, 1973, **11**, 189–198.

Isselbacher, K. J., Adams, R. D., Braunwald, E., Petersdorf, R. G., & Wilson, J. D. *Harrison's principles of internal medicine*. 9th ed. New York: McGraw-Hill, 1980.

Ivey, A. *Microcounseling: Interviewing skills manual*. 2nd ed. Springfield, Ill.: Charles C. Thomas, 1977.

Izard, C. E. *Human emotions*. New York: Plenum Press, 1977.

Janis, I. L. *Psychological stress: Psychoanalytic and behavioral studies of surgical patients*. New York: Wiley, 1958.

Jarvinen, K. A. J. Can ward rounds be a danger to patients with myocardial infarction? *British Medical Journal*, 1955, **1**, 318–320.

Johnson, D. W. *Reaching out: Interpersonal effectiveness and self-actualization*. Englewood Cliffs, N.J.: Prentice-Hall, 1972.

———. Attitude modification methods. In F. H. Kanfer & A. P. Goldstein (Eds.), *Helping people change*. 2nd ed. Elmsford, N.Y.: Pergamon Press, 1980, pp. 58–96.

Johnson, D. W. & Johnson, F. *Joining together: Group theory and group skills*. Englewood Cliffs, N.J.: Prentice-Hall, 1975.

Johnson, D. W. & Matross, R. P. Attitude modification methods. In F. H. Kanfer & A. P. Goldstein (Eds.), *Helping people change*. 1st ed. Elmsford, N.Y.: Pergamon Press, 1975, pp. 51–88.

Johnson, D. W., McCarty, K., & Allen, T. Congruent and contradictory verbal and nonverbal communications of cooperativeness and competitiveness in negotiations. *Communication Research*, 1976, **3**, 275–292.

Johnson, D. W. & Noonan, M. P. The effects of acceptance and reciprocation of self-disclosures on the development of trust. *Journal of Counseling Psychology*, 1972, **19**, 411–416.

Jourard, S. M. *Self disclosure: An experimental analysis of the transparent self*. New York: Wiley, 1971.

Kasteler, J., Kane, R. L., Olsen, D. M., & Thetford, C. Issues underlying prevalence of "doctor-shopping" behavior. *Journal of Health and Social Behavior*, 1976, **17**, 328–339.

Kincey, J., Bradshaw, P., & Ley, P. Patients' satisfaction and reported acceptance of advice in general practice. *Journal of the Royal College of General Practitioners*, 1975, **25**, 558–566.

King, S. H. *Perceptions of illness and medical practice*. New York: Russel Sage, 1962.

Kleck, R. Physical stigma and nonverbal cues emitted in face-to-face interaction. *Human Relations*, 1968, **21**, 119–128.

Knowles, J. H. The responsibility of the individual. *Daedalus*, 1977, **106**, 57–80.

Koos, E. "Metropolis"—what city people think of their medical services. *American Journal of Public Health*, 1955, **45**, 1551–1557.

Korsch, B. M., Gozzi, E. K., & Francis, V. Gaps in doctor-patient communication. I: Doctor-patient interaction and patient satisfaction. *Pediatrics*, 1968, **42**, 855–871.

LaCrosse, M. B. Nonverbal behavior and perceived counselor attractiveness and persuasiveness. *Journal of Counseling Psychology*, 1975, **22**, 563–566.

Langer, E. J., Janis, I. L., & Wolfer, J. A. Reduction of psychological stress in surgical patients. *Journal of Experimental Social Psychology*, 1975, **11**, 155–165.

Larsen, K. M. & Smith, C. K. Assessment of nonverbal communication in the patient-physician interview. *Journal of Family Practice*, 1981, **12**(3), 481–488.

Lazare, A., Eisenthal, S., Frank, A., & Stoeckle, J. Studies on a negotiated approach to patienthood. In E. B. Gallagher (Ed.), *The doctor-patient relationship in the changing health scene*. Washington, D.C.: DHEW Pub. # (NIH) 78-183, 1978, pp. 119–139.

Lazare, A. Eisenthal, S., Wasserman, L. et al. Patient requests in a walk-in clinic. *Comprehensive Psychiatry*, 1975, **16**, 467–477.

Lear, M. W. *Heartsounds*. New York: Simon and Schuster, 1980.

Lederer, H. How the sick view their world. *Journal of Social Issues*, 1952, **8**, 4–16.

Leigh, H. & Reiser, M. F. *The patient: Biological, psychological, and social dimensions of medical practice*. New York: Plenum, 1980.

Linn, L. S. & Wilson, R. M. Factors related to a communication style among medical house staff. *Medical Care*, 1980, **18**, 1013–1019.

Lorber, J. Good patients and problem patients: Conformity and deviance in a general hospital. *Journal of Health and Social Behavior*, 1975, **16**, 213–225.

Lynch, J. J., Thomas, S. A., Mills, M. E., Malinow, K., & Katcher, A. H. The effects of human contact on cardiac arrhythmia in coronary care patients. *The Journal of Nervous and Mental Disease*, 1974, **158**, 88–99.

Marsland, D. W., Wood, M. B., & Mayo, F. The databank for patient care, curriculum and research in family practice; 526,196 patient problems. *Journal of Family Practice*, 1976, **3**, 25–28.

Mayerson, E. W. *Putting the ill at ease*. New York: Harper & Row, 1976.

McDermott, W. Evaluating the physician and his technology. *Daedalus*, 1977, **106**(1), 135–158.

Mechanic, D. *Medical sociology: A selective view*. New York: The Free Press, 1968.

Milmoe, S., Rosenthal, R., Blane, H. T., Chafetz, M. L., & Wolf, I. The doctor's voice: Postdictor of successful referral of alcoholic patients. *Journal of Abnormal Psychology*, 1967, **72**, 78–84.

Montagu, A. *Touching*. New York: Harper and Row, 1978.

Murphy, K. C. & Strong, S. R. Some effects of similarity self-disclosure. *Journal of Counseling Psychology*, 1972, **19**, 121–124.

Nelson, A., Gold, B., Hutchinson, R., & Benezra, E. Drug default among schizophrenic patients. *American Journal of Hospital Pharmacy*, 1975, **32**, 1237–1242.

Nemiah, J. C. *Foundations of Psychopathology*. New York: Oxford University Press, 1961.

Ort, R. S., Ford, A. B., & Liske, R. E. The doctor-patient relationship as described by physicians and medical students. *Journal of Health and Human Behavior*, 1964, **5**, 25–34.

Osler, Sir W. Lecture to medical students. *Albany Medical Annals*, 1899, **20**, 307.

———. The master-word in medicine. *In Aequanimitas with other addresses to medical students, nurses, and practitioners of medicine*. Philadelphia: Blakiston Co., 1904, pp. 369–371.

Parsons, T. *The social system*. Glencoe, Ill.: The Free Press, 1951, pp. 428–479.

———. Definitions of health and illness in the light of American values and social structure. In E. G. Jaco (Ed.), *Patients, physicians and illness*. New York: The Free Press, 1958, pp. 165–187.

Pelletier, K. R. *Holistic medicine*. New York: Delacorte Press, 1979.

———. *Mind as healer, mind as slayer*. New York: Dell, 1977.

Pickering, Sir G. Medicine on the brink: The dilemma of a learned profession. *Perspectives in Biology and Medicine*, 1978, Summer, pp. 551–560.

Poole, A. D. & Sanson-Fisher, R. W. Understanding the patient: A neglected aspect of medical education. *Social Science and Medicine*, 1979, **13A**, 37–43.

Reader, G., Pratt, L., & Mudd, M. What patients expect from their doctors. *Modern Hospital*, July 1957, **89**, 88–94.

Richards, J., Taylor, C., & Price, P. The prediction of medical intern performance. *Journal of Applied Psychology*, 1962, **46**, 142–146.

Rickels, K., Lipman, R. S., Park, L. C., Covi, L., Uhlenhuth, E. H., & Mock, J. E. Drug, doctor warmth, and clinic setting in the symptomatic response to minor tranquilizers. *Psychopharmacologia*, 1971, **20**, 128–152.

Rogers, C. R. The necessary and sufficient conditions of therapeutic personality change. *Journal of Consulting Psychology*, 1957, **21**, 95–103.

Rosen, G. The evolution of social medicine. In H. E. Freeman, S. Levine, & L. G. Reeder (Eds.), *Handbook of medical sociology*, 2nd ed. Englewood Cliffs, N.J.: Prentice-Hall, 1972, pp. 30–60.

Rosenthal, R., Hall, J. A., DiMatteo, M. R., Rogers, P. L., & Archer, D. *Sensitivity to nonverbal communication: The PONS test*. Baltimore: Johns Hopkins University Press, 1979.

Rubin, J. Z. & Brown, B. R. *The social psychology of bargaining and negotiation*. New York: Academic Press, 1975.

Ryan, C. & Ryan, K. M. *A private battle*. New York: Fawcett Library, 1979.

Salzman, C., Shader, R., Scott, D. A., & Binstock, W. Interviewer anger and patient dropout in a walk-in clinic. *Comprehensive Psychiatry*, 1970, **11**, 267–273.

Segall, A. & Burnett, M. Patient evaluation of physician role performance. *Social Science and Medicine*, 1980, **14A**, 269–278.

Shapiro, A. K. A contribution to a history of the placebo effect. *Behavioral Science*, 1960, **5**, 109–135.

Shattuck, F. The science and art of medicine in some of their aspects. *Boston Medical and Surgical Journal*, 1907, **157**, 63–67.

Skipper, J. & Leonard, R. (Eds.) *Social interaction and patient care.* Philadelphia and Toronto: J. B. Lipincott, 1965.

Smith-Hanen, S. Effects of nonverbal behaviors on judged levels of counselor warmth and empathy. *Journal of Counseling Psychology*, 1977, **24**, 87–91.

Spiegel, P. & Machotka, P. *Messages of the body.* New York: The Free Press, 1974.

Stiles, W., Putnam, S., Wolfe, M., & James, S. Interaction exchange structure and patient satisfaction with medical interviews. *Medical Care*, 1979, **17**, 667–679.

Stimson, G. & Webb, B. *Going to see the doctor.* London: Routledge and Kegan Paul, 1975.

Stone, G. C. Patient compliance and the role of the expert. *Journal of Social Issues*, 1979, **35**(1), 34–59.

Strong, S. R. Counseling: An interpersonal influence process. *Journal of Counseling Psychology*, 1968, **15**, 215–224.

Strong, S. R. & Dixon, D. N. Expertness, attractiveness and influence in counseling. *Journal of Counseling Psychology*, 1971, **18**, 562–570.

Strupp, H. H. Toward a reformulation of the psychotherapeutic influence. *International Journal of Psychiatry*, 1973, **11**, 263–354.

Taylor, S. E. Hospital patient behavior: Reactance, helplessness or control? *Journal of Social Issues*, 1979, **35**(1), 156–184.

Thurlow, R. M. Malpractice: A growing threat to doctor-patient relations. *Medical Economics*, 1969, **46**, 212.

Truax, C. B. & Carkhuff, R. R. Client and therapist transparency in the psychotherapeutic encounter. *Journal of Counseling Psychology*, 1965, **12**, 3–9.

———. *Toward effective counseling and psychotherapy.* Chicago: Aldine, 1967.

Tumulty, P. A. What is a clinician and what does he do? *New England Journal of Medicine*, 1970, **283**, 20–24.

Vaccarino, J. M. Malpractice: The problem in perspective. *The Journal of the American Medical Association*, 1977, **238**, 861–863.

Ware, J. E., Davies-Avery, A., & Steward, A. L. The measurement and meaning of patient satisfaction. *Health and Medical Care Services Review*, 1978, **1**(1), 1–14.

Ware, J. E., Davies-Avery, A., & Stewart, A. L. The measurement and meaning of patient *of patient quality of care assessment.* Santa Monica, Calif.: The Rand Corporation, 1980.

Waterman, A. S. Individualism and interdependence. *American Psychologist*, 1981, **36**(7), 762–73.

Weiner, M. F. Personal openness with patients: Help or hindrance. *Texas Medicine*, February 1980, **76**(2), 60–62.

Woolfolk, A. Student learning and performance under varying conditions of teacher verbal and nonverbal evaluative communication. *Journal of Educational Psychology*, 1978, **70**, 87–94.

CHAPTER 4: PERCEPTIONS OF ILLNESS, PREVENTION, AND TREATMENT: THE PATIENT'S PERSPECTIVE

Ajzen, I. & Fishbein, M. Attitude-behavior relations: A theoretical analysis and review of empirical research. *Psychological Bulletin*, 1977, **84**, 888–918.

———. *Understanding attitudes and predicting social behavior.* Englewood Cliffs, N.J.: Prentice-Hall, 1980.

Alpert, J. J. Broken appointments. *Pediatrics*, 1964, **34**, 127–132.

Allport, G. W. Attitudes. In C. Murchinson (Ed.), *A handbook of social psychology.* Worcester, Mass.: Clark University Press, 1935, pp. 798–844.

Andersen, R. *A behavioral model of families' use of health services.* Research Series No. 25, Chicago Center for Health Administration Studies, University of Chicago, 1968.

Anderson, J. & Bartkus, D. Choice of medical care: A behavioral model of health and illness behavior. *Journal of Health and Social Behavior*, 1973, **14**, 348–362.

Antonovsky, A. & Hartman, H. Delay in the detection of cancer: A review of the literature. *Health Education Monographs*, 1974, **2**(2), 98–125.

Antonovsky, A. & Kats, R. The model dental patient: An empirical study of preventive health behavior. *Social Science Medicine*, 1970, **4**, 367–380.

Atkinson, J. W. & Feather, N. (Eds.). *A theory of achievement motivation*. New York: John Wiley and Sons, 1966.

Baekeland, F., Lundwall, L., & Shanahan, T. J. Correlates of patient attrition in the outpatient treatment of alcoholism. *Journal of Nervous and Mental Disease*, 1973, **157**, 99–107.

Bakker, C. B. & Dightman, C. R. Psychological factors in fertility control. *Fertility and Sterility*, 1964, **15**, 559–567.

Balch, P. & Ross, A. W. Predicting success in weight reduction as a function of locus of control: A unidimensional and multidimensional approach. *Journal of Consulting and Clinical Psychology*, 1975, **43**, 119.

Balint, M. *The doctor, his patient and the illness*. New York: International Universities Press, 1957.

Barnum, J. F. Outlook for treating patients with self-destructive habits. *Annals of Internal Medicine*, 1974, **81**, 387–393.

Battistella, R. M. Factors associated with delay in the initiation of physicians' care among late adulthood persons. *American Journal of Public Health*, 1971, **61**, 1348–1361.

Baumann, B. Diversities of conceptions of health and physical fitness. *Journal of Health and Human Behavior*, 1961, **2**, 39–46.

Becker, M. H. The health belief model and sick role behavior. *Health Education Monograph*, 1974, **2**, 409–419.

———. Understanding patient compliance: The contributions of attitudes and other psychosocial factors. In S. J. Cohen (Ed.), *New directions in patient compliance*. Lexington, Mass.: D. C. Heath, 1979, pp. 1–31.

Becker, M. H., Drachman, R. H., & Kirscht, J. P. Motivations as predictors of health behavior. *Health Services Reports*, 1972, **87**, 852–862.

Becker, M. H., Haefner, D. P., Kasl, S. V., Kirscht, J. P., Maiman, L. A., & Rosenstock, I. M. Selected psychosocial models and correlates of individual health related behaviors. *Medical Care Supplement*, 1979, **15**(5), 27–46.

Becker, M. H., Kabach, M. M., Rosenstock, I. M., & Ruth, M. Some influences on public participation in a genetic screening program. *Journal of Community Health*, 1975, **1**, 3–14.

Becker, M. H. & Maiman, L. A. Sociobehavioral determinants of compliance with health and medical care recommendations. *Medical Care*, 1975, **13**, 10–24.

Becker, M. H., Maiman, L. A., Kirscht, J. P., Haefner, D. P., & Drachman, R. H. The health belief model and prediction of dietary compliance: A field experiment. *Journal of Health and Social Behavior*, 1977, **18**, 348–366.

Becker, M. H., Nathanson, C. A., Drachman, R. H., & Kirscht, J. P. Mothers' health beliefs and children's clinic visits: A prospective study. *Journal of Community Health*, 1977, **3**, 125–135.

Becker, M. H., Radius, S. M., Rosenstock, I. M., Drachman, R. H., Schuberth, K. C., & Teets, K. C. Compliance with a medical regimen for asthma: A test of the health belief model. *Public Health Reports*, 1978, **93**, 268–277.

Beecher, H. K. *Measurement of subjective responses*. New York: Oxford University Press, 1959.

Bem, D. J. Self-perception: An alternative interpretation of cognitive dissonance phenomena. *Psychological Review*, 1967, **74**, 183–200.

Berkanovic, E. Behavioral science and prevention. *Preventive Medicine*, 1976, **5**, 92–105.

Caldwell, J. R., Cobb, S., Dowling, M. D. et al. The dropout problem in anti-hypertensive therapy. *Journal of Chronic Diseases*, 1970, **22**, 579–592.

Cohen, F. Personality, stress, and the development of physical illness. In G. C. Stone, F. Cohen, & N. E. Adler (Eds.), *Health psychology*. San Francisco: Jossey-Bass, 1979, Chap. 4.

Cohen, F. & Lazarus, R. S. Coping with the stresses of illness. In G. C. Stone, F. Cohen, & N. E. Adler (Eds.), *Health psychology*. San Francisco: Jossey-Bass, 1979, Chap. 9.

Corey, S. M. Professed attitudes and actual behavior. *Journal of Educational Psychology*, 1937, **28**, 271–280.

Cromwell, R. L., Butterfield, E. C., Brayfield, F. M., & Curry, J. J. *Acute myocardial infarction: Reaction and recovery*. St. Louis: C. V. Mosby, 1977.

Cummings, N. A. & Follette, W. T. Brief psychotherapy and medical utilization. In H. Dorken & Associates (Eds.), *The professional psychologist today: New developments in law, health insurance, and health practice*. San Francisco: Jossey-Bass, 1976.

Cummings, K. M., Becker, M. H., & Maile, M. C. Bringing the models together: An empirical approach to combining variables used to explain health actions. *Journal of Behavioral Medicine*, 1980, **3**(2), 123–145.

Czaczkes, J. W. & Kaplan, D. A. Selection of patients for renal haemodialysis. In J. S. Cameron (Ed.), *Dialysis and renal transplantation*. Proceedings of the Ninth Conference. Florence, Italy, 1972, pp. 167–172.

David, A. K. & Boldt, J. S. A study of preventive health attitudes and behaviors in a family practice setting. *The Journal of Family Practice*, 1980, **11**(1), 77–84.

Davis, M. S. Variations in patients' compliance with doctors' orders: Analysis of congruence between survey responses and results of empirical investigations. *Journal of Medical Education*, 1966, **41**, 1037–1048.

———. Physiologic, psychological and demographic factors in patient compliance with doctors' orders. *Medical Care*, 1968, **6**, 115–122.

Diamond, M. D., Weiss, A. J., & Grynbaum, B. The unmotivated patient. *Archives of Physical Medicine and Rehabilitation*, 1968, **49**, 281–284.

Donabedian, A. & Rosenfeld, L. S. Follow-up study of chronically ill patients discharged from hospital. *Journal of Chronic Diseases*, 1964, **17**, 847–862.

Edwards, W. Behavioral decision theory. *Annual Review of Psychology*, 1961, **12**, 473–498.

Elling, R., Whittemore, R., & Green, M. Patient participation in a pediatric program. *Journal of Health and Human Behavior*, 1960, **1**, 183–191.

Engel, G. L. The need for a new medical model: A challenge for biomedicine. *Science*, 1977 (April 8), **196**, 129–136.

Fabrega, H. Toward a model of illness behavior. *Medical Care*, 1973, **11**, 470–484.

Feinstein, A. R. "Compliance Bias" and the interpretation of therapeutic trials. In D. L. Sackett & R. B. Haynes (Eds.), *Compliance with therapeutic regimens*. Baltimore: Johns Hopkins University Press, 1976, pp. 152–156.

Festinger, L. *A theory of cognitive dissonance*. Stanford, Calif.: Stanford University Press, 1957.

Fink, R., Shapiro, S., & Roester, R. Impact of efforts to increase participation in repetitive screenings for early breast cancer detection. *American Journal of Public Health*, 1972, **62**, 328–336.

Fishbein, M. & Ajzen, I. Belief, attitude, intention, and behavior: An introduction to theory and research. Reading, Mass.: Addison-Wesley, 1975.

Fishbein, M., Jaccard, J. J., Davidson, A. R., Ajzen, I., & Token, B. Predicting and understanding family planning behaviors: Beliefs, attitudes, and intentions. In I. Ajzen & M. Fishbein, *Understanding attitudes and predicting social behavior*. Englewood Cliffs, N.J.: Prentice-Hall, 1980, pp. 131–147.

Flach, E. *Participation in case finding programs for cervical cancer*. Administrative Report, Cancer Control Program, United States Public Health Service. Washington, D.C.: Government Printing Office, 1960.

Follette, W. & Cummings, N. A. Psychiatric services and medical utilization in a prepaid health plan setting. *Medical Care*, 1967, **5**, 25–35.

Garfield, S. R. The delivery of medical care. *Scientific American*, 1970, **222**, 15–23.

Gentry, W. D. Preadmission behavior. In W. D. Gentry & R. B. Williams (Eds.), *Psychological aspects of myocardial infarction and coronary care*. 2nd ed. St. Louis: C. V. Mosby, 1979, Chap. 4.

Glasser, M. A. A study of the public's acceptance of the Salk vaccine program. *American Journal of Public Health*, 1958, **48**, 141.

Glick, B. S. Dropout in an outpatient, double-blind drug study. *Psychosomatics*, 1965, **6**, 44–48.

Gordis, L., Markowitz, M., & Lilienfeld, A. M. Why patients don't follow medical advice: A study of children on long-term antistreptococcal prophylaxis. *Journal of Pediatrics*, 1969, **75**, 957–968.

Green, L. W. Diffusion and adoption of innovations related to cardiovascular risk behavior in the public. In A. J. Enelow & J. B. Henderson (Eds.), *Applying behavioral science to cardiovascular risk—proceedings of a conference*. Washington, D.C.: American Heart Association, 1975.

Haefner, D. & Kirscht, J. P. Motivational and behavioral effects of modifying health beliefs. *Public Health Reports*, 1970, **85**, 478–484.

Hammel, R. W. & Williams, P. O. Do patients receive prescribed medication? *American Pharmacy Association Journal*, 1964, **4**, 331–334.

Hartman, P. E. & Becker, M. H. Noncompliance with prescribed regimen among chronic hemodialysis patients: A method of prediction and educational diagnosis. *Dialysis and Transplantation*, 1978, **7**, 978–989.

Haynes, R. B. Determinants of compliance: The disease and the mechanics of treatment. In R. B. Haynes, D. W. Taylor, & D. L. Sackett (Eds.), *Compliance in Health Care*. Baltimore: Johns Hopkins University Press, 1979, pp. 49–62.

Haynes, R. B., Taylor, D. W., & Sackett, D. L. (Eds.), *Compliance in health care*. Baltimore: Johns Hopkins University Press, 1979.

Heinzelmann, F. Factors in prophylaxis behavior in treating rheumatic fever: An exploratory study. *Journal of Health and Human Behavior*, 1962, **3**, 73–81.

Hochbaum, G. M. Why people seek diagnostic x-rays. *Public Health Reports*, 1956, **71**, 377–380.

———. *Public participation in medical screening programs: A sociopsychological study*. Public Health Service Publication 572. Washington, D.C.: Government Printing Office, 1958.

Hunter, R. C. A., Lohrenz, J. G., & Schwartzman, A. E. Nosophobia and hypochondriasis in medical students. *Journal of Nervous and Mental Disease*, 1964, **139**, 147–152.

Jacobs, M. The addictive personality: Prediction of success in a smoking withdrawal program. *Psychosomatic Medicine*, 1972, **34**, 30–38.

James, W. H., Woodruff, A. B., & Werner, W. Effect of internal and external control upon changes in smoking behavior. *Journal of Consulting Psychology*, 1965, **29**, 184–186.

Janis, I. L. & Rodin, J. Attribution, control, and decision making: Social psychology and health care. In G. C. Stone, F. Cohen, & N. E. Adler (Eds.), *Health psychology*. San Francisco: Jossey-Bass, 1979, pp. 487–521.

Janowski, C. B. & Drum, D. E. Diagnostic correlates of discharge against medical advice. *Archives of General Psychiatry*, 1977, **34**, 153–155.

Jessor, R., Graves, T. D., Hanson, R. C., & Jessor, S. L. *Society, personality, and deviant behavior: A study of a tri-ethnic community*. New York: Holt, Rinehart, and Winston, 1968.

Kaplan, D. A. & Czaczkes, J. W. Personality factors in chronic hemodialysis patients causing noncompliance with medical regimen. *Psychosomatic Medicine*, 1972, **34**, 333–344.

Kar, S. B. Consistency between fertility attitudes and behavior: A conceptual model. *Population Studies*, 1978, **32**, 173–185.

Kasl, S. & Cobb, S. Health behavior, illness behavior, and sick role behavior. I: Health and illness behavior. *Archives of Environmental Health*, 1966, **12**, 246–266. (a)

———. Health behavior, illness behavior, and sick role behavior. II: Sick role behavior. *Archives of Environmental Health*, 1966, **12**, 534–541. (b)

Kegeles, S. S. Why people seek dental care: A test of a conceptual formulation. *Journal of Health and Human Behavior*, 1963, **4**, 166–173.

———. A field experiment attempt to change beliefs and behavior of women in an urban ghetto. *Journal of Health and Social Behavior*, 1969, **10**, 115–124.

Kendall, P. L. & Reader, G. G. Contributions of sociology to medicine. In H. E. Freeman, S. Levine, & L. G. Reeder (Eds.), *Handbook of medical sociology*. 2nd ed. Englewood Cliffs, N.J.: Prentice Hall, 1972, pp. 1–29.

King, S. H. Social psychological factors in illness. In H. E. Freeman, S. Levine, & L. G. Reeder (Eds.), *Handbook of medical sociology*. 2nd ed. Englewood Cliffs, New Jersey: Prentice-Hall, 1972.

Kirscht, J. P., Becker, M. H., Haefner, D. P., & Maiman, L. A. Effects of threatening communications and mothers' health beliefs on weight change in obese children. *Journal of Behavioral Medicine*, 1978, **1**, 147–157.

Kirscht, J. P. & Rosenstock, I. M. Patient adherence to antihypertensive medical regimens. *Journal of Community Health*, 1977, **3**, 115–124.

Koos, E. *The health of Regionville*. New York: Columbia University Press, 1954.

Kosa, J. & Robertson, L. The social aspects of health and illness. In J. Kosa et al. (Eds.), *Poverty and health: A sociological analysis*. Cambridge, Mass.: Harvard University Press, 1969, 1975.

Langlie, J. K. Social networks, health beliefs, and preventive health behavior. *Journal of Health and Social Behavior*, 1977, **18**, 244–260.

———. Interrelationships among preventive health behaviors: A test of competing hypotheses. *Public Health Reports*, 1979, **94**(3), 216–225.

LaPiere, R. T. Attitudes *vs*. actions. *Social Forces*, 1934, **13**, 230–237.

Lazarus, R. S. *Psychological stress and the coping process*. New York: McGraw-Hill, 1966.

Leventhal, H., Hochbaum, G., & Rosenstock, I. *Epidemic impact on the general population in two cities: The impact of Asian influenza on community life: A study in five cities*. Public Health Service Publication 766. Washington, D.C.: Government Printing Office, 1960.

Lewin, K. The nature of field theory. In M. H. Marx (Ed.). *Psychological theory*. New York: Macmillan, 1951.

Ley, P. & Spelman, M. S. *Communicating with the patient*. London: Staples Press, 1967.

Lundy, J. R. Some personality correlates of contraceptive use among unmarried female college students. *Journal of Personality*, 1972, **80**, 9–14.

MacDonald, A. P., Jr. Internal-external locus of control and the practice of birth control. *Psychological Reports*, 1970, **27**, 206.

Maiman, L. A., Becker, M. H., Kirscht, J. P., Haefner, D. P., & Drachman, R. H. Scales for measuring health belief model dimensions: A test of predictive value, internal consistency, and relationships among beliefs. *Health Education Monographs*, 1977, **5**, 215–230.

Manno, B. & Marston, A. R. Weight reduction as a function of negative covert reinforcement (sensitization) versus positive covert reinforcement. *Behavior Research and Therapy*, 1972, **10**, 201–207.

Marsland, D. W., Wood, M. B., & Mayo, F. The databank for patient care, curriculum and research in family practice: 526,196 patient problems. *Journal of Family Practice*, 1976, **3**, 25–28.

Mechanic, D. *Medical sociology*. New York: The Free Press, 1968.

———. Social psychological factors affecting the presentation of bodily complaints. *New England Journal of Medicine*, 1972, **286**, 1132–1139.

———. The stability of health and illness behavior: results from a 16-year follow-up. *American Journal of Public Health*, 1979, **69**, 1142–1145.

Mechanic, D. & Volkart, E. H. Stress, illness behavior, and the sick role. *American Sociology Review*, 1961, **26**, 51–58.

O'Bryan, G. G. The relationship between an individual's I-E orientation and information-seeking, learning, and use of weight control relevant information. Dissertation Abstract Int.

33B:447B, 1972. (Univ. Microfilms no. 72-19:541.)

Ogionwo, W. Socio-psychological factors in health behavior: An experiment study on methods and attitude change. *International Journal of Health Education*, 1973, **16**, 1–16.

Parsons, T. *The social system*. Glencoe, Ill.: The Free Press, 1951.

Pervin, L. A. *Personality: Theory, assessment, and research*. 3rd ed. New York: John Wiley, 1980.

Phares, E. J. Locus of control in personality. Morristown, N.J. General Learning Press, 1976.

Phillips, D. L. Rejection: A possible consequence of seeking help for mental disorders. *American Sociological Review*, 1963, **28**, 963–972.

Radius, S. M., Becker, M. H., Rosenstock, I. M., Drachman, R. H., Schuberth, K. C., & Teets, K. C. *The Journal of Asthma Research*, 1978, **15**(3), 133–149.

Rosenberg, M. J. Cognitive structure and attitudinal affect. *Journal of Abnormal and Social Psychology*, 1956, **53**, 367–372.

Rosenstock, I. M. Why people use health services. *Milbank Memorial Fund Quarterly*, 1966, **44**, 94–127.

———. Historical origins of the health belief model. *Health Education Monographs*, 1974, **2**, 328–335.

Rosenstock, I. M. & Kirscht, J. P. Why people seek health care. In G. C. Stone, F. Cohen, & N. E. Adler (Eds.), *Health psychology*. San Francisco: Jossey-Bass, 1979, Chap. 7.

Rosenstock, I. M., Derryberry, M., & Carriger, B. K. Why people fail to seek poliomyelitis vaccination. *Public Health Reports*, 1959, **74**, 98–103.

Rotter, J. B. *Social learning and clinical psychology*. Englewood Cliffs, N.J.: Prentice-Hall, 1954.

———. Generalized expectancies for internal versus external control of reinforcement. *Psychological Monographs*, 1966, **80**(1), no. 609.

Saltzer, E. B. Cognitive moderators of the relationship between behavioral intentions and behavior. *Journal of Personality and Social Psychology*, 1981, **41**(2), 260–271.

———. Locus of control and the intention to lose weight. *Health Education Monographs*, 1978 (Spring), **6**(2), 118–128.

Seeman, M. & Evans, J. W. Alienation and learning in a hospital setting. *American Sociological Review*, 1962, **27**, 772–783.

Smetana, J. G. & Adler, N. E. Fishbein's value times expectancy model: An examination of some assumptions. *Personality and Social Psychology Bulletin*, 1980, **6**(1), 89–96.

Stang, D. J. & Wrightsman, L. S. *Dictionary of social behavior and social research methods*. Monterey, Calif.: Brooks-Cole, 1981.

Steele, J. L. & McBroom, W. H. Conceptual and empirical dimensions of health behavior. *The Journal of Health and Social Behavior*, 1972, **13**, 382–392.

Steffy, R. A., Meichenbaum, D. & Best, J. A. Aversive and cognitive factors in the modification of smoking behavior. *Behavior Research and Therapy*, 1970, **8**, 115–125.

Stone, G. C. Patient compliance and the role of the expert. *Journal of Social Issues*, 1979, **35**(1), 34–59.

Straits, B. & Sechrest, L. Further support of some findings about the characteristics of smokers and nonsmokers. *Journal of Consulting Psychology*, 1963, **27**, 282.

Suchman, E. A. Health orientation and medical care. *American Journal of Public Health*, 1966, **56**, 97–105.

———. Preventive health behavior: A model for research on community health campaigns. *Journal of Health and Social Behavior*, 1967, **8**, 197–209.

Tash, R. H., O'Shea, R. M., & Cohen, L. K. Testing a preventive-symptomatic theory of dental health behavior. *American Journal of Public Health*, 1969, **59**, 514–521.

Taylor, D. W. A test of the health belief model in hypertension. In R. B. Haynes, D. W. Taylor, & D. L. Sackett (Eds.), *Compliance in health care*. Baltimore: Johns Hopkins University Press, 1979, pp. 103–109.

Tolman, E. C. Principles of performance. *Psychological Review*, 1955, **62**, 315–326.

Waitzkin, H. & Waterman, B. *The exploitation of illness in capitalist society*. Indianapolis: Bobbs-Merrill, 1974.

Wallston, B. S. & Wallston, K. A. Locus of control and health: A review of the literature. *Health Education Monographs*, 1978 (Spring), **6**(2), 107–117.

Wallston, B. S., Wallston, K. A., Kaplan, G. D., & Maides, S. A. Development and validation of the health locus of control (HLC) scale. *Journal of Consulting and Clinical Psychology*, 1976, **44**, 580–585.

Wallston, K. A., Wallston, B. S., & DeVellis, R. Development of the multi-dimensional health locus of control (MHLC) scales. *Health Education Monographs*, 1978 (Spring), **6**(2), 160–170.

Weintraub, M., Wu, W., & Lasagna, L. Compliance as a determinant of serum digoxin concentration. *Journal of the American Medical Association*, 1973, **224**, 481–485.

West, D., Graham, S., Swanson, M., & Wilkinson, G. Five year follow-up of a smoking withdrawal clinic population. *American Journal of Public Health*, 1977, **67**, 536–544.

White, K. L., Williams, T. F., & Greenberg, B. G. The ecology of medical care. *New England Journal of Medicine*, 1961, **265**, 885–892.

Williams, A. F. Factors associated with seat belt use in families. *Journal of Safety Research*, 1972, **4**(3), 133–138. (a)

———. Personality characteristics associated with preventive dental health practices. *Journal of the American College of Dentistry*, 1972, **39**, 225–234. (b)

Wilson, R. N. *The sociology of health: An introduction*. New York: Random House, 1970.

Woods, S. M., Natterson, J., & Silverman, J. Medical students' disease: Hypochondriasis in medical education. *Journal of Medical Education*, 1966, **41**, 785–790.

Zola, I. K. Culture and symptoms—An analysis of patients' presenting complaints. *American Sociological Review*, 1966, **31**, 615–630.

———. Studying the decision to see a doctor: Review, critique, corrective. *Advances in Psychosomatic Medicine*, 1972, **8**, 216–236.

———. Pathways to the doctor—From person to patient. *Social Science and Medicine*, 1973, **7**, 677–689.

CHAPTER 5: NORMS AND COMPLIANCE: THE EFFECT OF THE PATIENT'S CULTURE

Aho, W. R. Relationship of wives' preventive health orientation to their beliefs about heart disease in husbands. *Public Health Reports*, January–February 1977, **92**(1), 65–71.

Ajzen, I. & Fishbein, M. *Understanding attitudes and predicting social behavior*. Englewood Cliffs, N.J.: Prentice-Hall, 1980.

Antonovsky, A. A model to explain visits to the doctor, with specific reference to the case of Israel. *Journal of Health and Social Behavior*, 1972, **13**, 446–454.

Antonovsky, A. & Hartman, H. The existing knowledge about delay. *Health Education Monographs*, Summer 1974, **2**(2), 99–129.

Antonovsky, A. & Kats, R. The model dental patient: An empirical study of preventive health behavior. *Social Science and Medicine*, 1970, **4**, 367–380.

Asch, S. E. *Social psychology*. Englewood Cliffs, N.J.: Prentice-Hall, 1952.

———. Effects of group pressure upon the modification and distortion of judgments. In E. E. Maccoby, T. M. Newcomb, & E. L. Hartley (Eds.), *Readings in social psychology*. New York: Holt, Rinehart and Winston, 1958.

Aslam, M., Davis, S. S., & Fletcher, R. Compliance in medication by Asian immigrants. *Nursing Times*, May 31, 1979, **75**(22), 931–932.

Bandura, A. & Walters, R. H. *Social learning and personality development*. New York: Holt, Rinehart and Winston, 1963.

Baric, L. Conjugal roles as indicators of family influence on health directed action. *International Journal of Health Education*, 1970, **13**, 58–65.

Becker, M. H. & Green, L. W. A family approach to compliance with medical treatment: A selective review of the literature. *International Journal of Health Education*, 1975, **18**, 173–182.

Becker, M. H. & Maiman, L. A. Strategies for enhancing patient compliance. *Journal of Community Health*, 1980, **6**(2), 113–135.

Bloom, S. W. *The doctor and his patient: A sociological interpretation*. New York: Russell Sage Foundation, 1963.

Bloom, S. W. & Wilson, R. N. Patient-practitioner relationships. In H. E. Freeman, S. Levine & L. G. Reeder (Eds.), *Handbook of medical sociology*. 2nd ed. Englewood Cliffs, N.J.: Prentice-Hall, 1972.

Blumer, H. *Symbolic Interactionism*. Englewood Cliffs, N.J.: Prentice-Hall, 1969.

Brim, O. G. & Wheeler, S. *Socialization after childhood: Two essays*. New York: John Wiley and Sons, 1966.

Bruhn, J. G. Culture, adaptation, and patterns of disease. *Southern Medical Journal*, September 1976, **69**(9), 1152–1156.

Bursten, B. & D'Esopo, R. D. The obligation to remain sick. *Archives of General Psychiatry*, 1965, **12**, 402–407.

Cartwright, A. *Patients and their doctors: A study of general practice*. London: Routledge and Kegan Paul, 1967.

Cassell, E. *The healer's art*. New York: Penguin Books, 1976.

Charon, J. M. *Symbolic interactionism*. Englewood Cliffs, N.J.: Prentice-Hall, 1979.

Childs, B. Genetic origin of some sex differences among human beings. *Pediatrics*, 1965, **35**, 798.

Clark, M. *Health in the Mexican-American culture*. Berkeley: University of California Press, 1970.

Cockerham, W. C. *Sociology of mental disorder*. Englewood Cliffs, N.J.: Prentice-Hall, 1981.

Coe, R. M. *Sociology of medicine*. New York: McGraw-Hill, 1978.

Cooley, C. H. *Human nature and the social order*. New York: Schocken Books, 1964.

Cummings, K. M., Becker, M. H., & Maile, M. C. Bringing the models together: An empirical approach to combining variables used to explain health actions. *Journal of Behavioral Medicine*, 1980, **3**(2), 123–145.

Davitz, L. L., Davitz, J. R., & Higuchi, Y. Cross-cultural inferences of physical pain and psychological distress—I. *Nursing Times*, April 14, 1977, **73**(15), 521–522. (a)

———. Cross-cultural inferences of physical pain and psychological distress—II. *Nursing Times*, April 21, 1977, **73**(16), 556–558. (b)

Davitz, L. J., Sameshima, Y. & Davitz, J. Suffering as viewed in six different cultures. *American Journal of Nursing*, 1976, **76**(8), 1296–1297.

Denzin, N. K. The methodologies of symbolic interaction: A critical review of research techniques. In, G. Stone & H. Farberman (Eds.), *Social psychology through symbolic interaction*. Waltham, Mass.: Ginn-Blaisdell, 1970.

Deutsch, M. & Gerard, H. B. A study of normative and informational social influence upon individual judgment. *Journal of Abnormal and Social Psychology*, 1955, **51**, 629–636.

DiMatteo, M. R. & Hays, R. The significance of patients' perceptions of physician conduct: A study of patient satisfaction in a family practice center. *Journal of Community Health*, Fall 1980, **6**(1), 18–34.

DiMatteo, M. R., Prince, L. M., & Taranta, A. Patients' perceptions of physicians' behavior: determinants of patient commitment to the therapeutic relationship. *Journal of Community Health*, 1979, **4**, 280–290.

Dingle, J. H. *An epidemiological study of illness in families*. New York: Academic Press, 1959.

Fabrega, H. The study of disease in relation to culture. *Behavior Science*, 1972, **17**, 183–203.

Festinger, L. Informal social communication. *Psychological Review*, 1950, **57**, 271–282.

———. A theory of social comparison processes. *Human Relations*, 1954, **7**, 117–140.

Fishbein, M. & Ajzen, I. *Belief, attitude, intention and behavior: An introduction to theory and research*. Reading, Mass.: Addison-Wesley, 1975.

Freidson, E. Client control and medical behavior. *American Journal of Sociology*, 1960, **65**, 377.

———. *Patients' views of medical practice*. New York: Russell-Sage Foundation, 1961.

Goldenberg, I. & Goldenberg, H. *Family therapy: An overview*. Monterey, Calif.: Brooks-Cole, 1980.

Gordon, N. B. & Kutner, B. Long-term and fatal illness and the family. *Journal of Health and Human Behavior*, 1965, **6**, 190.

Green, L. *Status identity and preventive health behavior*. Pacific Health Education Report No. 1. Berkeley: University of California, 1970.

Guttmacher, S. Commentary. *Man and Medicine*, 1980, **5**(1), 54–56.

Haggerty, R. J. Family diagnosis: Research methods and their reliability for studies of the medical social unit—the family. *American Journal of Public Health*, 1965, **55**, 1521.

Haggerty, R. J. & Alpert, J. J. The child, his family and illness. *Postgraduate Medicine*, 1963, **34**, 228.

Harvey, J. H. & Smith, W. P. *Social psychology: An attributional approach*. St. Louis: C. V. Mosby, 1977.

Haynes, R. B., Taylor, D. W., & Sackett, D. L. (Eds.). *Compliance in health care*. Baltimore: Johns Hopkins University Press, 1979.

Hertz, P. & Stamps, P. L. Appointment-keeping bevavior re-evaluated. *American Journal of Public Health*, November 1977, **67**(11), 1033–1036.

Hewitt, J. P. *Self and society: A symbolic interactionist social psychology*. 2nd ed. Boston: Allyn and Bacon, 1979.

Hill, R. R. Social stresses on the family. *Social Casework*, 1958, **39**, 142.

Hogan, R. Moral conduct and moral character: A psychological perspective. *Psychological Bulletin*, 1973, **79**, 217–232.

Horton, J. Time and cool people. *Transaction*, April 1967, **4**, 5–12.

Hunt, G. J. Social factors affecting health, illness and treatment. In G. U. Balis, L. Wurmser, & E. McDaniel (Eds.), *The behavioral and social sciences and the practice of medicine*. Boston: Butterworth, 1978.

Hyman, H. H. & Singer, E. An introduction to reference group theory and research. In E. P. Hollander & R. G. Hunt (Eds.), *Current perspectives in social psychology*. New York: Oxford University Press, 1971.

Kando, T. M. *Social interaction*. St. Louis: C. V. Mosby, 1977.

Kellner, R. *Family ill health: An investigation in general practice*. Springfield, Ill.: Charles C. Thomas, 1963.

Khasla, T. & Lowe, C. R. Obesity and smoking habits by social class. *Journal of Preventive Social Medicine*, 1972, **26**, 249–256.

Kiev, A. *Curanderismo: Mexican-American folk psychiatry*. New York: The Free Press, 1968.

Klein, R., Dean, A., & Bogdonoff, M. The impact of illness upon the spouse. *Journal of Chronic Disease*, 1968, **20**, 241.

Kleinman, A., Eisenberg, L., & Good, B. Culture, illness and care: Clinical lessons from anthropologic and cross-cultural research. *Annals of Internal Medicine*, 1978, **88**, 251–258.

Knapp, D. A., Knapp, D. E., & Engle, J. The public, the pharmacist and self medication. *Journal of the American Pharmacology Association*, 1966, **56**, 460.

Koos, E. L. *The health of Regionville*. New York: Columbia University Press, 1954.

Kosa, J., Alpert, J. J., & Haggerty, R. J. On the reliability of family health information. A comparative study of mothers: Reports on illness and related behavior. *Social Science and Medicine*, 1967, **1**, 165.

Langlie, J. K. Social networks, health beliefs, and preventive health behavior. *Journal of Health and Social Behavior*, 1977, **18**, 244–260.

Larson, R. & Sutker, S. Value differences and value consensus by socio-economic levels. *Social Forces*, 1966, **44**, 563–569.

Lin, T. & Lin, M. Service delivery issues in Asian-North American communities. *American Journal of Psychiatry*, April 1978, **135**(4), 454–456.

Litman, T. J. The family as basic unit in health and medical care: A social behavioral overview. *Social Science and Medicine*, 1974, **8**, 495–519.

Lynch, J. J., Flaherty, L., Emrich, C., Mills, M. E., & Katcher, A. Effects of human contact on the heart activity of curarized patients in a shock-trauma unit. *American Heart Journal*, 1974, **88**(2), 160–169.

Lynch, J. J., Paskewitz, D. A., Gimbel, K. S., & Thomas, S. A. Fundamentals of clinical cardiology. Psychological aspects of cardiac arrhythmia. *American Heart Journal*, 1977, **93**(5), 645–657.

Madigan, F. C. Are sex mortality differentials biologically caused? *Milbank Memorial Fund Quarterly*, 1957, **21**, 202.

Mathis, J. L. A sophisticated version of voodoo death. Report of a case. *Psychosomatic Medicine*, 1964, **26**(2), 104–107.

McKenzie, J. L. & Chrisman, N. J. Healing herbs, gods and magic: Folk health beliefs among Filipino-Americans. *Nursing Outlook*, May 1977, **25**(5), 326–329.

McKinlay, J. B. Social networks, lay consultation and help-seeking behavior. *Social Forces*, March 1973, **51**, 275–291.

Mead, G. H. *Mind, self, and society*. Chicago: University of Chicago Press, 1934.

Mechanic, D. Religion, religiosity, and illness behavior: The special case of the Jews. *Human Organization*, 1963, **22**, 202–208.

———. Influence of mothers on their children's health attitudes and behavior. *Pediatrics*, 1964, **33**, 444.

———. Response factors in illness: The study of illness behavior. *Social Psychiatry*, 1966, **1**, 11–20.

———. Illness behavior, social adaptation, and the management of illness: A comparison of educational and medical models. *Journal of Nervous and Mental Disease*, August 1977, **165**(2), 79–87.

———. *Medical sociology*. 2nd ed. New York: The Free Press, 1978.

———. Patient behavior, the provision of medical care, and medical-social policy. *Man and Medicine*, 1980, **5**(1), 13–23.

Merton, R. K. & Rossi, A. S. Contributions to the theory of reference group behavior. In R. K. Merton, *Social Theory and Social Structure*. Rev. and enlarged ed. Glencoe, Ill.: The Free Press, 1957.

Minuchin, S., Rosman, B. L., & Baker, L. *Psychosomatic families*. Cambridge, Mass.: Harvard University Press, 1978.

Morris, V., Hatch, M. H., & Chipman, S. S. Deterrants to well child supervision. *American Journal of Public Health*, 1966, **56**, 1232.

Muller, C. Income and the receipt of medical care. *American Journal of Public Health*, 1965, **55**, 510.

Nathanson, C. A. Illness and the feminine role: A theoretical review. *Social Science and Medicine*, 1975, **9**, 57–62.

Norman, J. C. (Ed.). *Medicine in the ghetto*. New York: Appleton-Century-Crofts, 1969.

Osterweis, M., Bush, P. J., & Zuckerman, A. E. Family context as a predictor of individual medicine use. *Social Science and Medicine*, 1979, **13A**, 287–291.

Parsons, T. Definitions of health and illness in the light of American values and social structure. In E. G. Jaco (Ed.), *Patients, physicians and illness*. New York: The Free Press, 1958, pp. 165–187.

Parsons, T. & Fox, R. Illness, therapy and the modern Urban American family. *Journal of Social Issues*, 1952, **8**, 31–44.

Pilowsky, I. & Spence, N. D. Ethnicity and illness behavior. *Psychological Medicine*, 1977, **7**, 447–452.

Pratt, L. The significance of the family in medication. *Journal of Comparative Family Studies*, 1973, **10**, 44.

———. *Family structure and effective health behavior: The energized family*. Boston: Houghton-Mifflin, 1976.

Primeaux, M. H. American Indian health care practices. *Nursing Clinics of North America*, 1977, **12**(1), 55–65.

Quesada, G. M. Language and communication barriers for health delivery to a minority group. *Social Science and Medicine*, 1976, **10**, 323–327.

Richardson, H. *Patients have families*. New York: Commonwealth Fund, 1945.

Richardson, W. Measuring the urban poor's use of physicians' services in response to illness episodes. *Medical Care*, 1970, **8**, 132.

Robinson, D. *The process of becoming ill*. London: Routledge and Kegan Paul, 1971.

Rokeach, M. *The nature of human values*. New York: The Free Press, 1973.

Rosenstock, I. M. Health behavior: Prevention and maintenance. In J. Kosa, A. Antonovsky, & I. K. Zola (Eds.), *Poverty and health: A sociological analysis*. Cambridge, Mass.: Harvard University Press, 1969.

Rosenstock, I. M. & Kirscht, J. P. Why people seek health care. In G. C. Stone, F. Cohen, & N. E. Adler (Eds.), *Health psychology*. San Francisco: Jossey-Bass, 1979, Chap. 7.

Rotter, J. B. Generalized expectancies for internal versus external control of reinforcement. *Psychological Monographs*, 1966, **80**(1), no. 609.

Rubel, A. J. Concepts of disease in Mexican-American Culture. *American Anthropologist*, 1960, **62**(5), 795–814.

Rundall, T. G. & Wheeler, J. R. C. The effect of income on use of preventive care: An evaluation of alternative explanations. *Journal of Health and Social Behavior*, 1979, **20**, 397–406.

Salk, L., Hilgartner, M., & Granich, B. The psychosocial impact of hemophilia on the patient and his family. *Social Science and Medicine*, 1972, **6**, 481.

Samora, J., Saunders, L., & Larson, R. Medical vocabulary knowledge among hospital patients. *Journal of Health and Human Behavior*, Summer 1961, **2**, 83–89.

Saunders, L. *Cultural differences and medical care*. New York: Russell-Sage Foundation, 1954.

Segall, A. The sick role concept: Understanding illness behavior. *Journal of Health and Social Behavior*, 1976, **17**, 163–170.

Shuval, J. T. *Social functions of medical practice: Doctor-patient relationships in Israel*. San Francisco: Jossey-Bass, 1970.

Suchman, E. Sociomedical variations among ethnic groups. *American Journal of Sociology*, 1964, **70**, 319–331.

———. Preventive health behavior: A model for research on community health campaigns. *Journal of Health and Social Behavior*, 1967, **8**, 197–209.

Surgeon General. *Healthy people: The Surgeon General's report on health promotion and disease prevention, 1979*. Washington, D.C.: Office of Assistant Secretary of Health, USDHEW, Public Health Service.

Syme, S. L. & Berkman, L. F. Reviews and commentary, social class, susceptibility and sickness. *Journal of Epidemiology*, July 1976, **104**(1), 1–8.

Torrens, P. R. *The American health care system: Issues and problems*. St. Louis: C. V. Mosby, 1978.

Triandis, H. C. *Interpersonal behavior*. Monterey, Calif.: Brooks/Cole, 1977.

Tucker, M. Effect of heavy medical expenditures on low income families, incidence and impact. *Public Health Reports*, 1970, **85**, 419.

Twaddle, A. C. Health decisions and sick role variations: An exploration. *Journal of Health and Social Behavior*, 1969, **10**, 105–115.

United States Department of Health, Education, and Welfare. *Adult Use of Tobacco, 1970*. Washington, D.C.: Publication No. HSM-73-8727, 1973.

Vogel, E. F. & Bell, N. W. The emotionally disturbed child as the family scapegoat. In N. W. Bell & E. F. Vogel (Eds.), *A modern introduction to the family*. New York: Free Press, 1968.

White, K. L., Williams, T. F., & Greenberg, B. G. The ecology of medical care. *New England Journal of Medicine*, 1961, **265**, 885–892.

Wingert, W. A. et al. The influence of familial organization on the utilization of pediatric emergency services. *Pediatrics*, 1968, **42**, 743.

Zborowski, M. Cultural components in responses to pain. *Journal of Social Issues*, 1952, **8**, 16–30.

Zola, I. K. Pathways to the doctor—From person to patient. *Social Science and Medicine*, 1973, **7**, 677–689.

CHAPTER 6: CHANGING BELIEFS AND ATTITUDES: THE FORMATION OF BEHAVIORAL INTENTIONS

Abelson, H. I. & Karlins, M. *Persuasion: How opinions and attitudes are changed*. 2nd rev. ed. New York: Springer, 1970.

Aday, L. A. & Anderson, R. A framework for the study of access to medical care. *Health Services Research*, 1974, **9**, 208–220.

Ajzen, I. & Fishbein, M. Factors influencing intention behavior relations. *Human Relations*, 1974, **27**, 1–15.

———. Acceptance, yielding, and impact: Cognitive processes in persuasion. In R. E. Petty, T. M. Ostrom, & T. C. Brock (Eds.), *Cognitive responses in persuasion*. Hillsdale, N.J.: Earlbaum, 1980.

———. *Understanding attitudes and predicting social behavior*. Englewood Cliffs, N.J.: Prentice Hall, 1980.

Applebaum, S. A. The refusal to take one's medicine. *Bulletin of the Menninger Clinic*, 1977, **41**, 511–521.

Aronson, E. The theory of cognitive dissonance: A current perspective. In L. Berkowitz (Ed.), *Advances in experimental social psychology*, 1969, **4**, 1–34.

Bandler, R. J., Madaras, G. R., & Bem, D. J. Self-observation as a source of pain perception. *Journal of Personality and Social Psychology*, 1968, **9**, 205–209.

Beck, K. H. & Frankel, A. A conceptualization of threat communications and protective health behavior. *Social Psychology Quarterly*, 1981, **44**(3), 204–217.

Becker, M. H. & Maiman, L. A. Strategies for enhancing patient compliance. *Journal of Community Health*, 1980, **6**, 113–135.

Bem, D. J. Self-perception: An alternative interpretation of cognitive dissonance phenomena. *Psychological Review*, 1967, **74**, 183–200.

———. Self-perception theory. In L. Berkowitz (Ed.), *Advances in experimental social psychology*. Volume 6, 1972.

Berkowitz, L. *A survey of social psychology*. 2nd ed. New York: Holt, Rinehart and Winston, 1980.

Bogart, L. *Strategy in advertising*. New York: Harcourt, 1967.

Brehm, J. W. *A theory of psychological reactance*. New York: Academic Press, 1966.

Brickman, P., Redfield, J., Harrison, A. A., & Crandall, R. Drive and predisposition as factors in the attitudinal effects of mere exposure. *Journal of Experimental Social Psychology*, 1972, **8**, 31–44.

Brock, T. C. Historical and methodological perspectives in the analysis of cognitive responses: An introduction. In R. E. Petty, T. M. Ostrom, & T. C. Brock (Eds.), *Cognitive responses in persuasion*. Hillsdale, N.J.: Lawrence Erlbaum, 1981.

Carnegie, D. *How to develop self-confidence and influence people by public speaking*. New York: Simon and Schuster, 1956.

Cook, T. & Flay, B. The temporal persistence of experimentally induced attitude change: An evaluative review. In L. Berkowitz (Ed.), *Advances in experimental social psychology*, Volume 11, 1978.

Croner, M. D. & Willis, R. H. Perceived differences in task competency and asymmetry of dyadic influence. *Journal of Abnormal and Social Psychology*, 1961, **62**, 705–708.

Davis, M. S. Physiologic, psychological and demographic factors in patient compliance with doctors' orders. *Medical Care*, 1968, **6**, 115–122.

DiMatteo, M. R. & Friedman, H. S. Interpersonal relations in health care. *Journal of Social Issues*, 1979, **35**(1), whole issue.

———. *Social psychology and medicine*. Cambridge, Mass.: Oelgeschlager, Gunn and Hain, 1982.

Eisenberg, L. The search for care. *Daedalus*, 1977, **106**, 235–246.

Festinger, L. A theory of cognitive dissonance. Evanston, Ill.: Row-Peterson, 1957.

———. Behavioral support for opinion change. *Public Opinion Quarterly*, 1964, **28**, 404–417.

Festinger, L. & Maccoby, N. On resistance to persuasive communications. *Journal of Abnormal and Social Psychology*, 1964, **68**, 359–366.

Fishbein, M. & Ajzen, I. *Belief, attitude, intention and behavior: An introduction to theory and research*. Reading, Mass.: Addison-Wesley, 1975.

French, J. R. P., Jr. & Raven, B. The bases of social power. In D. Cartwright (Ed.), *Studies in social power*. Ann Arbor: University of Michigan, Institute for Social Research, 1959, pp. 150–167.

Gerard, H. B., Conolley, E. S., & Wilhelmy, R. A. Compliance, justification, and cognitive change. In L. Berkowitz (Ed.), *Advances in experimental social psychology*, 1974, **7**, 217–247.

Goldstein, J. W., Gleason, T. C., & Korn, J. H. Whither the epidemic? Psychoactive drug use career patterns of college students. *Journal of Applied Social Psychology*, 1975, **5**, 16–33.

Gormeley, R. A. Note on seven brand rating scales and subsequent purchase. *Journal of Market Research Society*, 1974, **16**, 242–244.

Harrison, A. A. Mere exposure. In L. Berkowitz (Ed.), *Advances in experimental social psychology*, 1977, **10**, 39–83.

Haug, M. R. Issues of patient acceptance of physicians authority in Great Britain. In E. B. Gallagher (Ed.), *The doctor-patient relationship*. Washington, D.C.: DHEW Publication No. (NIH) 78-183, 1976.

Haug, M. R. & Lavin, B. Public challenge of physician authority. *Medical Care*, August 1979, **17**(8), 844–858.

Hertroijs, A. A study of some factors in a leprosy control scheme. *International Journal of Leprosy*, 1974, **42**, 419–427.

Hovland, C. I. Reconciling conflicting results derived from experimental and survey studies of attitude change. *American Psychologist*, 1959, **14**, 8–17.

Hovland, C. I., Janis, I. L., & Kelley, H. H. *Communication and persuasion*. New Haven: Yale, 1953.

Insko, C. I. *Theories of attitude change*. New York: Appleton-Century-Crofts, 1967.

Insko, C. I., Turnbull, W., & Yandell, B. Facilitative and inhibiting effects of distraction on attitude change. *Sociometry*, 1974, **37**, 508–528.

Janis, I. L. & King, B. T. The influence of role-playing on opinion change. *Journal of Abnormal and Social Psychology*, 1954, **49**, 211–218.

Janis, I. L. & Mann, L. Effectiveness of emotional role playing in modifying smoking habits and attitudes. *Journal of Experimental Research in Personality*, 1965, **1**, 84–90.

Johnson, D. W. Attitude modification methods. In F. H. Kanfer & A. P. Goldstein (Eds.), *Helping people change*. New York: Pergamon Press, 1980, Chap. 3.

Johnson, D. W. & Matross, R. P. Attitude modification methods. In F. H. Kanfer & A. P. Goldstein (Eds.), *Helping people change*. 1st ed. New York: Pergamon Press, 1975, pp. 51–88.

Kasteler, J., Kane, R. L., Olsen, D. M., & Thetford, L. Issues underlying prevalence of "doctor-shopping" behavior. *Journal of Health and Social Behavior*, 1976, **17**, 328–339.

Katz, D. & Stotland, E. A preliminary statement to a theory of attitude structure and change. In S. Koch (Ed.), *Psychology: A study of science*, Vol. 3, New York: McGraw-Hill, 1959.

Keating, J. P. & Brock, T. C. A myth about distraction. In Janis, L. (Ed.), *Current trends in Psychology*. Los Altos, Calif.: William Kaufmann, 1977, pp. 323-326.

Kelman, H. C. Compliance, identification, and internalization. Three processes of opinion change. *Journal of Conflict Resolution*, 1958, **2**, 51–66.

Kelman, H. C. Process of opinion change. *Public Opinion Quarterly*, 1961, **25**, 57–58.

Kiesler, C. A. *The psychology of commitment*. New York: Academic Press, 1971.

Kiesler, C. A. & Sakamura, J. A. A test of a model for commitment and dissonance. *Journal of Personality and Social Psychology*, 1966, **3**, 349–353.

Kipnis, D. *The powerholders*. Chicago and London: The University of Chicago Press, 1976.

Kirscht, J. P., Becker, M., & Eveland, J. Psychological and social factors as predictors of medical behavior. *Medical Care*, 1976, **14**, 422–431.

Levy, R. L. Relationship of an overt commitment to task compliance in behavior therapy. *Journal of Behavioral Therapy and Experimental Psychiatry*, 1977, **8**, 25–29.

Levy, R. L., Yamashita, D., & Pow, G. The relationship of an overt commitment to the frequency and speed of compliance with symptom reporting. *Medical Care*, 1979, **17**, 281–284.

London, H. *Psychology of the persuader*. Morristown, N.J.: General Learning Press, 1973.

Mann, L. & Janis, I. L. A follow-up study on the long-term effects of emotional role playing. *Journal of Personality and Social Psychology*, 1968, **8**, 339-342.

Marsland, D. W., Wood, M. B., & Mayo, F. The databank for patients' care, curriculum, and research in family practice: 526,196 patient problems. *Journal of Family Practice*, 1976, **3**, 25–28.

McGuire, W. J. The nature of attitudes and attitude change. In G. Lindzey & E. Aronson (Eds.), *Handbook of social psychology*. Vol. 3. Reading, Mass.: Addison-Wesley, 1969, pp. 136–314.

Miller, N., Maruyama, G., Beaber, R. J., & Valone, K. Speed of speech and persuasion. *Journal of Personality and Social Psychology*, 1976, **34**, 615–624.

Moreland, R. J. & Zajonc, R. B. Is stimulus recognition a necessary condition for the occurrence of exposure effects? *Journal of Personality and Social Psychology*, 1977, **35**, 191–199.

Osgood, C. E., & Tannenbaum, P. H. The principle of congruity in the prediction of attitude change. *Psychological Review*, 1955, **62**, 42–55.

Parsons, T. *The social system*. Glencoe, Ill.: The Free Press, 1951.

Pelletier, K. R. *Holistic medicine*. New York: Delacorte Press, 1979.

Raven, B. H. Patient-practitioner relationships. In A. Johnson, O. Grusky, & B. H. Raven (Eds.), *Contemporary health services: A social science perspective*. Boston: Auburn House, 1982, pp. 11–20.

Raven, B. H. The comparative analysis of power and influence. In J. T. Tedeschi (Ed.), *Perspectives on social power*. Chicago: Aldine, 1974.

Raven, B. H. The comparative analysis of power and influence. In J. T. Tedeschi (Ed.) *Perspectives on Social Power*. Chicago, Ill.: Aldine, 1974.

Reeder, L. The patient-client as a consumer: Some observations on the changing professional-client relationship. *Journal of Health and Social Behavior*, 1972, **13**, 406–413.

Rodin, J. Patient-practitioner relationships: A process of social influence. In A. Johnson, O. Grusky, & B. H. Raven (Eds.), *Contemporary health services: A social science perspective*. Boston: Auburn House, 1982, pp. 49–81.

Rodin, J. & Janis, I. L. The social power of health care practitioners as agents of change. *Journal of Social Issues*, 1979, **35**(1), 60–81.

Rodin, J. & Janis, I. L. The social influence of physicians and other health care practitioners as agents of change. In H. S. Friedman & M. R. DiMatteo (Eds.), *Interpersonal issues in health care*. New York: Academic Press, 1982.

Rosenberg, M. J. & Hovland, C. I. Cognitive, affective, and behavioral components of attitudes. In C. I. Hovland & M. J. Rosenberg (Eds.), *Attitude organization and change*. New Haven: Yale University Press, 1960.

Rosenstock, I. M. Patients' compliance with health regimens. *Journal of the American Medical Association*, 1975, **234**, 402–403.

Rosenstock, I. M. & Kirscht, J. P. Why people seek health care. In G. C. Stone, F. Cohen, & N. E. Adler (Eds.), *Health psychology*. San Francisco: Jossey-Bass, 1979, pp. 161–189.

Rosenthal, R. Interpersonal expectations. In R. Rosenthal & R. Rosnow (Eds.), *Artifact in behavioral research*. New York: Academic Press, 1969.

———. *Experimenter effects in behavioral research*. New York: Irvington Publishers, 1976.

Sejwacz, D., Ajzen, I., & Fishbein, M. Predicting and understanding weight loss: Intentions, behaviors and outcomes. In I. Ajzen & M. Fishbein (Eds.), *Understanding attitudes and predicting behavior*. New Jersey: Prentice Hall, 1980.

Seligman, M. E. *Helplessness*. San Francisco: W. H. Freeman, 1975.

Sherif, M. & Hovland, C. *Social judgment: Assimilation and contrast effects in communication and attitude change*. New Haven: Yale University Press, 1961.

Smetana, J. G. & Adler, N. E. Fishbein's value x expectancy model: An examination of some assumptions. *Personality and Social Psychology Bulletin*, 1980, **6**(1), 89–96.

Smith, B. L., Brown, B. L., Strong, W. J., & Rencher, A. C. Effects of speech rate on personality perception. *Language and Speech*, 1975, **18**, 145–152.

Stang, D. J. & Wrightsman, L. S. *Dictionary of social behavior and social research methods*. Monterey, Calif.: Brooks/Cole, 1981.

Stimson, G. V. Obeying doctors' orders: A view from the other side. *Social Science and Medicine*, 1974, **8**, 97–104.

Surgeon General. *Healthy people: The Surgeon General's report on health promotion and disease prevention, 1979*. Washington, D.C.: USDHEW Public Health Service, Office of Asst. Sec. Health & Surgeon General, 1979.

Triandis, H. C. *Interpersonal behavior*. Monterey, Calif.: Brooks/Cole, 1977.

Wallston, B. S. & Wallston, K. A. Toward a unified social psychological model of health behavior. In G. Sanders & J. Suls (Eds.), *Social psychology and illness*. Hillsdale, N.J.: Lawrence Erlbaum, 1981.

Wurtele, S. K., Galanos, A. N., & Roberts, M. C. Increasing return compliance in a tuberculosis detection drive. *Journal of Behavioral Medicine*, 1980, **3**, 311–318.

Zajonc, R. B. Attitudinal effects of mere exposure. *Journal of Personality and Social Psychology*, monograph supplement, 1968, **9**, Part 2, 1–27.

Zimbardo, P. G., Ebbesen, E. B., & Maslach, C. *Influencing attitudes and changing behavior*. 2nd ed. Reading, Mass.: Addison-Wesley, 1977.

Zimbardo, P. G., Snyder, M., Thomas, J., Gold, A., & Gurwitz, S. Modifying the impact of persuasive communications with external distraction. *Journal of Personality and Social Psychology*, 1970, **16**, 669–680.

CHAPTER 7: FROM INTENTIONS TO BEHAVIORS: SUPPORTS AND BARRIERS IN THE ACCOMPLISHMENT OF MEDICAL GOALS

Abernethy, J. D. The problem of noncompliance in long-term antihypertensive therapy. *Drugs*, 1976, **11**, 86–90.

Alderman, M. H. Organization for long-term management of hypertension. *Bulletin of the New York Academy of Medicine*, 1976, **52**, 697–717.

———. Three years of work-site based hypertensive treatment. Paper presented at the National Conference on High Blood Pressure Control, Washington, D.C., 1977.

Alderman, M. & Schoenbaum, E. Detection and treatment of hypertension at the work site. *New England Journal of Medicine*, 1975, **293**, 65–68.

Alpert, J. J. Broken appointments. *Pediatrics*, 1964, **34**, 127–132.

Antonovsky, A., Zola, I. K., & Kosa, J. *Poverty and health: A sociological analysis*. Cambridge, Mass.: Harvard University Press, 1969.

Atkins, C. J. Improving exercise compliance among chronic lung patients: a comparison of cognitive and behavioral approaches. Paper presented at the meeting of the Western Psychological Association, Los Angeles, April 12, 1981.

Azrin, N. H. & Powell, J. Behavioral engineering: The use of response priming to improve prescribed self-medication. *Journal of Applied Behavior Analysis*, 1969, **2**, 39–42.

Badgley, R. F. & Furnal, M. A. Appointment breaking in a pediatric clinic. *Yale Journal of Biology and Medicine*, 1961, **34**, 117–123.

Baekeland, F. & Lundwall, L. Dropping out of treatment: A critical review. *Psychological Bulletin*, 1975, **82**, 738–783.

Baekeland, F., Lundwall, L., & Shanahan, T. J. Correlates of patient attrition in the outpatient treatment of alcoholism. *Journal of Nervous and Mental Disorder*, 1973, **157**, 99–107.

Bandura, A. *Principles of behavior modification*. New York: Holt, Rinehart & Winston, 1969.

———. *Social learning theory*. Englewood Cliffs, N.J.: Prentice-Hall, 1977.

Bebbington, P. E. The efficacy of Alcoholics Anonymous: The elusiveness of hard data. *British Journal of Psychiatry*, 1976, **128**, 572–580.

Becker, H. S. & Geer, B. The fate of idealism in medical school. *American Sociological Review*, 1958, **23**, 50–56.

Becker, H. S., Geer, B., Hughes, E. C., & Strauss, A. M. *Boys in white: Student culture in medical school*. Chicago: University of Chicago Press, 1961.

Becker, M. H. & Green, L. W. A family approach to compliance with medical treatment—A selective review of the literature. *International Journal of Health Education*, 1975, **18**, 1–11.

Becker, M. H., Kaback, M. M., Rosenstock, I. M., & Ruth, M. V. Some influences on public participation in a genetic screening program. *Journal of Community Health*, 1975, **1**, 3–14.

Becker, M. H. & Maiman, L. A. Strategies for enhancing patient compliance. *Journal of Community Health*, 1980, **6**, 113–135.

Bellak, A. S., Rozensky, R., & Schwartz, J. A. A comparison of two forms of self-monitoring in a behavioral weight reduction program. *Behavior Therapy*, 1974, **5**, 523–530.

Bergman, A. B. & Werner, R. J. Failure of children to receive penicillin by mouth. *New England Journal of Medicine*, 1963, **268**, 1334–1338.

Bewley, B. & Bland, J. Academic performance and social factors related to cigarette smoking by school children. *British Journal of Preventive and Social Medicine*, 1977, **31**, 18–24.

Bigelow, G., Strickler, D., Leisbon, I., & Griffiths, R. Maintaining desulfiram ingestion among outpatient alcoholics: A security-deposit contingency contracting procedure. *Behavior Research Therapy*, 1976, **14**, 378–381.

Bonnar, J., Goldberg, A., Smith, J. A. Do pregnant women take their iron? *Lancet*, 1969, **1**, 457–458.

Bowen, R. G., Rich, R., Schlatfeldt, R. M. Effects of organized instruction for patients with the diagnosis of diabetes mellitus. *Nursing Research*, 1961, **10**, 151–159.

Bracken, M. B. The Jamaican family planning program: Clinic services and social support as factors in dropping out. *International Journal of Health Education*, 1977, **20**, 126–135.

Brand, F. & Smith, R. Medical care and compliance among the elderly after hospitalization. *International Journal of Aging Human Development*, 1974, **5**, 331–346.

Brand, F., Smith, R., & Brand, P. Effect of economic barriers to medical care on patients' noncompliance. *Public Health Reports*, 1977, **92**, 72–78.

Brigg, E. H. & Mudd, E. H. An exploration of methods to reduce broken first appointments. *Family Coordinator*, 1968, **17**, 41–46.

Caldwell, J. R., Cobb, S., Dowling, M. D., & De Jongh, D. The dropout problem in antihypertensive therapy. *Journal of Chronic Disease*, 1970, **22**, 579–592.

Caplan, R. Patient, provider, and organization: Hypothesized determinants of adherence. In S. J. Cohen (Ed.), *New directions in patient compliance*. Lexington, Mass.: D. C. Heath, 1979.

Caplan, R. D., Robinson, E. A. R., French, J. R. P., Caldwell, J. R., & Shinn, M. *Adhering to medical regimens: Pilot experiments in patient education and social support*. Ann Arbor: University of Michigan, 1976.

Carnahan, J. & Nugent, C. The effects of self monitoring by patients on the control of hypertension. *American Journal of Medical Science*, 1975, **269**, 69–73.

Carpenter, J. O. & Davis, L. J. Medical recommendations—followed or ignored? Factors influencing compliance in arthritis. *Archives of Physical Medicine and Rehabilitation*, 1976, **57**, 241–246.

Cartwright, L. K. Sources and effects of stress in health careers. In C. G. Stone, F. Cohen, & N. E. Adler (Eds.), *Health psychology*. San Francisco: Jossey-Bass, 1979.

Cassel, J. The contribution of the social environment to host resistance. *American Journal of Epidemiology*, 1976, **104**, 107–123.

Charney, E., Bynum, R., Eldredge, D., Frank, D., MacWhinney, J. B., & McNabb, N. How well do patients take oral penicillin? A collaborative study in private practice. *Pediatrics*, 1967, **40**, 188–195.

Christie, R. & Merton, R. K. Procedures for the sociological study of the value climate in medical schools. *Journal of Medical Education*, 1958, **33**, 125–133 (part 2).

Clinite, J. C. & Kabat, H. F. Prescribed drugs, errors during self administration. *Journal of the American Pharmaceutical Association*, 1969, **9**, 450–452.

Cobb, S. Social support as a moderator of life stresses. *Psychosomatic Medicine*, 1976, **38**(5), 300–314.

Cobb, B., Clark, R., McGuire, C., Howe, C. Patient-responsible delay of treatment in cancer. A social psychological study. *Cancer*, 1954, **7**, 920–926.

Cody, J. & Robinson, A. The effect of low-cost maintenance medication on the rehospitalization of schizophrenic outpatients. *American Journal of Psychiatry*, 1977, **134**, 73–76.

Cole, S. A., O'Connor, S., & Bennett, L. Self-help groups for clinical patients with chronic illness. *Primary Care*, June 1979, **6**(2), 325–339.

Colcher, I. S. & Bass, J. W. Penicillin treatment of streptococcal pharyngitis: A comparison of schedules and the role of specific counselling. *Journal of the American Medical Association*, 1972, **222**, 657–659.

Collette, J. & Ludwig, E. G. Patient compliance with medical advice. *Journal of the National Medical Association*, 1969, **61**, 408–411.

Cook, D., Morch, J., & Noble, E. Improving attendance at follow-up clinics. *Dimensions in Health Services*, 1976, **53**, 46–49.

Coplin, S., Hine, J., & Gormican, A. Out-patient dietary management in the Prader-Willi syndrome. *Journal of the American Diet Association*, 1976, **68**, 330–334.

Cornish, R. D. & Miller, M. V. Attitudes of registered nurses toward the alcoholic. *Journal of Psychiatric Nursing*, 1966, **14**, 69–78.

Crane, D. Physicians' attitudes toward the treatment of critically ill patients. *BioScience*, 1973, **23**, 471–474.

———. Decisions to treat critically ill patients: A comparison of social versus medical considerations. *Milbank Memorial Fund Quarterly*, 1975, **53**, 1–33. (a)

———. Controversy and the clinical mentality. In *The sanctity of social life: Physicians' treatment of critically ill patients*. New York: Russell Sage Foundation, 1975, pp. 17–32. (b)

Croog, S. H., Lipson, A., & Levine, S. Help patterns in severe illness: The roles of kin network, non-family resources, and institutions. *Journal of Marriage and the Family*, February 1972, pp. 32–41.

Cummings, K. M., Becker, M. H., & Maile, M. C. Bringing the models together: An empirical approach to combining variables used to explain health actions. *Journal of Behavioral Medicine*, 1980, **3**(2), 123–145.

Curtis, B. D., Simpson, D., & Steven, G. G. Rapid puffing as a treatment component of a community smoking program. *Journal of Community Psychiatry*, 1976, **4**, 186–193.

Daschner, F. & Marget, W. Treatment of recurrent urinary tract infection in children: Compliance of parents and children with antibiotic therapy regimen. *Acta Paediatriea Scandinavica*, 1975, **64**, 105–108.

Davidson, N., Hudson, B., & Parry, E.H.O. Defaults from follow-up after peripartum cardiac failure. *Tropical Geographical Medicine*, 1975, **27**, 109–114.

Davis, M. S. Variations in patients' compliance with doctors' orders: Analysis of congruence between survey responses and results of empirical investigations. *Journal of Medical Education*, 1966, **41**, 1037–1048.

Davis, M. & Eichhorn, R. L. Compliance with medical regimens: A panel study. *Journal of Health and Human Behavior*, 1963, **4**, 240–249.

Davison, G. C., Tsujimoto, R. N., & Galros, A. G. Attribution and the maintenance of behavior change in falling asleep. *Journal of Abnormal Psychology*, 1973, **82**, 124–133.

Davison, G. C. & Valins, S. Maintenance of self-attributed and drug attributed behavior change. *Journal of Personality and Social Psychology*, 1969, **11**, 25–33.

Diamond, M. D., Weiss, A. J., & Grynbaum, B. The unmotivated patient. *Archives of Physical Medicine Rehabilitation*, 1968, **49**, 281–284.

Dickinson, G. E. & Pearson, A. A. Differences in attitudes toward terminal patients among selected medical specialties of physicians. *Medical Care*, June 1979, **17**(6), 682–685.

DiMatteo, M. R. & Hays, R. Social support and serious illness. In B. Gottlieb (Ed.), *Social networks and social support*. Beverly Hills, Calif.: Sage Publications, 1981, pp. 117–148.

Dinoff, M., Rickard, N. C., & Colwick, J. Weight reduction through successive contracts. *American Journal of Orthopsychiatry*, 1972, **42**, 110–113.

Donald, C. A., Ware, J. E., Brook, R. H., & Davies-Avery, A. *Conceptualization and measurement of health for adults in the health insurance study: Volume IV, Social Health*. Santa Monica, Calif.: Publication No. R-1987, The Rand Corporation, 1978.

Duff, R. & Hollingshead, A. B. *Sickness and society*. New York: Harper & Row, 1968.

Dunbar, J. M., Marshall, G. D., & Hovell, M. F. Behavioral strategies for improving compliance. In R. B. Haynes, D. W. Taylor, & D. L. Sackett (Eds.). *Compliance in health care*. Baltimore: Johns Hopkins University Press, 1979, pp. 174–190.

Eichna, L. W. Medical school education, 1975–1979: A student's perspective. *New England Journal of Medicine*, 1980, **303**, 727–734.

Elling, R., Whittemore, R., & Green, M. Patient participation in a pediatric program. *Journal of Health and Human Behavior*, 1960, **1**, 183–189.

Epstein, L. H. & McCoy, J. F. Issues in smoking control. *Addictive Behaviors*, 1975, **1**, 65–72.

Eshelman, F. N. & Fitzloff, J. Effect of packaging on patient compliance with an antihypertensive medication. *Current Therapy Research*, 1976, **20**, 215–219.

Farquhar, J. W. *The American way of life need not be hazardous to your health*. New York: W. W. Norton, 1978.

Fass, M. F., Green, L. W., & Deeds, S. G. The effect of family education on patient adherence to antihypertensive regimens. Presented at the National Conference on High Blood Pressure Control, Washington, D.C., 1977.

Feinstein, A. R., Spagnuolo, M., Jonas, S., Kloth, H., Tursky, E., & Levitt, M. Prophylaxis of recurrent rheumatic fever. *Journal of the American Medical Association*, 1968, **206**, 565–568.

Fink, D., Malloy, M. J., Cohen, M., Greycloud, M. A., & Martin, F. Effective patient care in the pediatric ambulatory setting: A study of the acute care clinic. *Pediatrics*, 1969, **43**, 927–935.

Fink, D., Martin, F., Cohen, M., Greycloud, M., & Malloy, M. The management specialist in effective pediatric ambulatory care. *American Journal of Public Health*, 1969, **59**, 527–533.

Finnerty, F. A., Shaw, L. W., & Himmelsbach, C. K. Hypertension in the inner city. II: Detection and follow-up. *Circulation*, 1973, **47**, 76–78.

Francis, V., Korsch, B. M., & Morris, M. J. Gaps in doctor-patient communication. *New England Journal of Medicine*, 1969, **280**, 535–540.

Frank, A., Eisenthal, S., & Lazare, A. Are there social class differences in patients' treatment conceptions? *Archives of General Psychiatry*, 1978, **35**, 61–69.

Freidson, E. *Profession of medicine*. New York: Dodd, Mead, 1970.

Funkenstein, D. *Medical students, medical schools, and society during five eras*. Cambridge, Mass.: Ballinger, 1978.

Garb, J. R. & Stunkard, A. J. Effectiveness of a self-help group in obesity control: A further assessment. *Archives of Internal Medicine*, 1974, **134**, 716–720.

Geersten, H. R., Gray, R. M., Ward, J. R. Patient noncompliance within the context of seeking medical care for arthritis. *Journal of Chronic Disease*, 1973, **26**, 689–698.

Glick, B. S. Drop-out in an outpatient, double-blind drug study. *Psychosomatics*, 1965, **6**, 44–48.

Glogow, P. H. Noncompliance—A dilemma. *Sight-Saving Review*, Spring 1973, pp. 29–34.

Golden, K. M. The multiproblem patient: A goal-oriented approach. *Journal of the American Medical Association*, 1978, **240**(12), 1263–1264.

Goldfried, M. R. & Goldfried, A. P. Cognitive change methods. In F. H. Kanfer & A. P. Goldstein (Eds.), *Helping people change*. New York: Pergamon Press, 1975, pp. 89–116.

Goldiamond, T. Toward a constructionist approach to social problems: Ethical and constitutional issues raised by applied behavior analysis. *Behaviorism*, 1974, **2**, 1–84.

Goldstein, A. P. & Kanfer, F. H. (Eds.). *Maximizing treatment gains: Transfer enhancement in psychotherapy*. New York: Academic Press, 1979.

Gordis, L. & Markowitz, M. Evaluation of the effectiveness of comprehensive and continuous pediatric care. *Pediatrics*, 1971, **48**, 766–776.

Gordis, L., Markowitz, M., & Lilienfeld, A. M. Why patients don't follow medical advice: A study of children on long-term antistreptococcal prophylaxis. *Journal of Pediatrics*, 1969, **75**, 957–968.

Gordon, B. G. & Kutner, B. Long term and fatal illness and the family. *Journal of Health and Human Behavior*, 1965, **6**(4), 190–196.

Gottlieb, B. H. The development and application of a classification scheme of informal helping behaviors. *Canadian Journal of Behavioural Science*, 1978, **10**, 105–115.

Gray, P. M., Kesler, J. P., Moody, P. M. Effects of social class and friends' expectations on oral polio vaccination participation. *American Journal of Public Health*, 1966, **56**, 2028–2032.

Gussow, Z. & Tracy, G. S. The role of self-help clubs in adaptation to chronic illness and disability. *Nursing Digest*, 1978, pp. 23–31.

Hamilton, S. H. & Borstein, P. H. Broad-spectrum behavioral approach to smoking cessation: Effects of social support and paraprofessional training on the maintenance of treatment effects. *Journal of Consulting and Clinical Psychology*, 1979, **47**(3), 598–600.

Haney, C. A. Psychosocial factors involved in medical decision making. In R. Coombs & C. Vincent (Eds.), *Psychosocial aspects of medical training*. Springfield, Ill.: Thomas, 1971.

———. Psychosocial factors involved in medical decision making. In T. Millon (Ed.). *Medical behavioral science*. Philadelphia: W. B. Saunders, 1975, pp. 420–432.

Hansen, A. Broken appointments in a child health conference. *Nursing Outlook*, 1953, **1**, 417–419.

Harfouche, J., Abi-Yaghi, M., Melidossian, A., & Azouri, L. Factors associated with broken appointments in an experimental family health center. *Tropical Doctor*, 1973, **3**, 128–133.

Harris, M. D. & Bruner, C. G. A comparison of a self-control and a contract procedure for weight control. *Behavioral Research Therapy*, 1971, **9**, 347–354.

Haynes, R. B. Determinants of compliance: The disease and the mechanics of treatment. In R.

B. Haynes, D. W. Taylor, & D. L. Sackett (Eds.), *Compliance in health care*. Baltimore: Johns Hopkins University Press, 1979, pp. 49–62. (a)

———. Strategies to improve compliance with referrals, appointments, and prescribed medical regimens. In R. B. Haynes, D. W. Taylor, & D. L. Sackett (Eds.), *Compliance in health care*. Baltimore: Johns Hopkins University Press, 1979, pp. 121–143. (b)

Haynes, R. B., Sackett, D. L., Gibson, E. S., Taylor, B. W., Hackett, B. C., Roberts, R. S., & Johnson, A. L. Improvement of medication compliance in uncontrolled hypertension. *Lancet*, 1976, **1**, 1265–1268.

Haynes, R., Sackett, D., Gibson, E., Taylor, D., Roberts, R., & Johnson, A. Manipulation of the therapeutic regimen to improve patient compliance. Conceptions and misconceptions. *Clinical Pharmacology and Therapeutics*, 1977, **22**, 125–130.

Haynes, R. B., Taylor, D. W., & Sackett, D. L. *Compliance in Health Care*. Baltimore: Johns Hopkins University Press, 1979.

Heinzelmann, F. & Bagley, R. W. Response to physical activity programs and their effects on health behavior. *Public Health Reports*, 1970, **85**, 905–911.

Hemminki, E. & Heikkila, J. Elderly people's compliance with prescriptions and quality of medication. *Scandanavian Journal of Social Medicine*, 1975, **3**, 87–92.

Hoenig, P. & Ragg, N. The non-attending psychiatric outpatient: An administrative problem. *Medical Care*, 1966, **4**, 96–100.

Hollingshead, A. B. & Redlich, F. C. Class and the prevalence of disorders. In *Social class and mental illness*. New York: John Wiley & Sons, 1958, pp. 194–219.

Hudson, L. D. & Sbarboro, J. A. Twice weekly tuberculosis chemotherapy. *Journal of the American Medical Association*, 1973, **223**, 139–143.

Hulka, B., Kupper, L., Cassel, J., Efird, R., & Burdette, J. Medication use and misuse: Physician-patient discrepancies. *Journal of Chronic Disease*, 1975, **28**, 7–21.

Hurtado, A., Greenlick, M., & Columbo, T. Determinants of medical care utilization: Failure to keep appointments. *Medical Care*, 1973, **11**, 189–198.

Ireland, H. D. Outpatient chemotherapy for tuberculosis. *American Review of Respiratory Disease*, 1960, **82**, 378–383.

Johnson, S. M. & White, G. Self-observation as an agent of behavioral change. *Behavior Therapy*, 1971, **2**, 488–497.

Jones, E. E. How do people perceive the causes of behavior? In I. L. Janis (Ed.), *Current trends in psychology*, Readings from the *American Scientist*. Los Altos, Calif.: Wm. Kaufman, 1977, pp. 317–332.

Jones, E. E. & Nisbett, R. E. *The actor and the observer: Divergent perceptions of the causes of behavior*. New York: General Learning Press, 1971.

Kanfer, F. H. Self-monitoring: Methodological limitations and clinical applications. *Journal of Consulting and Clinical Psychology*, 1970, **35**, 148–152.

———. Self management methods. In F. H. Kanfer & A. P. Goldstein (Eds.), *Helping people change*. 2nd ed. New York: Pergamon Press, 1980.

Kanfer, F. H. & Phillips, J. S. *Learning foundations of behavior therapy*. New York: Wiley, 1970.

Kaplan, B. H., Cassel, J. C., & Gore, S. Social support and health. *Medical Care*, 1977, **15**(5), 47–58.

Karoly, P. Operant methods. In F. H. Kanfer & A. P. Goldstein (Eds.), *Helping people change*. 2nd ed. New York: Pergamon Press, 1980.

Kasl, S. V. Issues in patient adherence to health care regimens. *Journal of Human Stress*, 1975, **1**, 5–17.

Katz, R. C. & Zlutnick, S. *Behavior therapy and health care: Principles and applications*. New York: Pergamon Press, 1975.

Kincey, J., Bradshaw, P., & Ley, P. Patients' satisfaction and reported acceptance of advice in general practice. *Journal of the Royal College of General Practitioners*, 1975, **25**, 558–566.

King, H. Health in the medical and other learned professions. *Journal of Chronic Diseases*, 1970, **23**, 257–281.

Kiritz, S. & Moos, R. H. Physiological effects of social environments. *Psychosomatic Medicine*, 1974, **36**(2), 96–114.

Knowles, J. H. The responsibility of the individual. *Daedalus,* 1977, **1061**, 57–80.

Kramer, M. *Reality shock: Why nurses leave nursing.* St. Louis: Mosby, 1974.

Lane, M. F., Barbarite, R. V., Bergner, L., & Harris, D. Child resistant medicine containers: Experience in the home. *American Journal of Public Health*, 1971, **61**, 1861–1868.

Langlie, J. K. Social networks, health beliefs, and preventive health behavior. *Journal of Health and Social Behavior*, 1977, **18**, 244–260.

Latiolais, C. J. & Berry, C. C. Misuse of prescription medications by outpatients. *Drug Intelligence: Clinical Pharmacy*, 1969, **3**, 270–277.

Lee, S. D. & Tenerlin, M. K. Social class, diagnosis and prognosis for psychotherapy. *Psychotherapy: Theory, Research & Practice*, 1970, **7**, 181–185.

Lewis, C. E. & Michnich, M. Contracts as a means of improving patient compliance. In I. Barofsky (Ed.), *Medication compliance: A behavioral management approach.* Thorofare, N.J.: Charles B. Slack, 1977, pp. 69–75.

Lima, J., Nazarian, L., Charney, E., & Lahti, C. Compliance with short term antimicrobial therapy. Some techniques that help. *Pediatrics*, 1976, **57**, 383–386.

Linkewich, J. A., Catalano, R. B., & Flack, H. C. The effect of packaging and instruction on outpatient compliance with medication regimens. *Drug Intelligence: Clinical Pharmacy*, 1974, **8**, 10–15.

Linn, L. S. Interns' attitudes and values as antecedents of clinical performance. *Journal of Medical Education*, 1979, **54**, 238–241.

Linn, L. S. & Lewis, C. E. Attitudes toward self-care among practicing physicians. *Medical Care*, 1979, **17**(2), 183–189.

Lipman, R. S., Rickels, K., Uhlenhuth, E. H., Park, L. C., & Fisher, S. Neurotics who fail to take their drugs. *British Journal of Psychiatry*, 1965, **3**, 1043–1049.

Lipowski, Z. J. Psychosocial aspects of disease. *Annals of Internal Medicine*, 1969, **71**, 1197–1206.

Litwak, E. & Szelenyi, I. Primary group structures and their functions: Kin, neighbors, and friends. *American Sociological Review*, 1969, **34**, 465.

Lorber, J. Good patients and problem patients: Conformity and deviance in a general hospital. *Journal of Health and Social Behavior*, 1975, **16**, 213–225.

Ludwig, E. G. & Gibson, G. Self perception of sickness and the seeking of medical care. *Journal of Health and Social Behavior*, 1969, **10**, 125–133.

Ludy, J., Gagon, J., & Caiola, S. The patient-pharmacist interaction in two ambulatory settings—Its relationship to patient satisfaction and drug misuse. *Drug Intelligence: Clinical Pharmacy*, 1977, **11**, 81–89.

MacDonald, M. E., Hagberg, K. L., & Grossman, B. J. Social factors in relation to participation in follow-up care of rheumatic fever. *Journal of Pediatrics*, 1963, **62**, 503–513.

MacElveen, P. M. Cooperative triad in hemodialysis care and patient outcomes. *Communicating Nursing Research*, 1972, **5**, 134–147.

MacHann, W. A community hypertension-control program: Follow-up and patient compliance. *Bulletin of the New York Academy of Medicine*, 1976, **52**, 665–670.

Mahoney, M. J. Self-reward and self monitoring techniques for weight control. *Behavior Therapy*, 1974, **5**, 48–57.

Mahoney, M. J. & Mahoney, K. *Permanent weight control: A total solution to the dieter's dilemma*. New York: W. W. Norton, 1976.

Mahoney, M. J., Moura, N. G. M., & Wade, T. C. The relative efficacy of self-rewards, self-punishment, and self monitoring techniques for weight loss. *Journal of Consulting and Clinical Psychology*, 1973, **40**, 404–407.

Mahoney, M. J. & Thoresen, C. E. *Self-control: Powr to the person.* Monterey, Calif.: Brooks/Cole, 1974.

Malahy, B. The effect of instruction and labeling on the number of medication errors made by patients at home. *American Journal of Hospital Pharmacy*, 1966, **23**, 283–292.

Maletzky, B. M. Behavior recording as treatment: A brief note. *Behavior Therapy*, 1974, **5**, 107–111.

Mann, R. A. The behavior-therapeutic use of contingency contracting to control an adult-behavior problem: Weight control. *Journal of Applied Behavioral Analysis*, 1972, **5**, 99–109.

Martin, R. A. & Poland, E. Y. *Learning to change.* New York: McGraw-Hill, 1980.

Maslach, C. Burned-out. *Human Behavior*, 1976, **5**(9), 16–22.

Mattar, M. E., Markello, J., & Yaffe, S. J. Inadequacies in the pharmacologic management of ambulatory children. *Journal of Pediatrics*, 1975, **87**, 137–141. (a)

———. Pharmaceutic factors affecting pediatric compliance. *Pediatrics*, 1975, **55**, 101–108. (b)

Matthews, D. & Hingson, R. Improving patient compliance: A guide for physicians. *Medical Clinics of North America*, 1977, **61**, 879–889.

Mattsson, A. Long-term physical illness in childhood: A challenge to psychosocial adaptation. *Pediatrics*, 1972, **50**, 801–811.

McAlister, A. L., Farquhar, J. W., Thorensen, C. E., et al. Behavioral science applied to cardiovascular health: Progress and research needs in the modification of risk-taking habits in adult populations. *Health Education Monographs*, 1976, **4**, 75–94.

McInnis, J. K. Do patients take antituberculosis drugs? *American Journal of Nursing*, 1970, **70**, 2152–2153.

McKenney, J. M., Slining, J. M., Henderson, H. R., Devins, D., & Barr, M. The effect of clinical pharmacy services on patients with essential hypertension. *Circulation*, 1973, **48**, 1104–1111.

Mealey, S. A. Navajos can and do keep appointments. *Nursing Practice*, 1975, **1**, 13–15.

Meichenbaum, D. H. *Cognitive behavior modification.* Morristown, N.J.: General Learning Press, 1977.

Meichenbaum, D. & Genest, M. Cognitive behavior modification: An integration of cognitive and behavioral methods. In F. H. Kanfer & A. P. Goldstein (Eds.), *Helping people change.* 2nd ed. New York: Pergamon Press, 1980, pp. 390–422.

Meller, W. & Anderson, A. Medical compliance, the effect of appointment reminders on keeping appointments in a core city pediatric outpatient department. *Minnesota Medicine*, 1976, **59**, 625–626.

Milmoe, S., Rosenthal, R., Blane, H. T., Chafetz, M. L., & Wolf, I. The doctor's voice: Postdictor of successful referral of alcoholic patients. *Journal of Abnormal Psychology*, 1967, **72**, 78–84.

Modlin, H. C. & Montes, A. Narcotics addiction in physicians. *American Journal of Psychiatry*, 1964, **121**, 358–369.

Moulding, T., Onstad, G. D., & Sbarbaro, J. A. Supervision of outpatient drug therapy with the medication monitor. *Annals of Internal Medicine*, 1970, **73**, 559–564.

Mumford, E. *Interns: From student physicians.* Cambridge, Mass.: Harvard University Press, 1970.

Murthy, R. S., Ghosh, A., & Wig, N. Drop-outs from psychiatric walk-in clinic. *Indian Journal of Psychiatry*, 1977, **19**, 11–17.

Nazarian, L., Mechaber, J., Charney, E., & Coulter, M. Effect of a mailed appointment reminder on appointment keeping. *Pediatrics*, 1974, **53**, 349–352.

Neely, E. & Patrick, M. L. Problems of aged persons taking medications at home. *Nursing Research*, 1968, **17**, 52–55.

Nelson, A., Gold, B., Hutchinson, R., & Benezra, E. Drug default among schizophrenic patients. *American Journal of Hospital Pharmacy*, 1975, **32**, 1237–1242.

Nelson, R. O., Lipinski, D. P., & Black, J. L. The relative reactivity of external observations and self-monitoring. *Behavior Therapy*, 1976, **7**, 314–321.

Nordholm, L. A. Beautiful patients are good patients: Evidence for the physical attractiveness stereotype in first impressions of patients. *Social Science and Medicine*, 1980, **14A**, 81–83.

Norman, J. C. (Ed.), *Medicine in the ghetto*. New York: Appleton-Century-Crofts, 1969.

Oakes, T. W., Ward, J. R., Gray, R. M., Klauber, M. R., & Moody, P. M. Family expectations and arthritis patient compliance to a hand resting splint regimen. *Journal of Chronic Disease*, 1970, **22**, 757–764.

Oh, S. B. A clinical and sociomedical study for defaulting tuberculosis treatment. *International Union against Tuberculosis Bulletin*, 1974, **47**, 223–224.

Onstad, G. D., Sbarboro, J. A., & Rotenberg, L. Post hospital chemotherapy of the unreliable patient. *American Review Respiratory Disease*, 1970, **101**, 258–263.

Ort, R. S., Ford, A. B., & Liske, R. E. The doctor-patient relationship as described by physicians and medical students. *Journal of Health and Human Behavior*, 1964, **5**, 25–34.

Packard, V. *The people shapers*. Boston: Little, Brown, 1977.

Pam, A., Bryskin, L., Rachlin, S., Rosenblatt, A. Community adjustment of self-discharged patients. *Psychiatric Quarterly*, 1973, **47**, 175–183.

Parkes, C. M., Brown, G. W., & Monck, E. M. The general practitioner and the schizophrenic patient. *British Medical Journal*, 1962, **1**, 972–976.

Pilisuk, M. & Froland, C. Kinship, social networks, social support and health. *Social Science and Medicine*, 1978, **12B**, 273–280.

Piper, G., Jones, J., & Matthews, V. The Saskatoon smoking study: Results of the second year. *Canadian Journal of Public Health*, 1974, **65**, 127–129.

Pratt, L. Optimism-pessimism about helping the poor with health problems. *Social Work*, 1970, **15**(2), 29–33.

Raynes, A. E. & Warren, G. Some characteristics of "drop-outs" at first contact with a psychiatric clinic. *Community Mental Health Journal*, 1971, **7**, 144–150.

Rezler, A. G. Attitude change during medical school: A review of the literature. *Journal of Medical Education*, 1974, **49**, 1023–1030.

Rickels, K., Anderson, J., & Howard, K. Dropout contact by mail: A useful research tool. *Diseases of the Nervous System*, 1968, **29**, 545–548.

Rickels, K., Boren, R., & Stuart, H. M. Controlled psychopharmacological research in general practice. *Journal of New Drugs*, 1964, **4**, 138–147.

Rimanczyk, R. G. Self-monitoring in the treatment of obesity: Parameters of reactivity. *Behavior Therapy*, 1974, **5**, 531–540.

Rimm, D. C. & Masters, J. C. *Behavior therapy: Techniques and empirical findings*. New York: Academic Press, 1974.

Roemer, M. I. On paying the doctor and the implications of different methods. *Journal of Health and Human Behavior*, 1962, **3**, 4–14.

Rogers, C. R. The necessary and sufficient conditions of therapeutic personality change. *Journal of Consulting Psychology*, 1957, **21**, 95–103.

Rogoff, N. The decision to study medicine. In R. K. Merton, G. G. Reader & P. L. Kendall (Eds.), *The student physician*. Cambridge, Mass.: Harvard University Press, 1957, pp. 109–129.

Romm, F. J., Armstrong, P. S., & Prior, A. P. A comparison of program and contraceptive use continuation rates in a family planning clinic. *American Journal of Public Health*, 1975, **65**, 693–699.

Rose, K. D. & Rosow, F. Physicians who kill themselves. *Archives of General Psychiatry*, 1973, **29**, 800–805.

Rosenberg, P. P. Catch 22—The medical model. In E. C. Shapiro & L. M. Lowenstein (Eds.), *Becoming a physician*. Cambridge, Mass.: Ballinger, 1979.

Rosenstock, I. M. & Kirscht, J. P. Why people seek health care. In G. C. Stone, F. Cohen, & N. E. Adler (Eds.), *Health psychology*. San Francisco: Jossey-Bass, 1979, pp. 161–189.

Russell, M., Wilson, C., Feyerabend, C., & Cole, P. V. Effect of nicotine chewing gum on smoking behavior and as an aid to cigarette withdrawal. *British Medical Journal*, 1976, **2**, 391–393.

Salzman, C., Shader, R., Scott, D. A., & Binstock, W. Interviewer anger and patient dropout in a walk-in clinic. *Comprehensive Psychiatry*, 1970, **11**, 267–273.

Seeman, M. & Evans, J. W. Stratification and hospital care. Part 1: The performance of the medical intern. *American Sociological Review*, 1961, **26**, 67–80. (a)

———. Stratification and hospital care. Part 2: The objective criterion of performance. *American Sociological Review*, 1961, **26**, 193–204. (b)

Schwartz, D., Wang, M., Zeitz, L., & Goss, M. E. Medication errors made by elderly, chronically ill patients. *American Journal of Public Health*, 1962, **52**, 2018–2029.

Shader, R. I., Binstock, W. A., Ohly, J. I., & Scott, D. Biasing factors in diagnosis and disposition. *Comprehensive Psychiatry*, 1969, **10**, 81–89.

Shepard, D. S. & Moseley, T. A. Mailed versus telephoned appointment reminders to reduce broken appointments in a hospital outpatient department. *Medical Care*, 1976, **14**, 268–273.

Silverstone, J. T. & Solomon, T. The long-term management of obesity in general practice. *British Journal of Clinical Practice*, 1965, **19**, 395–398.

Skinner, B. H. *The behaviors of organisms: An experimental analysis*. New York: Appleton-Century-Crofts, 1938.

Stamler, R., Stamler, J., Civinelli, J., Pritchard, D., Gosch, F., Ticho, S., Restivo, B., & Fine, D. Adherence and blood-pressure response to hypertension treatment. *Lancet*, 1975, **2**, 1227–1230.

Staudenmayer, H. & Lefkowitz, M. S. Physician-patient psychosocial characteristics influencing medical decision-making. *Social Science and Medicine*, 1981, **15**, 77–81.

Storms, M. D. Videotape and the attribution process: Reversing actors' and observers' points of view. *Journal of Personality and Social Psychology*, 1973, **27**, 165–175.

Stuart, R. B. & Davis, B. *Slim chance in a fat world: Behavioral control of obesity*. Champaign, Ill.: Research Press, 1972.

Suchman, E. A. Preventive health behavior: A model for research on community health campaigns. *Journal of Health and Social Behavior*, 1967, **8**, 197–209.

Sudnow, D. *Passing on*. Englewood Cliffs, N.J.: Prentice-Hall, 1967.

Sussman, M. B. Relationships of adult children with their parents in the United States. In E. Shanas & G. Streib (Eds.), *Social structure and family generational relations*. Englewood Cliffs, N.J.: Prentice-Hall, 1965, pp. 91–93.

Taylor, S. E. Hospital patient behavior: Reactance helplessness, or control? *The Journal of Social Issues*, 1979, **35**(1), 156–184.

Tischler, G. L. Decision-making process in the emergency room. *General Psychiatry*, 1966, **14**, 69–78.

Thoresen, C. E. & Mahoney, M. J. *Behavioral self-control*. New York: Holt, Rinehart, & Winston, 1974.

Tolsdorf, C. C. Social networks, support and coping: An exploratory study. *Family Process*, 1976, **15**, 407–417.

Tuomilehto, J., Rajala, A., Puska, P. A study on the drop-outs of the hypertension register of the North Karelia Project. *Community Health*, 1976, **7**, 149–152.

Vertinsky, P. A., Yang Cung-Fang, Macleod, P. J. M., & Hardwick, D. F. A study of compliance factors in voluntary health behaviors. *International Journal of Health Education*, 1976, **19**, 3–15.

Weintraub, M., Au, W. Y., & Lasagna, L. Compliance as a determinant of serum digoxin concentration. *Journal of the American Medical Association*, 1973, **224**, 481–485.

Willcox, D. R., Gillan, R., Hare, E. H. Do psychiatric outpatients take their drugs? *British Medical Journal*, 1965, **2**, 790–792.

Williams, A. & Duncan, B. A commercial weight reducing organization: A critical analysis. *Medical Journal of Australia*, 1976, **1**, 781–785.

Williams, W. & Lee, J. Methadone maintenance: A comparison of methadone treatment subjects and methadone treatment dropouts. *International Journal of the Addictions*, 1975, **10**, 599–608.

Wills, T. A. Perceptions of clients by professional helpers. *Psychological Bulletin*, 1978, **85**(5), 968–1000.

Wilson, G. T. Cognitive factors in lifestyle changes: A social learning perspective. In P. O. Davidson & S. M. Davidson (Eds.), *Behavioral medicine: Changing health lifestyles*. New York: Brunner-Mazel, 1980.

Wolpe, J. *Psychotherapy by reciprocal inhibition*. Stanford, Calif.: Stanford University Press, 1958.

Zifferblatt, S. M. Increasing patient compliance through the applied analysis of behavior. *Preventive Medicine*, 1975, **4**, 173–182.

Zola, I. K. Problems of communication, diagnosis, and patient care: The interplay of patient, physician and clinic organization. *Journal of Medical Education*, 1963, **38**, 829–838.

CHAPTER 8: IMPLICATIONS OF A SOCIAL-PSYCHOLOGICAL APPROACH TO COMPLIANCE

Anderson, W. T. & Helm, D. T. The physician-patient encounter: A process of reality negotiation. Paper presented at the meeting of the American Sociological Association, September 1977.

Antonovsky, A. *Health, stress, and coping*. San Francisco: Jossey-Bass, 1979.

Arluke, A. Medicine under capitalism. *Social Science and Medicine*, 1978, **12A**, 437–438.

Bloom, S. W. & Summey, P. Models of the doctor-patient relationship: A history of the social system concept. In E. B. Gallagher (Ed.), *The doctor-patient relationship in the changing health scene*. publication no. NIH 78-183. Washington, D.C.: Department of Health, Education and Welfare, 1978, pp. 17–41.

Callahan, D. Shattuck lecture—Contemporary biomedical ethics. *New England Journal of Medicine*, 1980, **302**, 1228–1233.

Carlson, R. J. *The end of medicine*. New York: Wiley, 1975.

Cassell, E. J. Review of "Communication and awareness in a cancer ward." *Social Science and Medicine*, 1978, **12**, 318.

Cobb, B. Why do people detour to quacks? *The Psychiatric Bulletin*, 1954, **3**, 66–69.

Collins, B. E. & Hoyt, M. F. Personal responsibility for consequences: An integration and extension of the forced compliance literature. *Journal of Experimental Social Psychology*, 1972, **8**, 558–593.

Conrad, P. & Kern, R. (Eds.) *The sociology of health and illness*. New York: St. Martin's Press, 1981.

Corcoran, A. C. *A mirror up to medicine*. New York: J. B. Lippincott, 1961.

Crawford, R. Individual responsibility and health politics. In P. Conrad & R. Kern (Eds.), *The sociology of health and illness*. New York: St. Martin's Press, 1981, pp. 468–481.

Danziger, S. K. The uses of expertise in doctor-patient encounters during pregnancy. *Social Science and Medicine*, 1978, **12**, 359–367.

Davis, A. The motivation of the underprivileged worker. In W. F. White (Ed.), *Industry and society*, New York: McGraw-Hill, 1946, pp. 84–106.

De Charms, R. *Personal causation: The internal affective determinants of behavior*. New York: Academic Press, 1968.

Deci, E. L. *Intrinsic motivation*. New York: Plenum, 1975.

DeVries, A. Health care responsibility. *Metamedicine*, 1980, **1**, 95–106.

Dubos, R. *Mirage of health*. New York: Harper & Row, 1959.

Eisenberg, L. The search for care. *Daedalus*, 1977, **106**, 235–246.

Eisenthal, S., Emery, R., Lazare, A., & Udin, H. "Adherence" and the negotiated approach to patienthood. *Archives of General Psychiatry*, 1979, **36**, 393–398.

Festinger, L. *A theory of cognitive dissonance*. Evanston, Ill.: Row, Peterson, 1957.

Fox, R. C. The medicalization and demedicalization of American society. *Daedalus*, 1977, **106**, 9–22.

Frank, J. D. *Persuasion and healing*. Baltimore: Johns Hopkins University Press, 1961.

Freidson, E. *Patients' views of medical practice*. New York: Russell Sage Foundation, 1961.

———. *Profession of medicine*. New York: Dodd, Mead, 1970.

Fuchs, V. *Who shall live*? New York: Basic Books, 1975.

Haney, C. A. & Colson, A. C. Ethical responsibility in physician-patient communication. *Ethics in Science and Medicine*, 1980, **7**, 27–36.

Harvey, J. H. & Smith, W. P. *Social psychology: An attributional approach*, St. Louis: Mosby, 1977.

Haug, M. R. The erosion of professional authority: A cross-cultural inquiry in the case of the physician. *Health and Society*, Winter 1976, pp. 83–106.

Haug, M. R. & Lavin, B. Practitioner or patient—Who's in charge? *Journal of Health and Social Behavior*, 1981, **22**, 212–229.

Haynes, R. B. Introduction. In R. B. Haynes, D. W. Taylor, & D. L. Sackett (Eds.), *Compliance in health care*. Baltimore: Johns Hopkins University Press, 1979, pp. 1–7.

Hippocrates. *Volume II. On decorum* (with English translation by W. H. S. Jones). London: William Heinemann, 1923.

Hofstadter, R. *Anti-intellectualism in American life*. New York: Alfred Knopf, 1962.

Horton, J. Time and cool people. *Trans-Action*, April 1967, pp. 5–12.

Illich, I. *Medical nemesis*. New York: Pantheon, 1976.

Ingelfinger, F. J. Medicine: Meritorious or meretricious? *Science*, 1978, **200**, 942–946.

Jonsen, A. R. Ethical issues in compliance. In R. B. Haynes, D. W. Taylor, & D. L. Sackett (Eds.), *Compliance in health care*. Baltimore: Johns Hopkins University Press, 1979, pp. 113–120.

Kass, L. R. Ethical dilemmas in the care of the ill. I. What is the physician's service? *Journal of the American Medical Association*, 1980, **244**, 1811–1816.

Ketchum, S. A. & Pierce, C. Rights and responsibilities. *The Journal of Medicine and Philosophy*, 1981, **6**, 271–280.

Kiesler, C. A. *The psychology of commitment: Experiments linking behavior to belief*. New York: Academic Press, 1971.

Knowles, J. H. The responsibility of the individual. *Daedalus*, 1977, **106**, 57–80.

Kronenfeld, J. J. Self care as a panacea for the ills of the health care system: An assessment. *Social Science and Medicine*, 1979, **13A**, 263–267.

Lasch, C. *The culture of narcissism*. New York: Warner Books, 1979.

Lerner, M. J. The justice motive in social behavior. *Journal of Social Issues*, 1975, **31**, 1–20.

Lorber, J. Good patients and problem patients: Conformity and deviance in a general hospital. *Journal of Health and Social Behavior*, 1975, **16**, 213–225.

MacIntyre, A. Patients as agents. In S. F. Spicker, H. T. Englehardt, & D. Dordrecht, *Philosophical medical ethics: Its nature and significance*. New York: Reidel, 1977.

Maddison, D. Professionalism and community responsibility. *Social Science and Medicine*, 1980, **14A**, 91–96.

Marsh, F. H. The "deeper meaning" of confidentiality within the physician-patient relationship. *Ethics in Science and Medicine*, 1976, **6**, 131–136.

Marshall, V. W. Physician characteristics and relationships with older patients. In M. R. Haug (Ed.), *Elderly patients and their doctors*. New York: Springer, 1981.

Masters, R. D. Is contract an adequate basis for medical ethics? *Hastings Center Report*, 1975, **5**, 24–28.

McKeown, G. *The role of medicine: Dream, mirage, or nemesis*. London: Blackwell, 1976.

Minnick, W. C. *The art of persuasion*. 2nd ed. Boston: Houghton Mifflin, 1968.

Navarro, V. *Medicine under capitalism*. New York: Prodist, 1976.

Newton, L. A framework for responsible medicine. *The Journal of Medicine and Philosophy*, 1979, **4**, 57–69.
Parsons, T. *The social system*. Glencoe, Ill.: The Free Press, 1951.
———. Definitions of health and illness in the light of American values and social structure. In E. G. Jaco (Ed.), *Patients, physicians and illness*. New York: The Free Press, 1958, pp. 165–187.
———. The sick role and the role of the physician reconsidered. *Milbank Memorial Fund Quarterly/Health and Society*, 1975, **53**, 257–278.
Pellegrino, E. D. Toward an expanded medical ethics: The Hippocratic ethic revisited. In J. Bulger (Ed.), *Hippocrates revisited*. New York: Medcom, 1973, pp. 133–147.
———. Protection of patients' rights and the doctor-patient relationship. *Preventive Medicine*, 1975, **4**, 398–403.
Pranulis, L. V., Dabbs, M. J., & Johnson, J. General anesthesia and the patient's attempts at control. *Social Behavior and Personality*, 1975, **3**, 49–54.
Pratt, L. V. Reshaping the consumer's posture in health care. In E. B. Gallagher (Ed.), *The doctor-patient relationship in the changing health scene*. Washington, D.C.: DHEW publication no. NIH 78-183, 1978, pp. 197–214.
Rodin, J. Patient-practitioner relationships: A process of social influence. In A. W. Johnson, O. Grusky, & B. H. Raven (Eds.), *Contemporary health services: Social science perspectives*. Boston: Auburn House, 1982, pp. 49–81.
Roth, J. *Timetables*. Indianapolis: Bobbs-Merrill, 1963.
Sackett, D. L. Future applications and hypotheses from old research. Conference on New Directions in Patient Compliance, August 8–10, 1978, French Lick, Indiana.
———. A compliance practicum for the busy practitioner. In R. B. Haynes, D. W. Taylor, & D. L. Sackett (Eds.), *Compliance in health care*. Baltimore: Johns Hopkins University Press, 1979, chap. 18.
Shaw, G. B. Preface to *The doctor's dilemma*. Baltimore: Penguin, 1911.
Siegler, M. A physician's perspective on a right to health care. *Journal of the American Medical Association*, 1980, **244**, 1591–1596.
Silver, G. A. The "care" in self-care. In *Consumer Self-Care in Health*. Research proceedings series, National Center for Health Services Research, U.S. Department of Health, Education and Welfare, Public Health Service, August 1977, p. 10.
Sontag, S. *Illness as metaphor*. New York: Vintage, 1978.
Starr, P. The politics of therapeutic nihilism. In P. Conrad & R. Kern (Eds.), *The sociology of health and illness*. New York: St. Martin's Press, 1981, pp. 334–348.
Stimson, G. & Webb, B. *Going to see the doctor*. London: Routledge & Kegan Paul, 1975.
———. The face-to-face interaction and after the consultation. In D. Tuckett & J. M. Kaufert (Eds.), *Basic readings in medical sociology*. London: Tavistock, 1978, pp. 144–152.
Stone, G. C. Patient compliance and the role of the expert. *Journal of Social Issues*, 1979, **35**(1), 34–59.
Strauss, M. B. *Familiar medical quotations*. Boston: Little Brown, 1968.
Szasz, T. S. & Hollender, M. H. A contribution to the philosophy of medicine. The basic models of the doctor-patient relationship. *Archives of Internal Medicine*, 1956, **97**, 585–592.
Taylor, S. E. Hospital patient behavior: Reactance, helplessness, or control? *Journal of Social Issues*, 1979, **35**(1), 156–184.
Thomas, L. *The Medusa and the snail*. New York: Viking Press, 1979.
Vaccarino, J. M. Malpractice: The problem in perspective. *The Journal of the American Medical Association*, 1977, **238**, 861–863.
Veatch, R. Models for ethical medicine in a revolutionary age. *Hastings Center Report*, 1972, **2**, 5.

Waitzkin, H. & Waterman, B. *The exploitation of illness in capitalist society*. Indianapolis: Bobbs-Merrill, 1974.
Wilson, R. N. *The sociology of health: An introduction*. New York: Random House, 1970.

Author Index*

* Due to the large number of authors' works cited in this book, the author index contains only the names of senior authors (first authors) of the research reports.

Subject Index

About the Authors

M. Robin DiMatteo is Associate Professor of Psychology at the University of California, Riverside. She received her Ph.D. in social psychology from Harvard University (1976). Her dissertation, *The Sensitive Physician*, focused on physicians' nonverbal communication skills and their relationship to patient satisfaction with medical care. Her research has been funded by grants from the Massachusetts Mental Health Center, the Kellogg Foundation, and the National Institute of Mental Health. She is the author of numerous research papers and theoretical articles in journals such as *Health Psychology* and *Professional Psychology*. She is also co-author of *Social Psychology and Medicine* (Oelgeschlager, Gunn, and Hain, 1982) and co-editor of *Interpersonal Issues in Health Care* (Academic Press, 1982).

D. Dante DiNicola will receive his M.D. from the University of California, Los Angeles, School of Medicine in Spring 1983, and will begin residency training in psychiatry. He received his B.S. degree from the University of California, Riverside, where he was a Regents Scholar. His research on physician performance assessment is published in *Medical Care* and in *Behavioral Medicine*, and he has published several articles on patient resistance to therapeutic regimens.